CARDIOVASCULAR NURSING

- **Standard care** ■ **Care plans**
- **Teaching plans**

CARDIOVASCULAR NURSING
▪ Standard care ▪ Care plans
▪ Teaching plans

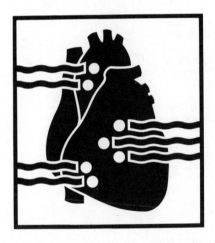

Karen Majorowicz, RN, MSN
Instructor
Sante Fe Community College
Gainesville, Florida

Carol V. Hayes-Christiansen, RN, MEd
Associate Professor Emeritus
University of Florida, College of Nursing
Gainesville, Florida

Springhouse Corporation
Springhouse, Pennsylvania

STAFF FOR THIS VOLUME

Executive Director, Editorial
Stanley E. Loeb

Executive Director, Creative Services
Jean Robinson

Director of Trade and Textbooks
Minnie Bowen Rose, RN, BSN, MEd

Art Director
John Hubbard

Editors
Bernadette Glenn (associate acquisitions editor), Diane Labus

Copy Editors
David Prout (manager), Diane Armento, Jane V. Cray, Keith de Pinho, Elizabeth Kiselev

Designers
Stephanie Peters (associate art director), Elaine Ezrow, Lesley Weissman Cook, Darcey Feralio

Art Production
Robert Perry (manager), Anna Brindisi, Loretta Caruso, Donald Knauss, Catherine Mace, Robert Wieder

Typography
David Kosten (manager), Diane Paluba (assistant manager), Joyce Rossi Biletz, Brenda Mayer, Robin Rantz, Brent Rinedoller, Valerie Rosenberger

Manufacturing
Deborah Meiris (manager), T.A. Landis

Production Coordination
Aline S. Miller (manager), Laurie J. Sander

© 1989 by Springhouse Corporation, 1111 Bethlehem Pike, Springhouse, Pa., 19477. All rights reserved. Reproduction in whole or part by any means whatsoever without written permission of the publisher is prohibited by law. Authorization to photocopy any items for internal or personal use, or the internal or personal use of specific clients, is granted by Springhouse Corporation for users registered with the Copyright Clearance Center (CCC) Transactional Reporting Service, provided that the base fee of $.75 per page is paid directly to CCC, 27 Congress St., Salem, Mass. 01970. For those organizations that have been granted a license by CCC, a separate system of payment has been arranged. The fee code for users of the Transactional Reporting Service is 0874341671/89 $00.00 + $.75. Printed in the United States of America.

CARDCP010389

Library of Congress Cataloging-in-Publication Data
Majorowicz, Karen.
  Cardiovascular nursing/ Karen Majorowicz,
Carol V. Hayes-Christiansen
  p. cm.
  Includes bibliographies and index.
  1. Cardiovascular system—Diseases—
Nursing—Handbooks, manuals, etc.
  I. Hayes-Christiansen, Carol V. Title.
  [DNLM: 1. Cardiovascular Diseases—nursing.
WY 152.5 M234c]   RC674.M24   1989
610.73'691—dc19   DNLM/DLC
for Library of Congress   88-38915
ISBN 0-87434-167-1   CIP

DEDICATION

To Dorothy M. Smith, who first helped me believe in myself; to John and Elaine, who helped me deepen and sustain that belief; and to Ken, my husband, who supported me during the moments of doubt.

Carol V. Hayes-Christiansen

To my Wednesday Night Group for their day-to-day support, and to my family for their encouragement throughout this project.

Karen Majorowicz

TABLE OF CONTENTS

PREFACE

In today's health care system, increasing numbers of nurses are confronted with the responsibility of caring for patients with some type of cardiovascular disease. To meet this responsibility, nurses need specific information about the nursing and medical management of patients with cardiovascular disease.

This book, organized into three sections of alphabetically arranged entries, provides essential information in a quick-reference format that medical-surgical nurses will find useful in the clinical setting.

Section I, "Nursing Diagnosis Care Plans," focuses on the independent functions of nurses working with patients with cardiovascular disease. It consists of a series of care plans for selected diagnostic categories from the list approved by the North American Nursing Diagnosis Association (NANDA) that authors have identified as commonly seen in patients with cardiovascular disease. For each diagnostic category, sample etiologies, and supporting data have been provided. Each care plan includes outcome criteria and suggested interventions that the nurse may use in treating that diagnosis.

Nurses working with patients with cardiovascular disease also practice in an interdependent dimension in which the responsibility for the care of the patient is shared with the doctor. In this dimension, major nursing responsibilities include assessment, monitoring, and implementing prescribed medical orders. Section II, "Standard Care Plans," focuses on these functions. Organized by disease process, this section consists of a series of care plans that give specific information nurses need when caring for patients with cardiovascular disease. Selected care plans also include an overview of commonly prescribed classes of medications. Cardiovascular pharmacology is changing rapidly; the reader is urged to consult current product information and a pharmacology textbook for complete information on specific drugs prescribed.

Section III, "Teaching Plans," focuses on the third major area of responsibility for nurses working with cardiovascular patients—teaching. This section, which consists of a series of teaching plans specifically designed with cardiovascular patients in mind, is prefaced by a knowledge-deficit care plan that offers a brief overview of teaching-learning principles. Each subsequent teaching plan is directed to the nurse and includes suggestions for assessment data, teaching strategies, and evaluation methods as well as an outline of recommended content and outcome criteria. Each teaching plan also includes one or more patient-teaching aids, written specifically for patients, which may be photocopied and distributed to individual patients.

Because the authors feel strongly that effective patient education in cardiovascular disease requires more than simply giving information, the teaching plans and patient-teaching aids emphasize a problem-solving approach. The reader is urged to use this approach to assist patients and their families in developing specific, realistic plans for incorporating prescribed measures into their individual life-styles.

The teaching plans and patient-teaching aids are designed to be complete and comprehensive. Because some patients will not need or be able to use all of the material provided, the reader is encouraged to adapt the materials to meet the specific needs of individual patients and families.

In the interest of brevity and clarity, the authors have chosen to use "she" and "her" when referring to the nurse and "he," "his," and "him" when referring to the patient.

K.M.
C.H.C.

ACKNOWLEDGMENTS

Our sincere thanks to our friends and families, who encouraged and supported us consistently throughout the writing and publishing processes; to Susan Taddei and the other editorial and publishing staff at Springhouse Corporation, for their assistance and guidance; and to our nursing colleagues, who helped us identify the need for this book and provided suggestions for its development based on their experience in the clinical setting.

Special thanks to Janice Allen-Kelsey, RN, MSN, a doctoral student and former instructor in the College of Nursing at the University of Florida, Gainesville, for contributing the sections on essential hypertension and peripheral vascular bypass surgery and for teaching plans on blood pressure measurement and hypertension management.

Karen Majorowicz
Carol V. Hayes-Christiansen

SECTION I: NURSING DIAGNOSIS CARE PLANS

Activity Intolerance

Activity Intolerance related to decreased cardiac output and decreased skeletal muscle perfusion secondary to congestive heart failure

SUPPORTING DATA
• Dyspnea with exertion
• Dyspnea at rest
• Orthopnea
• Paroxysmal nocturnal dyspnea
• Tachycardia at rest or with activity
• Hypotension at rest
• Drop in systolic blood pressure with activity
• Fatigue with minimal activity
• Increased fatigue without increased activity

PLAN OF CARE
Outcome criteria
• Patient performs planned amount of activity with no increased dyspnea or undue fatigue.
• Patient increases amount of activity performed with no increased dyspnea or undue fatigue.

Interventions and rationales
☑ **Intervention 1**
In collaboration with the doctor, limit patient's activity during the acute phase of congestive heart failure (CHF). Restrictions may include:
• bed rest with bathroom privileges
• chair rest
• strict bed rest.
Rationale and comments: Limited activity during the acute phase of CHF decreases the demand for cardiac output and promotes excretion of retained fluid. Unless CHF is severe, patients are usually not placed on strict bed rest because of the complications associated with immobility.

☑ **Intervention 2**
Provide adequate rest.
• Alternate periods of activity with periods of rest, including:
 —rest after visitors
 —rest before and after diagnostic tests that require patient to travel to another department
 —rest between self-care activities

—rest before and after ambulating
—rest before and after meals.
• Implement measures to promote sleep at night (see "Sleep-Pattern Disturbance" in this section).

☑ Intervention 3

Implement measures to decrease factors contributing to patient's activity intolerance, including:
• dyspnea and fluid retention
• patient's emotional response to his diagnosis and prognosis
• inadequate sleep and rest.

Rationale and comments: Patients with CHF experience decreased activity tolerance because:
• cardiac output drops when the heart's pumping action is compromised
• skeletal muscle perfusion decreases as a result of a hemodynamic compensatory mechanism that causes a shift in blood flow from the periphery to more vital organs
• hypoxia results from impaired gas exchange that occurs as a result of fluid accumulation in the alveoli and interstitial tissue of the lung.

☑ Intervention 4

Administer the prescribed medications to improve the heart's effectiveness as a pump. Commonly prescribed classes of medication include:
• cardiac glycosides
• diuretics
• vasodilators
• angiotensin-converting enzyme inhibitors.

Rationale and comments: The patient's activity tolerance will improve as the heart's effectiveness as a pump improves. (For additional information on these medications, see "Congestive Heart Failure" in Section II.)

☑ Intervention 5

In collaboration with the health care team, assess the patient's readiness to progress his activity level; look for the following:
• decreased dyspnea at limited activity level
• stable pulse rate and blood pressure with limited activity
• improved arterial blood gas levels
• decreased pulmonary congestion on chest X-ray
• decreased rales in lung fields
• decreased edema in dependent sites
• fluid weight loss as reflected by daily weight.

Rationale and comments: These signs and symptoms indicate that the heart is pumping more effectively and that the patient's activity level may be slowly, carefully increased.

☑ Intervention 6

In collaboration with the health care team, increase the patient's activity level and monitor his response.

• Increase the amount of time the patient spends out of bed in a chair.
• Increase the amount of time the patient ambulates in his room.
• Have the patient ambulate for short distances in the hall at a slow pace (with oxygen, if necessary); increase the distance gradually.

Rationale and comments: A patient's activity level may be increased by changing the type of activity permitted, increasing the length of time that the patient engages in activity, or increasing the frequency of activity.

☑ Intervention 7
Monitor the patient at all levels of activity for any signs of intolerance with increased activity (see "Supporting Data" above for details).

Rationale and comments: Each patient will increase his activity level at a different speed; careful assessment of the patient's individual response at each activity level can assist the health care team in pacing the patient's activity appropriately.

☑ Intervention 8
If signs and symptoms of activity intolerance develop:
• Have the patient stop the activity and rest.
• Administer oxygen, if available, as prescribed.
• Position the patient with the head of the bed elevated and his feet dependent.
• Decrease the patient's activity to a level below the level at which symptoms appeared.
• Assess the patient for probable causes of activity intolerance, and implement appropriate interventions:
  —Assess for signs indicative of worsening CHF.
  —Assess the type, amount, and pace of activity that precipitated symptoms.
  —Assess for other factors as outlined in Intervention 3 above.

Rationale and comments: Signs and symptoms of activity intolerance may develop because the activity was too strenuous for the patient, the patient's CHF has worsened or become more acute, or other factors have decreased the patient's activity tolerance. Appropriate interventions depend on the underlying cause.

☑ Intervention 9
Explain the activity plan and restrictions to the patient and his family.

Rationale and comments: Explaining the activity plan and restrictions to the patient and family helps to promote compliance.

☑ Intervention 10
Teach the patient and family how to manage activity plans (see "Congestive Heart Failure: Disease Process and Home Care" in Section III).

Activity Intolerance related to decreased myocardial reserve secondary to myocardial infarction, myocardial ischemia secondary to coronary artery disease, or cardiovascular and systemic stresses associated with open-heart surgery

SUPPORTING DATA
• Dyspnea at rest
• Dyspnea that increases with activity
• Feelings of excessive fatigue with activity
• Palpitations with activity
• Dizziness with activity
• Changes in vital signs with activity, including:
  —significant increase in respiratory rate
  —weak pulse
  —abrupt onset of tachycardia or bradycardia
  —pulse rhythm that becomes significantly irregular
  —pulse rate that exceeds preset, individualized limit
  —systolic blood pressure that falls or fails to rise with activity
• Diaphoresis with activity
• Unsteady gait

PLAN OF CARE
Outcome criteria
• Patient experiences decreased signs and symptoms of activity intolerance.

Interventions and rationales
☑ **Intervention 1**
Assess the patient for signs and symptoms of activity intolerance during activity or exercise (see "Supporting Data" above).

☑ **Intervention 2**
If patient develops signs or symptoms of activity intolerance:
• have him stop the activity immediately and rest
• administer oxygen as ordered if dyspnea is present
• if patient experiences angina, follow the interventions outlined in "Angina Pectoris" in Section II.

Rationale and comments: Signs or symptoms of activity intolerance indicate that the exercise is imposing too much stress on the myocardium.

☑ **Intervention 3**
If any of the following symptoms occur, consult the doctor before the patient resumes exercise:
• abrupt onset of bradycardia
• abrupt onset of tachycardia
• significantly irregular pulse rhythm
• new or more severe chest pain

• dizziness or diaphoresis
• pulse rate that consistently exceeds preset limits (even with decreased activity)
• change in overall cardiovascular status.

Rationale and comments: Managing these signs and symptoms often requires medical intervention. Continued exercise may result in excessive myocardial stress.

✓ Intervention 4
If any of the following milder signs or symptoms occur, decrease the patient's exercise level:
• pulse rate that exceeds preset limits during exercise
• pulse rate that exceeds preset limits for 10 or more minutes after the end of exercise
• dyspnea persisting for 10 minutes or more after the end of exercise
• unusual fatigue the day after exercise
• episode of "usual" chest pain that occurs with exertion.

Rationale and comments: Milder symptoms suggest that the exercise has been too strenuous. In many cases, reducing the amount of exercise will eliminate the symptoms.

✓ Intervention 5
To reduce the patient's exercise level:
• instruct him to perform exercise at a slower pace
• have him perform exercises for a shorter period of time; for example, reduce the time spent with stretching exercises and walking
• instruct him to perform one or two less repetitions of each stretching exercise
• tell him to walk a shorter distance
• decrease the total number of exercise periods per day
• assess his overall activity level and implement strategies to reduce the level, if indicated. Consider the following:
   —the number and frequency of visitors as well as the length of visits and phone calls
   —activities of daily living
   —scheduled diagnostic tests
   —frequency and adequacy of rest periods
   —cardiac rehabilitation classes or other scheduled activities.

✓ Intervention 6
Assess the patient's response to decreased activity (see "Supporting Data" above for details).
• If signs of activity intolerance continue with decreased activity, notify the doctor.
• If no signs of activity intolerance are present, continue the patient's activity at the current level; gradually increase the activity as indicated by the patient's condition.

Rationale and comments: Medical interventions may be required to manage continued activity intolerance.

Activity Intolerance related to ischemia in exercising muscles of lower extremities secondary to decreased arterial blood flow secondary to atherosclerosis

SUPPORTING DATA
• Pain in calf of leg that occurs with walking and disappears with rest (no position change required for relief)
• Arterial occlusion as documented by angiography, Doppler ultrasound, or plethysmography
• Diminished or absent peripheral pulses in affected extremity

PLAN OF CARE
Outcome criteria
• Patient increases distance walked before experiencing intermittent claudication.
• Patient experiences fewer episodes of intermittent claudication during exercise period.

Interventions and rationales
☑ **Intervention 1**
Collaborate with the doctor about the patient's readiness to engage in a planned activity program.

Rationale and comments: Not all patients with occlusive arterial disease will benefit from a planned activity program. Usually, patients with severe, unrelieved rest pain; infected ulcers; or gangrene are on limited activity and are not started on a planned activity program.

☑ **Intervention 2**
In collaboration with the doctor, develop an activity plan using the following guidelines:
• Assess the distance the patient can walk before experiencing intermittent claudication to provide baseline data about the severity of his disease and current functional capacity.
• Instruct the patient to exercise daily using the following protocol:
  —Walk at a slow to moderate pace on a level surface until intermittent claudication occurs.
  —When intermittent claudication occurs, stop walking, rest, and allow the pain to disappear.
  —When the pain disappears, resume walking on a level surface at the same pace until intermittent claudication recurs.
  —When intermittent claudication recurs, stop and rest again until the pain disappears.
  —Continue the same pattern for a prescribed time period (usually 30 to 60 minutes).

Rationale and comments: The above protocol increases development of collateral circulation in the lower extremities. Collateral circulation increases blood flow to the affected tissue, thus compensating for the atherosclerotic occlusion of the involved artery.

☑ **Intervention 3**

Assess the patient for effectiveness of the activity program. Note the following:

• the distance walked before pain develops; compare this with the baseline distance

• the number of times during the exercise period the patient stops to allow pain to disappear.

Rationale and comments: Increased collateral circulation results in decreased ischemia. With improved collateral circulation, the patient will be able to walk longer periods before developing pain and will have fewer episodes of pain during the exercise period.

Increased ischemia (as evidenced by increased episodes of pain or decreased distance walked before pain develops) indicates progressive disease; notify the doctor if this occurs.

☑ **Intervention 4**

If the patient experiences signs of decreased ischemia, collaborate with the doctor about increasing the length or frequency of activity.

Activity Intolerance, Potential for

Potential for Activity Intolerance related to decreased myocardial reserve secondary to myocardial infarction, myocardial ischemia secondary to coronary artery disease, or cardiovascular and systemic stresses associated with open-heart surgery

SUPPORTING DATA
• Diagnosis of acute myocardial infarction (MI)
• Diagnosis of angina pectoris
• Postoperative condition after coronary artery bypass grafting (CABG) surgery
• Postoperative condition after valve replacement surgery

PLAN OF CARE
Outcome criteria
• Patient has no symptoms of activity intolerance.
• Patient increases activity, as planned, while meeting the following criteria:
—maintains vital signs within preset parameters
—experiences no undue fatigue
—reports no angina with activity.

Interventions and rationales
☑ Intervention 1
In collaboration with the health care team, determine whether the patient is ready to increase activity by assessing for the following:
• presence, extent, and location of MI
• complications such as congestive heart failure (CHF); dysrhythmias; or uncontrolled, persistent, or recurrent ischemic chest pain
• left ventricular ejection fraction
• coexisting diseases; for example, chronic respiratory diseases (such as chronic obstructive pulmonary disease), musculoskeletal disorders (such as arthritis), or neuromuscular disorders (such as cerebrovascular accident)
• patient's physical condition before hospitalization
• patient's response to low-level activities.

Rationale and comments: When planning activity for any patient, consider the following factors:
• Generally, MI patients should progress their activity more slowly than patients who have not had an MI. The infarct's size and location may affect the patient's activity tolerance.

• Uncontrolled CHF, dysrhythmias, or ischemic chest pain are major contraindications for increasing a patient's activity level. When such complications are controlled, however, the patient's activity level may be increased.
• Left ventricular ejection fraction provides some prognostic information about the patient's condition. Generally, an ejection fraction of > 40% indicates that the patient will tolerate activity progression well. An ejection fraction of 35% to 40% indicates that he may need to progress more slowly and that he should be observed closely for CHF or dysrhythmias. An ejection fraction of < 35% is associated with high risk of complications and occurrence of a second cardiac event. In such a case, the patient's activity tolerance usually is limited and the rehabilitation period extended.
• Coexisting diseases can increase the amount of energy required to perform a given activity, thereby increasing myocardial oxygen demand. Certain diseases also can limit the activity level a patient can achieve and should be considered when setting realistic goals for the patient.
• The patient's usual level of fitness influences how rapidly and to what extent his activity level increases.

☑ Intervention 2
Assess for and reduce factors that may decrease the patient's activity tolerance level, including the following:
• postoperative incisional pain
• fatigue
• emotional response to diagnosis, prognosis, and surgery
• atelectasis.

☑ Intervention 3
Begin the patient's activity at a low level and assess his response using the parameters outlined in intervention 5 below (see *Recommended low-level activities* for examples of low-level activities).

Rationale and comments: Low-level activities are usually begun in the intensive care unit when the patient's cardiovascular status stabilizes. Signs of activity intolerance at this level indicate that the patient is not yet ready to advance.

☑ Intervention 4
In collaboration with the health care team, develop a specific activity plan for each patient.
• Determine acceptable vital sign parameters for beginning and continuing the prescribed activity.
• Consider activities of daily living, such as bathing, eating, visiting with family or friends, and using the toilet or bedside commode, in the activity plan.
• Do not schedule exercise activities immediately after meals.
• Include sufficient rest periods in the prescribed plan, and alternate periods of activity with periods of rest.
• Develop a specific exercise prescription that includes the following:
   —stretching and warm-up exercises (See *Examples of stretching exercises,* page 12)

RECOMMENDED LOW-LEVEL ACTIVITIES

Any activity that requires the use of one to two times the amount of energy used by the body at rest is considered a low-level activity. Examples of low-level activities include the following:

For myocardial infarction (MI) patients (after transfer from the intensive care unit [ICU]):	• Feeding self • Assisting with bed bath • Watching television or reading for pleasure • Performing active range-of-motion (ROM) exercises of the arms, legs, and ankles • Sitting for short periods in a chair (<15 minutes) • Visiting for short periods with friends or family • Using a bedside commode *Note:* Using a bedside commode requires the use of about three times the amount of energy used by the body at rest, which is less than that needed to use a bedpan.
For patients with uncomplicated coronary artery bypass grafting (CABG) (after transfer from the ICU):	• Assisting with bed bath • Sitting in chair for 30 minutes three times a day • Ambulating in room • Performing active ROM exercises of the arms, legs, and ankles
For patients with complications after CABG surgery (after transfer from the ICU):	• See the activities for MI patients above.
For valve-replacement surgery patients (after transfer from the ICU):	• For those with such significant complications as congestive heart failure or dysrhythmias, see the activities for MI patients above. • For those with no complications, see the activities for patients who have undergone uncomplicated CABG above.
For patients with angina:	• Activities will vary depending on the patient's condition and doctor's orders.

—planned walking
—a cool-down period
—a plan for increasing activity and exercise when the patient shows no sign of activity intolerance at current activity level.
• Share the activity and exercise prescription with the patient and his family. *Note:* If the hospital has a formal cardiac rehabilitation program, use the guidelines for in-hospital cardiac rehabilitation (usually called Phase I guidelines). If formal guidelines are unavailable, consult the doctor regarding choice of exercises and distances to walk. (For more information on an exercise prescription, *see Guidelines: Exercise prescription for in-hospital use,* page 13.)

Rationale and comments: Vital sign parameters should be individualized based on the patient's condition. Currently, several methods exist for setting upper pulse-rate limits, including setting an arbitrary limit of <120 beats/

EXAMPLES OF STRETCHING EXERCISES

Instruct the patient to perform the following exercises.

Lying in bed	• Flex and extend the wrist, elbow, shoulder, hip, knee, and ankle, alternating the use of right and left extremities (for example, first the left wrist, then the right wrist).
Sitting in a chair	• With knees bent, raise one knee to the chest, then lower it slowly to a resting postion. Alternate right and left knees. • With knees bent and feet flat on the floor, raise one foot until the knee and leg are straight, then lower the foot until the knee is bent and the foot is flat on the floor. Alternate right and left legs.
Standing	• With hands on hips (resting position), bend the upper trunk slightly to the left, then return to the resting position. Then bend toward the right, and return to the resting position. • With hands on hips (resting position), bend the upper trunk slightly to the left, then forward, to the right, and finally back to the resting position. • With arms at the sides, twist the trunk first to the left, then to the right. • Extend and straighten both arms, then make large circles with the arms. • With arms at the sides, raise the arms to shoulder level, then above the head, keeping the arms straight. Return arms to shoulder level, then back to the sides. • Standing flat on the floor, raise up on tiptoes briefly, then return to standing flat.

minute; taking the patient's resting heart rate, then adding an additional 20 beats/minute; or setting an individualized limit based on the results of a low-level exercise test.

When considering activities of daily living in the activity plan, keep in mind that even routine activities involve expending energy and that they may increase myocardial work load and oxygen demand. The amount of energy expended with each activity as well as the total amount of energy expended during the day must be considered. The number and type of activities permitted each day will vary, depending on the patient's condition.

If a patient performs numerous activities consecutively (such as eating breakfast, bathing, shaving, and getting out of bed), the total amount of energy expended at one time may be too high. Alternating rest with activity helps to limit the stress on the heart.

Exercise performed immediately after meals increases myocardial work load and stress.

☑ Intervention 5
Assess the patient's response to activity.
• Check vital signs:
—before beginning exercise

GUIDELINES: EXERCISE PRESCRIPTION FOR IN-HOSPITAL USE

Have the patient begin by exercising once or twice a day; this may be increased to three or four times a day if indicated by patient response. Also have him ambulate (without performing stretching exercises) once or twice a day in addition to other exercises.

Stretching and warm-up exercises

Length of time	15 to 20 minutes
Number of repetitions	Begin with 5 repetitions done slowly (instruct patient to avoid holding his breath and to use diaphragmatic breathing while performing exercises); may increase 1 repetition every 1 to 2 days as indicated by patient response.
Specific exercises	Consult doctor or physical therapist. (See *Examples of stretching exercises* for specific exercises.)

Walking program

Length of time	Begin with 5 to 10 minutes per walk; may increase up to 30 minutes per walk before discharge if indicated by patient response.
Distance	Variable, depending on patient status. Usual initial distance for patient with uncomplicated myocardial infarction is 100 feet per walk; usual distance for patient with uncomplicated coronary artery bypass grafting is 100 to 200 feet per walk.
Plan for increasing walking	• Walk the prescribed distance at a slow pace. • Walk the same distance at a faster pace. • Increase the distance and walk at a slow pace. • Walk the increased distance at a faster pace. • Repeat. • May increase distance by 25 to 100 feet per walk. • Increase pace, distance, or both only when indicated by patient's response. *Note:* How often walking can be increased will vary among patients. Some will need to stay at one level (pace and distance) for several days. Others may be able to increase distance and pace each day.

Cool-down exercises

Length of time	Proportional to length of exercise period (for example, 1 to 2 minutes for an exercise period of 5 to 10 minutes; 5 to 10 minutes for an exercise period of 20 to 30 minutes).
Type of exercise	Walking at a pace slower than the pace used for the walking program above.

—in the middle of stretching exercises
—before beginning ambulation
—in the middle of ambulation
—at the end of ambulation
—10 minutes after completing ambulation.
• Observe the patient throughout the activity or exercise for signs of activity intolerance, such as:
—pulse rate exceeding preset limits
—abrupt onset of tachycardia or bradycardia
—pulse rhythm that becomes extremely irregular
—complaints of dizziness
—diaphoresis
—systolic blood pressure that falls or fails to rise with activity.

☑ Intervention 6

Have the patient stop the activity or exercise when he:
• achieves the preset prescribed level
• complains of fatigue
• develops signs of activity intolerance.

Rationale and comments: Patients may feel that they can engage in activity that exceeds planned levels; however, prescribed activity is carefully planned on the basis of energy consumption and myocardial work load. Alternating periods of increased work load with periods of rest is vital for satisfactory recovery.

Activity should cease before the patient becomes excessively fatigued. Complaint of fatigue may be the initial clue that the patient needs to stop and rest.

☑ Intervention 7

If the patient develops signs of activity intolerance, implement the interventions outlined in "Activity Intolerance" in this section.

☑ Intervention 8

Teach the patient and family how to manage activities.

☑ Intervention 9

Suggest that the patient consider participating in an outpatient cardiac rehabilitation program after discharge.

Rationale and comments: Participating in a cardiac rehabilitation program can help patients increase activity tolerance.

Anxiety

Anxiety related to dyspnea

SUPPORTING DATA
• Statements about feeling short of breath
• Use of accessory muscles during breathing
• Increased respiratory rate
• Fear of being unable to breathe
• Increased pulse rate
• Restlessness
• Asking not to be left alone

PLAN OF CARE
Outcome criteria
• Patient's respiratory rate returns to his previous usual rate.
• Patient breathes abdominally or thoracically without using accessory muscles or returns to his normal pattern.
• Patient reports feeling less short of breath.
• Patient states feeling safe enough to be left alone.

Interventions and rationales
☑ **Intervention 1**
Stop the present activity and intervene as follows:
• If patient is out of bed, have him sit in a chair with a back support, with his feet down.
• If patient is in bed, raise the head of the bed.

Rationale and comments: The patient needs all of his resources for breathing. A back support allows the patient to relax against the back rather than having to use energy to support his weight. Blood can pool in the feet if they are in a dependent position, which reduces venous return to the heart and thus to the lungs. Raising the head of the bed allows the abdominal contents to drop, putting less pressure on the diaphragm and providing more room for chest expansion.

☑ **Intervention 2**
Administer oxygen, as ordered.

Rationale and comments: Feeling short of breath can be frightening to the patient. Administering oxygen, which is necessary for the myocardium, helps reduce the patient's feelings of anxiety by reassuring him that something is being done to help him.

☑ Intervention 3
Take vital signs.

Rationale and comments: Shortness of breath may be caused by factors that can be identified by changes in vital signs, such as a dysrhythmia or a drop in blood pressure. Taking vital signs provides baseline data in case other changes occur later.

☑ Intervention 4
Stay with the patient.

Rationale and comments: Fear is less stressful when it does not have to be experienced alone. Staying with a patient provides an opportunity to observe the effect of current interventions and to determine the need for others.

☑ Intervention 5
Use touch.
• Place your hand on the patient's shoulder.
• Hold the patient's hand if he seems to indicate this is appropriate.
• Place your hand where the patient can take it if he desires.
• Remove your hand if the patient seems uninterested.

Rationale and comments: Not all patients feel comforted by touch. Placing a hand within the patient's reach allows him to take it if he wishes. If he puts pressure on your hand when you take his, chances are the touch is comforting. If he releases pressure, chances are he has had enough.

☑ Intervention 6
When the patient's breathing is more comfortable and he is ready:
• use therapeutic communication techniques to talk about the experience (see *Therapeutic communication techniques*).
• try to determine the precipitating cause or event.

Rationale and comments: Talking during the acute dyspnea attack is inappropriate as it takes the patient's energy and delays the onset of treatment. Discussing the experience after it is over helps to reduce its frightening aspects and allows the patient to put it into perspective. Identifying the precipitating event can provide clues to the patient's activity tolerance. It also may affect medical treatment and assist the patient to develop awareness of the effects of his behavior.

☑ Intervention 7
Carry out any doctor's orders for treating the cause of dyspnea.

Rationale and comments: Fluid volume excess, atelectasis, anxiety, hypoxemia, and pain are some of dyspnea's causes.

THERAPEUTIC COMMUNICATION TECHNIQUES

Technique	Definition	Example
Closed question	Narrow, restricted question, giving the patient the least amount of freedom and the nurse the most control; often can be answered by "yes" or "no"	"Have you felt frightened since you've had your heart attack?"
Open question	Broad, unrestricted question or statement that establishes a topic and lets the patient structure an answer	"Tell me about the feelings you've been having since your heart attack."
Direct question	Question that is straight and to the point; may be open or closed	"What kinds of feelings have you been having since your heart attack?"
Indirect question	Question or statement that allows the nurse to elicit a response from the patient without seeming to have posed a question	"I've been wondering what thoughts and feelings you've been having since you transferred from the coronary care unit."
Primary question	Any question used to introduce a new topic to elicit new information; may be open or closed, direct or indirect	Nurse: "What activities do you understand you'll be able to do or not do when you go home?" Patient: "I shouldn't lift anything heavy."
Secondary question	Any question that elicits more fully the desired information	"How many pounds does 'heavy' mean to you?"
Clarification	Any question or statement that seeks to elucidate replies that are vague, incomplete, or meaningless	"I don't quite understand what you mean when you say, 'I'm not good for anything anymore.' "
Focusing statement or question	Technique used to control the interaction or conversation between the nurse and patient by centering it on content objectives or a particular topic or question	"You've told me how your wife and daughter feel about your heart attack; I was wondering if you had some of the same feelings."

(continued)

THERAPEUTIC COMMUNICATION TECHNIQUES (continued)

Technique	Definition	Example
Reflection	Reflection encompasses two techniques: echoing and mirroring. • *Echoing,* or restating the content, can be accomplished in one of two ways: —repeating (reflecting) exactly certain words or phrases, changing only the pronoun —restating part of what the patient said, thus allowing him to hear what he just said; this may help him to continue discussing the subject and lets him know that the nurse heard what he said and is willing to explore it further.	*Patient:* "I'm so worried about what is going to happen..." *Nurse:* "You're so worried..." *Patient:* "I'm scared I'm not going to make it through the operation." *Nurse:* "Scared?"
	• *Mirroring* is a way of sending back to the patient his feelings, attitudes, and the nurse's impressions of his behavior. With this technique, the nurse observes a particular behavior of the patient and verbalizes her impression of what the behavior seems to be communicating. Promoting a feeling that the patient has been understood, this technique requires that the nurse have a certain degree of sensitivity in recognizing and stating the patient's feelings and attitudes as soon as he has completed his statements. However, the nurse must remember to reflect the patient's feelings, not her own.	*Nurse:* "You seem more pensive and thoughtful today. Want to share your thoughts?" (The nurse may follow this reflection with silence, allowing the patient to decide whether to continue.)

THERAPEUTIC COMMUNICATION TECHNIQUES *(continued)*

Technique	Definition	Example
Summarizing	Technique that allows patient to hear succinctly what the nurse has understood him to say; patient can then verify correctness or can reword what he intended so that he can be understood	"As I understand it then, your chest pain began about 2 hours ago and only now is beginning to lessen."
Silence	This technique may be used: • to indicate to the patient that the nurse expects him to speak • to give the patient an opportunity to organize thoughts, consider alternative actions, explore his feelings, or make decisions • to allow the patient to take initiative for the conversation or to discover that he can be accepted even though he doesn't feel like talking.	The nurse can break the tension by gently asking the patient what he's thinking about at the moment. *Note:* The nurse needs to recognize when the patient is using silence constructively and when he is becoming tense by the situation.

Adapted from Becknell, E., and Smith, D., *System of Nursing Practice*. Philadelphia: F.A. Davis Co., 1975. Used with permission.

Anxiety related to fear of dying and/or powerlessness or loss of control in response to a diagnosis of chronic cardiovascular disease

SUPPORTING DATA

• Complains about food, delays in scheduled activities, room temperature, and personnel

• Repeats the same story or complaint (Use of therapeutic communication techniques seems to have no effect; patient retells the story to the next person.)

• Talks constantly, but not about anything in particular (The purpose of the talking is to prevent close inspection of feelings, to maintain control, or to keep the nurse at his bedside.)

• Changes the subject when asked about his feelings

• Uses such phrases as "I probably won't even be here tomorrow"; talks about others who have died; asks questions about how he is doing; speaks frequently about what he'll have to give up or what he will no longer be able to do

• Asks for his spouse or others to stay with him continuously
• Asks for lights to be left on or doors left open
• Reports having nightmares, either spontaneously or when asked
• Uses the call light frequently, especially to request things he is capable of getting himself
• Visits the nurses' station frequently when allowed out of bed
• Fails to establish eye contact, turns away from the nurse, uses a loud tone of voice, or answers in monosyllables
• Scratches himself constantly; doesn't get any sleep or sleeps all the time; or tosses, turns, or talks in his sleep
• Talks about various fears
• Refuses to adhere to any restrictions placed on activities, diet, or smoking
Note: Conversation with the patient may be nonspecific for anxiety, dying, or loss of control. You'll need to rely on your own knowledge base and empathetic feelings along with the therapeutic communication techniques mentioned in this section to assist patients and families in recognizing and identifying feelings so that they may accept them and deal with them accordingly.

PLAN OF CARE
Outcome criteria
• Patient, family, and/or caregiver expresses feelings to the nurse.
• Patient, family, and/or caregiver states increased comfort with feelings experienced.
• Patient, family, and/or caregiver states ways in which each can reduce discomfort of feelings experienced.

Interventions and rationales
☑ Intervention 1
Plan for at least 15 minutes of uninterrupted time with the patient, family, and/or caregiver; 30 minutes is even better. Ask the unit clerk to take phone messages so that you won't be interrupted. The patient may need daily sessions for several days.

Rationale and comments: You can probably safely assume that each patient with a myocardial infarction (MI), congestive heart failure, or stable or unstable angina will have anxiety. Part of the nurse's responsibility involves helping patients to express feelings; patients require time to become comfortable expressing feelings.

☑ Intervention 2
Besides listening to the patient during scheduled sessions, listen to his comments during all contacts and respond as mentioned in the interventions below.

Rationale and comments: The expression of feelings cannot always wait for a scheduled session. All contacts with the patient provide an opportunity to assist him to express his feelings.

☑ Intervention 3

Use therapeutic communication techniques as discussed in *Therapeutic communication techniques,* pages 17 to 19.

Rationale and comments: Nurses cannot depend on patients to volunteer all necessary information. Part of the nurse's responsibility includes helping patients to identify, explore, and express their fears and to give information and assistance that will help them face these fears. To help the patient face his feelings, the nurse must overcome her own anxiety concerning death.

☑ Intervention 4

Avoid the use of communication blocks (see *Blocks to communication,* page 22).

Rationale and comments: Like most other people, patients find talking about dying and feeling out of control difficult. However, when given the opportunity to express such feelings, they may be relieved to be able to talk about them with a nonjudgmental person, such as a nurse.

☑ Intervention 5

Explain all procedures, delays, and changes in schedule to the patient.

Rationale and comments: Surprises and unusual events create stress that produces physiologic effects in the body, such as increased heart rate, increased atherogenesis, and even ventricular dysrhythmias. Type A individuals experience time urgency.

☑ Intervention 6

If time permits and you feel comfortable with the technique, ask the patient to draw human figures (including one of himself). Ask him to include what he thinks is wrong with his heart. Also ask him to interpret the drawings.

Rationale and comments: Even to those uninitiated in the interpretation of psychological tests, human figure drawings can be exceedingly useful when hypothesizing about a patient's state of mind.

☑ Intervention 7

Administer medications for anxiety, as ordered.

Rationale and comments: A high percentage of hospitalized patients with MI suffer from depression and anxiety.

☑ Intervention 8

Stay with the patient or family member as much as possible if either is in a state of panic, or attempt to contact a friend or clergy to be with the family.

Rationale and comments: Individuals face fear easier in the company of someone else, rather than alone.

☑ Intervention 9

Leave lights on or doors open as requested by the patient.

Rationale and comments: Darkness can be frightening and increases the feeling of being alone.

BLOCKS TO COMMUNICATION

Block	Definition	Example
Value judgment	Moralizations by the nurse that imply or state directly how she feels the patient should feel or act; causes patient to fear disapproval or lack of care from nurse and to not express any more feelings	"How could you have gained so much weight?" "I don't see how you can feel that way!"
False or inappropriate reassurance	Comments made by the nurse that imply or state directly her feeling that everything will be all right when, in fact, it may not be true; causes the patient to stop expressing his feelings	"You don't need to worry about that!"
Advice and opinions	Comments or statements the nurse makes to inform the patient about what she thinks he should do in a particular situation or how she feels about a given subject; prevents patient from exploring his own ideas and coming to his own conclusions	"I think you should give up your job now that you've had a heart attack."
Leading questions	Questions posed by the nurse that imply a particular answer; inhibits the patient from stating his true thoughts or feelings because he finds it difficult to contradict a nurse	"You aren't having any pain now, are you?" "You don't eat a lot of eggs or red meat, do you?" "You aren't worried about that, are you?"
"Why" questions	Questions the nurse asks that require the patient to give a specific reason even if he is unlikely to know the answer; forces the patient to invent reasons to please the nurse or to give incomplete answers *Note:* "What" questions are considered the better approach.	"Why are you so upset over this test?" "Why aren't you taking your blood pressure pills?"

Adapted from Becknell, E., and Smith, D., *System of Nursing Practice.* Philadelphia: F.A. Davis Co., 1975. Used with permission.

✔ Intervention 10

Listen carefully during each contact with the patient for clues that feelings are either diminishing in intensity or continuing to exist. Continue listening, clarifying, and reflecting as often as necessary.

Rationale and comments: Fear of dying does not necessarily disappear after only one opportunity to discuss it. Patients differ in their ability to identify or name feelings and in their ability to express them to someone else.

✔ Intervention 11

Be as matter-of-fact as possible when identifying changes in the patient's condition. If the patient asks questions about his condition, answer as truthfully as possible, per your institution's policy.

Rationale and comments: Patients are sensitive to nurses' nonverbal cues and may misinterpret them to mean that their condition is not improving. Answering questions truthfully avoids the trap of lying and helps promote a trusting relationship between nurse and patient. Agencies and doctors differ regarding the amount of information patients can be told and by whom.

✔ Intervention 12

After a relationship with the patient or family is developed and conversation about feelings is flowing rather easily, suggest to the patient or family ways other than talking that may be used to reduce the intensity of anxious feelings, including:
• deep breathing
• using guided imagery
• exercising (within physical tolerance and medical orders)
• participating in arts and crafts
• watching television
• reading or doing puzzles.

Rationale and comments: Being able to employ his own methods of anxiety reduction can give a patient a feeling of mastery or control. Because someone may not always be available to discuss his feelings when anxiety arises, the patient may need to rely on other activities to divert the energy produced by such feelings.

✔ Intervention 13

Ask the patient or family every 3 or 4 days (at times other than during scheduled sessions) how they are feeling.

Rationale and comments: Evaluating the effect of nursing interventions on patients is important. If questions are posed and comments solicited only at the time of scheduled sessions, they may appear like leading questions and a true picture will not be obtained.

Anxiety related to impending cardiac surgery

SUPPORTING DATA

• Expresses fear of not surviving surgery
• Wonders about decision to have surgery
• Asks questions about the procedure, particularly about how long it will take, what he will be able to do afterward, and how long he will be in the intensive care unit or hospital
• May express one or more of the following either verbally or behaviorally:
—speaks in terms of fate or God's will
—uses precise technical language when discussing the illness
—discusses everything but his illness and the impending procedure or changes the subject if the nurse mentions it
—sleeps excessively or is unable to sleep, paces the floor, and has either a reduced appetite or an increased one
• Displays increased frequency of angina
• Cannot concentrate on any activity for any length of time

PLAN OF CARE
Outcome criteria

• Patient and family state their feelings about surgery.
• Patient states his role, the sensations he will experience, and the sequence of events for the day of surgery.
• Patient states he feels ready to go to surgery.
• Patient demonstrates a deep, forceful cough when asked.
• Patient participates in postoperative care when asked.

Interventions and rationales

☑ Intervention 1

Use therapeutic communication techniques any time the patient or family alludes to or directly states feelings of distress related to surgery (see *Therapeutic communication techniques,* pages 17 to 19).

Rationale and comments: Because patients often have fears, misconceptions, and concerns about future functioning, nurses inquire about these concerns. However, discussing uncomfortable feelings can be difficult for many patients; therefore, nurses rely on therapeutic techniques to help patients be more specific and discharge the energy created by anxiety.

☑ Intervention 2

Do preoperative teaching at a time convenient for the patient and family.

Rationale and comments: Unless a specific time is established, other activities may push aside the time necessary to prepare the patient for surgery. Sometimes, knowledge about an event helps reduce the associated anxiety. Including the family in the patient-teaching session lets them hear the same information as the patient, gives them a chance to ask questions, facilitates their relationship with the nurse, and gives the nurse the opportunity to enlist their aid and emotional support for the patient during the preoperative and postoperative periods.

☑ **Intervention 3**

Plan to allow for at least 30 minutes of uninterrupted time with the patient.

Rationale and comments: Sufficient time is needed for the patient and family to express their feelings and to ask questions.

☑ **Intervention 4**

Try to do the teaching the day before surgery. Ask the evening nurse to ask the patient if he has more questions and how he feels since hearing the information.

Rationale and comments: Teaching the patient during the early part of the day, not later in the evening, gives him a chance to ask the evening nurse further questions or to talk about the feelings he experienced during the patient-teaching session. Teaching the patient earlier than 2 days before surgery gives him too much time to dwell on the surgery, thereby contributing to his anxiety.

☑ **Intervention 5**

Provide the patient with the following information:

• *Patient's role.* The patient needs to know what he can and must do to help himself in the following areas:

—Coughing. Ask the patient to cough, and determine that he can cough deeply and forcefully. (Teaching a patient who is in pain to cough deeply is impossible. The patient's ability to cough effectively must be determined and obtained preoperatively when he is not in pain so that he may produce an effective cough postoperatively when he is in pain.)

If the patient is unable to produce a deep cough, work with him until he is able to do so by asking him to do the following: take a deep breath, exhale through the mouth, then cough from deep within the lung.

Show the patient how to use a pillow, bath blanket, or his hands to splint the sternum. (Having a method to reduce pain may help him do the task more easily.)

Explain to the patient that, although it will hurt to cough, he will be asked to do so anyway. Also explain that he will have pain medication available to help him and that he can use the above methods to splint his incision to reduce the pain. (Patients find it difficult to believe that they are asked to do something that is so painful for them. By acknowledging the patient's pain, you help him to feel less alone in performing such a difficult task.)

—Deep breathing. Important because it opens the alveoli and moves mucus, which stimulates a cough, deep breathing can also be used as a relaxation technique. Suggest that the patient practice these skills two or three times an hour during the remainder of his waking day. (Practicing these skills preoperatively emphasizes their importance and provides an outlet for anxious feelings as well as a distraction from them.)

—Asking for pain medication. Inform the patient that he should request pain medication when he needs it, not to wait for the nurse to administer it as ordered. (In some institutions, nurses offer medication as often as

ordered; in others, the nurse waits for the patient to ask for medication. The important thing is that the patient knows how to obtain medication.)
—Ambulating when asked. Explain to the patient that he may be asked to begin ambulating sooner than he expects. (Some patients think that they will be on bed rest until they feel well enough to get up.) Explain that walking will help prevent deep vein thrombosis, assist with deep breathing and hence coughing, promote peristalsis, and promote a feeling of improvement.

• *Sensations.* Unexplained and unexpected sensations can be extremely frightening to the patient. Therefore, it is important to prepare the patient to expect to feel certain new sensations associated with the surgery. Advise the patient to anticipate the following:
—Pain caused by incisions, chest tubes, or coughing. Emphasize that the tubes will be inserted after he is asleep (if applicable to your institution's policy) and that they will be removed as soon as possible.
—Inability to talk, but ability to hear, if endotracheal tube is left in place after anesthesia. Explain to the patient that the tube will be removed as soon as he is able to breathe on his own. Tell him that, not only are nurses expert at nonverbal communication and will understand what he is trying to communicate, but that he will be able to write when awake. (Patients need to know that they will have a way to communicate with the nurses and that the nurses will be able to understand what they are trying to say.)
—Feeling of having to void related to indwelling (Foley) catheter. Explain that this feeling may go away and that the tube will be removed as soon as possible. (Having a catheter inserted may make the patient feel uncomfortable and may be the the only thing on which he can focus. Having been informed about the catheter preoperatively and reminded of it postoperatively, he may be able to tolerate it better.)
—Feeling restrained upon awakening from anesthesia. Warn the patient that it may be necessary to restrain him before he awakens from anesthesia after surgery. Explain that the restraints may be applied until he is awake enough to follow commands so that he does not inadvertently pull on any of his I.V. lines. (When patients are awakening from anesthesia, they may be restless and unable to follow directions. Being warned about the restraints may help the patient not fight against them.)
—Soreness at the back of the throat or in the nose from the nasogastric tube. Explain to the patient that this tube will be removed when he no longer needs the breathing tube and has peristalsis again. Also explain that the endotracheal tube may also produce soreness at the back of his throat. (Many patients with endotracheal tubes get air in their stomachs, which the nasogastric tube removes. Again, being warned about the sensation may help the patient tolerate it and can even be reassuring because he remembers being told that this might occur.)
—Feeling of confinement because of numerous I.V. lines and monitors. Warn the patient that he may feel a sense of being confined and entangled. Remind him about the lines postoperatively (after he recovers from the anesthesia) so that he doesn't pull on them.

• *Sequence of events.* Telling the patient the sequence in which he can expect things to happen gives him a sense of predictability. Because institutions differ in their methods, the following plans should be adapted to the setting in which they will be used.

—Activities in the room the night before surgery and the morning of surgery, including the following:

(1) Shaving the skin. Advise the patient that he may be shaved the night before surgery or while he is asleep in the operating room the day of surgery to avoid bacteria growing overnight in any scratches or cuts.

(2) Showering with antiseptic solution both the evening before and the morning of surgery. Tell him that, if he cannot tolerate a shower, he may wash his skin with a cloth and antiseptic solution.

(3) Taking vital signs the morning of surgery. (Surgery cannot be performed if he has a fever. Also, if any new cardiac dysrhythmias are detected, surgery may be postponed.)

(4) Removal of false teeth and jewelry. If the patient desires, and the institution's policy allows, jewelry can be taped so it cannot be easily removed or catch on anything.

(5) Taping of medals (religious or other). Advise the patient not to pin any medals to his gown because the gown will be discarded when he is anesthetized and the medals will be lost. Tape medals to his abdomen or back as long as they will not interfere with placement of a cautery pad or other aspects of surgery. Put a note on the chart indicating the location of such medals.

(6) Administration of sleeping pills and preoperative sedation. (Sleep the night before surgery helps time pass more quickly, provides rest, and reduces awareness of anxiety. Institutions differ on the amount of medication that is given to patients preoperatively.)

(7) Transport to surgery. Depending on your institution's policy, inform the patient that he may have to wait in a holding area with other preoperative patients until the anesthesiologist is ready for him in the operating room or that he may remain in his room until the specific operating room is ready.

—Activities in the operating room or holding area. Advise the patient to expect to have at least one I.V. line started and a blood pressure cuff and cardiac monitor attached before surgery begins. (All patients receiving anesthetics are required to have at least one I.V. line in place in case emergency drugs need to be administered should the patient have an adverse reaction to the anesthetic. Usually more than one line is started, but only the first one may be started before the patient is put to sleep. A blood pressure cuff and cardiac monitor are required because the patient's blood pressure and cardiac rhythms can be altered by anesthesia and need to be watched closely during induction.)

Inform the patient that the anesthesiologist will tell him that he is putting him to sleep and that he may ask him to breathe oxygen through a mask even though the anesthetic is being given intravenously. (Anesthetics can cause respiratory depression, so oxygen is given to help prevent hypoxia.)

Note: Avoid telling the patient what will happen during the surgery itself unless he presses you for details. He won't have any control over the events, and the knowledge of what will be happening may be distressing to him.

—Activities after surgery. Depending on the institution's policy, inform the patient that he will awaken from surgery in an intensive care unit (ICU). (Some institutions require that patients go first to a recovery room, then to the ICU. The patient should know where he will be after surgery so that, after he awakens, he can begin his orientation process.) Also inform the patient's family so that they know where he will be and when.

Inform the patient that, as he is recovering from the anesthesia, he may hear much activity going on around him, some of which relates directly to him and much of which does not. Explain that, as the anesthesia wears off, he will be able to identify many of the sounds and will soon be able to discern those that belong to him.

• *Other information to cover.* If the patient expects to see his family before surgery, give a time by which they should arrive. Explain that the scheduled time for surgery refers to the actual procedure—when the surgeon begins to make an incision. (Sometimes the family misinterprets the surgery time to mean the time at which the patient leaves his room and, consequently, arrives too late.)

Tell the family where to wait during the surgery and whether they can expect to hear a progress report during the actual procedure. Also tell the family where to meet the doctor after surgery so that they can discuss the outcome. Avoid mentioning a specific length of time for the procedure; the family may hold this as absolute and worry if the procedure takes longer, even if the delay has nothing to do with the patient's condition.

Tell the family what the ICU visiting hours are and where the ICU and its waiting room are located. (Knowing this helps the family maintain contact with the patient despite their separation from him. It also lets them go directly to the waiting room when they come to visit rather than worry about getting lost and missing the visiting time.)

☑ Intervention 6
Tell the patient and family that anxiety is a normal feeling in their situation.

Rationale and comments: Acknowledging the normality of anxiety may assist both the patient and family to discuss the feeling and not believe they are going crazy or are abnormal in any way.

☑ Intervention 7
Ask the patient and family if they have any questions.

Rationale and comments: Nurses sometimes forget or fail to cover the very thing the patient or family wants to know. Being able to ask questions lets the family participate more than just listening does.

☑ Intervention 8
An hour later or on the next shift, ask the patient to tell the nurse what he knows about his role, the sensations he might experience, and what

things he expects to happen to him. Clarify any confusion and answer any questions he may still have.

Rationale and comments: Questioning the patient after a period of time is a way to evaluate the effectiveness of teaching. The patient may have forgotten the content, may have some confusion, or may have thought of more questions.

✓ Intervention 9

Ask the patient how he feels about the operation now that he has had the preoperative teaching (see *Therapeutic communication techniques,* pages 17 to 19).

Rationale and comments: The patient may know the facts; however, he may have more anxiety because of them and need an opportunity to talk about his feelings.

✓ Intervention 10

Anticipate that the patient may have increased anxiety, and ask if he needs help with some distraction techniques, such as:
• practicing coughing and deep breathing
• ambulating around the unit
• watching television
• reading
• visiting the hospital gift shop
• walking around outdoors (if hospital policy allows).

Rationale and comments: Talking about surgery can increase the patient's anxiety and only surgery can make the anxiety go away. Mild to moderate anxiety can be relieved for a while by distraction; however, severe anxiety cannot.

✓ Intervention 11

Note on a checklist or chart what the patient's and family's reaction is to the preoperative teaching, the questions they ask, and what the nurse on the next shift needs to do.

Rationale and comments: Documentation is essential for continuity of patient care. Using a checklist eliminates the need for writing the content to be covered in each separate chart and thereby allows more time to note responses to the teaching.

✓ Intervention 12

Postoperatively, ask the patient and family the following questions:
• Did they feel adequately prepared for the surgery experience?
• Do they have suggestions to offer other patients in similar situations?
• Can they offer any suggestions to nurses for improving the preoperative teaching they received?
• Do they wish to share any feelings about the experience now that it is over?

Rationale and comments: These questions serve as an evaluation of preoperative teaching and as a way to assist the patient and family to incorporate the experience into their present lives.

Anxiety related to lack of knowledge of procedures

SUPPORTING DATA
• Patient states he does not know what is going to happen to him during the procedure.
• Patient asks questions about the procedure, what it will feel like, how long it will take, and what he will have to do afterward.
• Patient states feeling fear, concern, or anxiety about the procedure itself, any pain that might be involved, or any complications that can occur.
• Family states the same things as above.

PLAN OF CARE
Outcome criteria
• Patient states feelings before and after procedure.
• Patient states the sensations, his role, and the sequence of events for each procedure he expects.
• Patient states he felt prepared for the procedure.
• Patient participates in preprocedural and postprocedural activities.

Interventions and rationales
☑ **Intervention 1**
Use the methods outlined in *Therapeutic communication techniques,* pages 17 to 19, any time the patient or family alludes to or states directly feelings of concern, fear, or anxiety about the upcoming procedure.

☑ **Intervention 2**
Ask the patient or family about their feelings or concerns if not stated spontaneously.

Rationale and comments: Unexpressed feelings create tension that could alter a patient's response to some diagnostic procedures, such as serial blood pressure measurements, or result in such complications as dysrhythmias. Not all patients can express themselves easily. Some may need the assistance of another person to put their feelings into words. If the nurse brings up the subject, she indicates it is an acceptable topic for discussion.

☑ **Intervention 3**
Set aside a specific time to talk with the patient and family about the procedure he will undergo. Ideally, this time should be uninterrupted and far enough in advance of the procedure so that they have enough time to absorb the information, think of further questions, and discuss any additional feelings the explanation may have aroused.

If time permits, schedule a follow-up session. If this is impossible, try to cover all of the areas mentioned in the following interventions during your initial explanation.

Rationale and comments: Setting a specific time to explain the procedure ensures that this task is awarded the same status as that of other scheduled nursing tasks.

✅ Intervention 4

Accompany the doctor when he visits the patient to explain the procedure.
• Listen for questions the patient asks the doctor and observe his nonverbal behavior.
• Use the patient's questions as a beginning point for your initial explanation session (if the doctor's session preceded yours), or use them as part of the follow-up session (if your session preceded the doctor's).
• Ask the patient to repeat what the doctor told him to ensure that he fully comprehended the explanation. If he has further questions, contact the doctor again.

Rationale and comments: The patient may not have heard correctly what the doctor said or, if his anxiety level was too high during the explanation, may not have really heard anything. Many cardiovascular diagnostic procedures have potentially life-threatening risks that can be frightening to patients and families. By accompanying the doctor, the nurse can assess the patient's comprehension firsthand and begin discussing the patient's feelings and concerns as soon as the doctor leaves.

✅ Intervention 5

Organize explanations into the following categories:
• patient's role during and after the procedure
• sensations he's likely to experience during and after the procedure
• sequence of events.

Rationale and comments: Research has shown that, if he is prepared in these three categories, the patient can better tolerate feelings of anxiety about the procedure and participate in the procedure and aftercare more easily.

✅ Intervention 6

When the patient returns to his room after the procedure, and the immediate postprocedural care has been implemented, ask him the following:
• how he is feeling
• how he thought the procedure went
• whether he felt adequately prepared for what he experienced.

Rationale and comments: The nurse's first priority after the patient returns to his room is to provide postprocedural care; however, taking time to discuss the event with the patient is also important. Asking the patient to express his feelings gives him permission to discuss them. The patient can also assist the nurse to evaluate the patient-teaching session and to improve professional behavior. For example, the nurse may discover that the explanation failed to cover a particular aspect of the procedure that was, in fact, most important to the patient. Knowing this, the nurse can then incorporate it into future explanations of that procedure.

Anxiety related to transfer from intensive or coronary care unit

SUPPORTING DATA

• Spontaneous or evoked feelings of fear or insecurity about transfer:
—Patient asks many questions about the nurses and the unit to which he is going.
—Patient asks if spouse or other persons will be able to stay with him in his new room.
—Patient even states that he wishes he could stay in the coronary or intensive care unit, where he knows everyone.
• Tachycardia
• Diaphoresis

PLAN OF CARE
Outcome criteria

• Patient's vital signs remain within his normal range.
• Patient and family state they are comfortable with the transfer process.
• Patient exhibits no complications that can be traced to the stress of transfer.
• Patient states he feels he slept well the night of transfer.

Interventions and rationales
☑ **Intervention 1**

Two days before the anticipated transfer, inform the patient and family that he will be transferred to a general medical unit.

Rationale and comments: The patient needs time to adjust to the idea of transfer but not such a long time as to build fears.

☑ **Intervention 2**

Arrange for a receiving nurse to visit the coronary care unit (CCU) to meet the patient and family.

Rationale and comments: Research has shown that transfer is a critical period, producing much stress. During this period, the nurse should focus interventions specifically on reducing stress. Beginning a nurse-patient relationship, a person-to-person orientation, is one way to reduce such stress.

☑ **Intervention 3**

If possible, take the patient to the new unit the day before transfer to introduce him to the staff and familiarize him with the new unit.

Rationale and comments: Familiarity helps reduce fear. The patient can see that nurses are available to help him and that he will not be alone. This is a person-to-space orientation.

☑ **Intervention 4**

Discuss the upcoming transfer with the family, and ask them to arrange to be present when it occurs. Also ask them to plan to spend time with the patient in his new room.

Rationale and comments: Strengthening the patient's support systems helps reduce the potential negative effects of stress during the transfer period. The family serves as a bridge between the constant care available in the CCU and the intermittent care available on a general unit.

☑ Intervention 5
Use therapeutic communication techniques (see *Therapeutic communication techniques,* pages 17 to 19) when listening and talking with the patient about the transfer so that he can identify his fears and understand them.

Rationale and comments: Feelings such as fear create energy, which increases the heart's work load. When expressed, these feelings are usually less frightening to the patient.

☑ Intervention 6
If possible, check the patient hourly on the day of transfer and especially during the first night. If hourly checks are impossible, tell the patient when you will return and then do so. If the patient is unable to sleep, see "Sleep-Pattern Disturbance" in this section.

Rationale and comments: Paying such frequent attention to the patient helps him to feel secure and less stressful, which reduces the heart's work load. Anxiety often interferes with sleep, and the inability to sleep increases anxiety.

☑ Intervention 7
Ask the patient about his feelings the day after the transfer.

Rationale and comments: Discussing his feelings the next day helps the patient to provide closure for the experience.

Bowel Elimination, Alteration in: Constipation

Alteration in Bowel Elimination: Constipation related to reduced activity, activity intolerance, restricted fluid intake per doctor's orders, insufficient food intake secondary to dislike of diet or poor appetite, psychological factors (such as fear of lack of privacy), inability to use or dislike of bedpan, difficulty asking for help, lack of a routine, or use of drugs (especially morphine sulfate)

SUPPORTING DATA
• Passage of small, hard, dry stools
• No stool for 2 or more days with oral intake and active bowel sounds
• Urge to defecate but inability to pass stool
• Headache
• Lack of appetite
• Sluggish, lethargic, bloated feeling
• Abdominal pain
• Frequent passage of liquid stool

PLAN OF CARE
Outcome criteria
• Passage of soft, formed stools per patient's usual schedule
• No discomfort in abdomen or rectum
• No reliance on laxatives, enemas, or suppositories

Interventions and rationales
☑ Intervention 1
Upon admission or as soon after as patient's condition allows, obtain the following information:
• frequency of bowel movements
• usual time(s) of day for defecation
• patient's definitions of constipation and diarrhea (Individuals have personal definitions for these two conditions, and then they act on these definitions.)
• patient's usual ways to prevent constipation (Part of the nurse's responsibilities involves helping patients to maintain habits during their hospitalization.)
• frequency of constipation and how patient usually treats it. (Some patients are stressed if they don't have a bowel movement every day.)

Rationale and comments: Constipation may result in the use of Valsalva's maneuver, which is dangerous to a patient with heart disease. Exhalation against a closed glottis results in decreased venous blood return to the heart, a slowed pulse rate, decreased cardiac output, and reduced coronary artery perfusion. When the patient then exhales, intrathoracic pressure drops and pulse rate increases. A patient with a damaged heart should avoid this additional stress.

Note: Some patients, especially those with low exercise tolerance or fluid restriction, may require the use of stool softeners.

☑ Intervention 2

Using the data obtained above, establish a scheduled time for the patient to sit on the bedside commode. Provide as much privacy as possible.

Rationale and comments: Even if no bowel movement occurs each time, the body responds to the regularity of this action; as other etiologic factors are overcome, bowel movements are likely to occur. The bedside commode provides a more natural position for defecation than the bedpan and therefore requires less energy. Lack of privacy alone can prevent successful elimination.

☑ Intervention 3

Prepare a fluid plan that is within doctor's orders for diet and fluid restrictions. Consider the following:

• Patient's preferences for kinds of fluids within diet order. (Keep in mind that, even if caffeine intake is unrestricted, all caffeine-containing drinks act as diuretics and thus defeat the purpose of the fluid intake plan. Also, some commercial sodas and juices have a high sodium component. Remember that diabetic patients will require sugar-free drinks.)

• Patient's preferences for amounts to drink at one time. (Because patients differ in the amount of fluid they can consume at one time, insisting that a patient drink more than he is willing to creates a power struggle and a stressful atmosphere that should be avoided. Adhering as much as possible to the patient's wishes gives him a feeling of being in control and of being cared for.)

• Rest and sleep periods. (The patient must have time to rest and sleep when he is not being asked to do anything for cardiac and psychological well-being.)

• Mealtimes. (If the patient's appetite is poor, he may be able to drink instead of eat. However, keep in mind that fluids can cause feelings of fullness rapidly and may interfere with the ingestion of food.)

• Medications. (A large amount of fluid can be consumed with oral medications; however, if the patient's fluid intake is restricted to less than 1,000 ml/day, the amount he takes with his medications should be carefully planned to get the pills down and still have fluids left for mealtimes and during the night.)

• Diet order. (A regular diet, regardless of sodium restriction, affords the patient numerous selections of foods appropriate to assist in bowel elimination. This type of diet provides foods that are high in fiber, including whole grain foods and raw fruits and vegetables.) If any other diet is ordered, assist the patient to choose the appropriate foods from the selections offered.

• Fluid plan goals. (Informing the patient and family about what the total daily fluid intake should be [if unrestricted, the patient should drink at least 2,000 ml/day] and planning the scheduled intake with them enhances adherence to the plan.)

Rationale and comments: Fluid is one of the main lubricants that assists passage of stool. If the patient is on a fluid-restricted diet, the nurse needs to ensure that he drinks the appropriate amount of fluid by developing an effective care plan—one that includes the patient's preferences and medical orders as well as the patient's and family's participation.

☑ Intervention 4

Write down the fluid plan and place it at the patient's bedside. Also place a copy in the patient's record.

Rationale and comments: Making the plan accessible to all health care personnel fosters compliance. Also, it should be made available to the family so they can assist the patient to follow it. The copy included in the patient's record can be used as a reference for subsequent admissions.

☑ Intervention 5

Explain to the patient which foods on the menu are the most appropriate to assist with elimination. If he has no clear preferences among the choices, select the foods for him.

Rationale and comments: Not all patients are equally informed about which foods are best to eat for easier bowel elimination. Sometimes, patients are willing to allow the nurse to make the decision for them, especially if choosing is a difficult or tiring task. Also, patients may be willing to eat foods and drink fluids that are beneficial to improving their condition, even those not among their favorites.

☑ Intervention 6

Ask the patient to exercise as much as he can tolerate or doctor's orders allow.

Rationale and comments: Exercise increases peristalsis and improves and helps maintain muscle tone.

☑ Intervention 7

Incorporate into the plan the patient's own rituals for assisting with a bowel movement, for example:

• drinking a glass of warm water or coffee upon arising
• eating particular cereals, fruits, or other foods at particular times.

Rationale and comments: Personal rituals provide a feeling of comfort and safety important to enhancing elimination.

☑ Intervention 8

Record the patient's bowel movements on the appropriate hospital records.

Rationale and comments: A record helps to measure success of interventions and provides data by which further decisions can be made.

☑ Intervention 9

Administer stool softeners or other prophylactic medications, as ordered.

Rationale and comments: Some institutions have standard protocols for cardiac patients that include medications to prevent constipation. If bulk-forming laxatives are used, they must be followed by a full glass of water or juice to remove all substance from the esophagus. Also, the patient must have a high fluid intake to keep material from forming a solid bolus in the intestine. However, these measures will be impossible if the patient's fluid intake is restricted.

☑ Intervention 10

If prophylactic measures are unsuccessful and no bowel movement occurs for 2 days, administer laxatives or enemas as ordered.

Rationale and comments: The patient should avoid performing Valsalva's manuever if at all possible. Parasympathetic nerve stimulation can occur in the rectum with the presence of stool, resulting in susceptibility to bradycardia.

☑ Intervention 11

Assess the patient for impaction if he has no bowel movement in 3 to 5 days; if he reports pressure in the rectum but is unable to pass stool; or if he has frequent, liquid stools. Perform a digital examination or report to the doctor per the institution's policy.

Rationale and comments: Mucosal irritation caused by stool in the rectum produces a liquid stool, which is the only thing that can get by the obstructing hard mass.

Note: Although morphine sulfate is an excellent analgesic for myocardial infarction pain or anginal pain not relieved by nitrates, it has constipating effects. The measures mentioned in the interventions above should be instituted upon admission to prevent constipation. Also, the patient may require more frequent use of laxatives than that ordinarily ordered during the acute phase to counteract the morphine and to avoid difficult passage of stool.

Comfort, Alteration in: Acute Pain

Alteration in Comfort: Acute Pain related to tissue trauma caused by surgery for coronary artery bypass grafting (CABG), valve replacement, peripheral arterial bypass, or leg amputation

SUPPORTING DATA
• Complaint of pain
• Tachycardia
• Elevated blood pressure (over patient's normal pressure)
• Shallow respirations
• Pallor and diaphoresis
• Anorexia
• Refusal to move, turn in bed, cough, deep-breathe, get out of bed, ambulate, or participate in prescribed exercises
• Insomnia
• Inability to concentrate
• Crying
• Irritability
• Withdrawal

PLAN OF CARE
Outcome criteria
• Patient reports that pain has decreased or disappeared.
• Patient experiences fewer episodes of acute pain.
• Patient moves, turns, and exercises as directed.

Interventions and rationales
☑ Intervention 1

Assess the patient for signs or symptoms of pain every few hours (see "Supporting Data" above). Keep the following points in mind.
• For patients who have undergone amputation, determine whether the patient's pain is incisional pain, phantom limb sensation, or phantom limb pain. Choice of interventions may vary depending on type of pain.
—Incisional pain, which is localized in the area of the surgical incision, is common postoperatively and usually responds to mild analgesics.
—Phantom limb sensation, a painless awareness of the amputated limb, is a common postoperative phenomenon. Patients rarely require analgesics and in many cases find distraction techniques and other nonpharmacologic means of pain relief effective.

—Phantom limb pain may range from uncomfortable cramping to excruciating, severe pain. Occurring in some patients, not all, it may develop immediately after surgery or after the patient is discharged. Various treatment methods are used; however, their effectiveness varies among patients.

• For patients who have undergone CABG surgery, determine whether the patient is having incisional pain or anginal pain.

—Incisional pain, which is aggravated by movement, respiration, coughing, or bending, is frequently located in the midsternal region and does not radiate.

—Anginal pain, which occurs rarely after CABG surgery, suggests a serious complication involving graft closure. If the patient develops signs of angina, notify the doctor immediately. (For information about characteristics of angina, see "Angina Pectoris" in Section II.)

• For patients who have undergone peripheral arterial bypass surgery, determine if the patient is having incisional pain or a recurrence of ischemic pain. Recurrent ischemic pain can be caused by an abrupt occlusion of the graft. Abrupt occlusions are characterized by pain in the affected extremity; loss of peripheral pulses distal to the occlusion; and change in skin temperature from warm to cold and skin color to pale, cyanotic, or mottled below the level of the occlusion. If the patient is experiencing recurrent ischemic pain resulting from the abrupt occlusion of an arterial graft, he'll require immediate medical intervention to prevent serious complications.

Rationale and comments: Each patient's pain experience is unique and is mediated by physiologic, emotional, cognitive, sociocultural, and behavioral factors. Because some patients don't report pain, nurses need to anticipate that each patient will experience pain postoperatively and require assistance to obtain pain relief.

☑ Intervention 2
Administer pain medication, as indicated by the patient's condition and within the legal parameters set by doctor's orders. Keep in mind the following points.

• Administer pain medication before the pain becomes severe.

—Tell the patient to report pain before it becomes severe.

—Because some patients deny they're in pain, assess the patient for such nonverbal signs of pain as refusal to move or exercise or to perform other activities. (When pain is allowed to build to a severe level, it is often difficult to relieve and frequently requires higher doses of medication.)

• Offer pain medication at regular intervals. (Administering medication at regular intervals is more effective.)

• Medicate the patient for pain before having him turn, cough, deep-breathe, perform prescribed exercises, or get out of bed. (Such activities tend to increase pain in postoperative patients.)

• Administer pain medication at night when the patient is preparing for sleep. (Pain seems more intense at night because the patient is less dis-

tracted and tends to focus more on the pain. Keep in mind that, if the patient is in pain, sleeping medications will be ineffective.)
• Observe the patient for adverse reactions to analgesics; consult the doctor for revised orders, when needed. If the following adverse reactions occur, notify the doctor immediately because the dosage may need to be adjusted or the medication changed:
—hypotension or dizziness
—confusion or hallucinations
—excessive sedation.
Note: Elderly patients are at particular risk for developing serious adverse reactions to pain medications.

☑ Intervention 3
Use the following nonpharmacologic means to obtain pain relief.
• Distraction. The following distraction techniques may decrease the patient's pain by drawing his attention away from it:
—watching television or listening to the radio
—visiting with family or friends
—playing games or working on hobbies
—reading.
• Physical relaxation or comfort. Relaxation that decreases muscle tension and stiffness associated with pain can be achieved by:
—a back rub
—position changes
—deep-breathing exercises.
• Decreased external stimuli. An environment that is perceived by the patient as calm and restful can facilitate pain relief. External stimuli can be decreased by:
—turning the lights down or off
—reducing or eliminating unpleasant sights or odors
—reducing the noise level in the patient's room by closing the door or turning off the television.

☑ Intervention 4
Develop with the patient a plan for achieving pain control. Be sure to cover the following:
• Discuss the role of pain relief in the recovery process. Explain that pain interferes with activity and exercise; this slows the patient's rehabilitation and increases the risk of complications related to immobility, including atelectasis, deep vein thrombosis, and constipation. Also explain that pain triggers a stress response, which increases myocardial work load and oxygen demand, and that pain relief prevents that response and lessens stress on the heart.
• Tell the patient which medications are available and how they can best be used.
• Advise the patient about which nonpharmacologic pain relief measures he may use.

Rationale and comments: Giving the patient some control over his pain decreases the associated distress. Some patients are concerned about taking pain medications unnecessarily and think they should avoid taking them for as long as possible. Providing information about the role of pain relief in facilitating recovery can help to allay this fear.

☑ Intervention 5

Evaluate the effectiveness of the interventions for relieving the patient's pain, and revise the interventions as needed. Evaluation techniques include:
• asking the patient if his pain is relieved or lessened
• observing the patient's ability or willingness to move, turn, or exercise as directed
• assessing the patient's vital signs for a drop in elevated blood pressure or for slowing of tachycardia.

☑ Intervention 6

If pain control is not achieved, consider:
• adjusting the administration of analgesics, as permitted within the legal parameters of the doctor's orders
• assessing for factors that may decrease effectiveness of pain control measures and intervening appropriately. Factors include:
—emotional response to surgery or condition
—anxiety
—inadequate sleep and rest.

Rationale and comments: The effectiveness of pain medication can be assessed by the patient's subjective report, physiologic parameters, or an increase in functional ability.

☑ Intervention 7

Additional interventions for patients who have undergone amputation include the following.
• If the patient's pain continues or increases despite interventions, implement the following:
—Assess the incision site for signs of infection and notify the doctor if any are present.
—Assess the residual limb for increased edema and notify the doctor if present.
—Assess for an incorrectly applied dressing; reapply the dressing, if needed.
• If the patient reports continued or increased phantom limb pain, consult the doctor about additional interventions to control the pain.

Rationale and comments: Although no single method has proved universally effective in relieving phantom limb pain, various methods have proved effective in some cases. They include antidepressant and neuroleptic medications, transcutaneous electrical nerve stimulation, local heat application, and surgical revision of the stump.

Alteration in Comfort: Acute Pain related to edema that occurs secondary to venous congestion caused by the occlusion of a vein by a thrombus

SUPPORTING DATA
• Pain, frequently described as dull and aching, in the affected extremity that is unaffected by rest
• Edema in the extremity

PLAN OF CARE
Outcome criteria
• Patient states that pain has lessened or is relieved.
• Patient's affected extremity is less edematous.

Interventions and rationales
☑ Intervention 1

Assess the patient every few hours for signs of pain.

Rationale and comments: Pain can result from edema, which results from vascular congestion that occurs when the lumen of a vein is narrowed by a thrombus.

☑ Intervention 2

Implement the following measures to reduce edema:
• Elevate the foot of the bed 30 degrees (unless contraindicated).
• Apply warm, moist heat, as ordered. Be sure to follow your institution's policy and the manufacturer's instructions for this.
• Administer anticoagulants as prescribed.

Rationale and comments: Elevating the foot of the bed facilitates venous return and decreases venous pooling, which helps decrease edema. However, this may be contraindicated for patients with severe arterial occlusive disease of the legs or severe congestive heart failure.

Applying warm, moist heat decreases pain by relieving venospasm and increasing the reabsorption of edema.

Administering anticoagulant therapy prevents any additional occlusion of the lumen of the vein by preventing growth of the thrombus.

☑ Intervention 3

Administer prescribed analgesics, as indicated by the patient's condition and within the legal parameters established by doctor's orders. (See the nursing diagnosis "Alteration in Comfort: Acute Pain related to tissue trauma" in this care plan for principles of analgesic administration.)

Rationale and comments: Use of mild analgesics may be required to control pain during the acute phase of deep vein thrombosis.

☑ Intervention 4

Use nonpharmacologic means to relieve the patient's pain. (See the nursing diagnosis "Alteration in Comfort: Acute Pain related to tissue trauma" for more information.)

☑ **Intervention 5**
Evaluate the effectiveness of measures used to decrease the patient's pain. Consider:
• the patient's statement of the type and nature of pain
• the amount of edema in the affected extremity.
Rationale and comments: The effectiveness of pain relief may be assessed by the patient's subjective report. Because pain and edema are closely related in patients with deep vein thrombosis, assessing for changes in the amount of edema present is also important.

Alteration in Comfort: Acute Pain related to ischemia that results when the blood flow to a lower extremity drops below the amount needed for the metabolic activities of the tissue at rest

SUPPORTING DATA
• Pain in feet or toes while at rest
• Tachycardia
• Elevated blood pressure (over the patient's normal pressure)
• Rapid respirations
• Pallor and diaphoresis
• Anorexia
• Refusal to move in bed
• Insomnia
• Crying
• Irritability
• Withdrawal

PLAN OF CARE
Outcome criteria
• Patient reports relief of pain.

Interventions and rationales
☑ **Intervention 1**
Assess the patient for signs of ischemic rest pain every few hours (see "Supporting Data" above).
Rationale and comments: Ischemic rest pain results when the blood flow to the leg drops below the level needed by the tissues for metabolic activities at rest.

☑ **Intervention 2**
Administer pain medication, as indicated by the patient's condition and within the legal parameters set by doctor's orders. (See "Alteration in Comfort: Acute Pain related to tissue trauma" in this care plan for principles of analgesic administration.)

Rationale and comments: Because ischemic pain is often quite severe, analgesics are prescribed.

☑ Intervention 3

Implement measures to promote blood flow to the affected extremity, including:

• Position the patient with the head of the bed elevated 30 degrees. (This position facilitates blood flow to the legs, which may help to decrease ischemia and its associated pain.)

• Keep the patient's legs warm by following these procedures. (Cold can cause vasoconstriction, which decreases blood flow and increases ischemia.)

—Avoid applying any form of heat directly to the legs. (Direct application of heat increases the tissues' oxygen demands by increasing its metabolic activity. In occlusive arterial disease, the diseased arteries cannot respond to this increased demand and ischemia results.)

—Keep the room temperature comfortably warm.

—Instruct the patient to wear cotton or wool socks to keep his feet warm.

—Use a bed cradle to keep covers off the patient's legs and feet if desired. (The weight of bed covers may increase pain.)

• Instruct the patient to refrain from smoking. (Smoking causes increased vasoconstriction and leads to increased ischemia by decreasing the blood flow.)

☑ Intervention 4

Use nonpharmacologic means of pain relief to supplement other measures. (See "Alteration in Comfort: Acute Pain related to tissue trauma" in this care plan for techniques to use.)

Rationale and comments: Improving blood flow can help to decrease ischemia and its associated pain.

☑ Intervention 5

Develop with the patient a plan for controlling ischemic pain. (Giving him some control decreases the distress associated with pain and can facilitate more effective relief.)

Depression, Reactive: Situational*

Reactive Situational Depression related to fatigue, pain, feelings of powerlessness, guilt, or anger, secondary to cardiac or peripheral vascular disease

SUPPORTING DATA
• Weakness, increased heartbeat, or lethargy
• Boredom
• Loss of appetite or weight or, conversely, increased appetite and weight gain†
• Difficulty sleeping, especially early in the morning, or sleeping excessively
• Statements about feeling worthless, sad, depressed, or unable to do anything
• Inappropriate guilt feelings
• Loss of interest in usual activities, family life, or sexual activity
• Decreased ability to concentrate or indecisiveness
• Agitation or hypoactivity
• Talk about dying or wishing for death, perhaps even of suicide; attempted suicide
• Irritability or outbursts of anger
• Refusal to participate in prescribed medical care plan; statements of "What's the use? It doesn't do any good anyway."
• Lack of desire to learn posthospital care
• Feelings of sadness or frequent crying episodes

PLAN OF CARE
Outcome criteria
• Patient eats and drinks according to collaborative plan.
• Patient has bowel movements according to prehospital or usual pattern.
• Patient reports feeling rested after naps and nighttime sleeping.
• Patient participates in all activity orders, increasing time and distance according to his physical ability and doctor's orders.
• Patient discusses his feelings with the nurse when asked.
• Patient states his plans for dealing with depression after hospitalization.
• Patient abides by prescribed treatment.

*Diagnosis not in NANDA classification at the time of writing. Used by permission of Dr. Marjory Gordon.
†Must be distinguished from weight gain caused by fluid retention.

Interventions and rationales
☑ **Intervention 1**

Observe the patient for signs of depression on the 3rd or 4th day after myocardial infarction (MI) or cardiac surgery. Signs include:
• lack of appetite
• questions about what he can do or expressions of fear about trying to increase activity
• slow verbal response
• irritable outbursts toward family members and nursing staff
• refusal to get out of bed.

☑ **Rationale and comments:** Depression is a universal response to MI and often begins in the coronary care unit after the initial anxiety and fear associated with heart attack subside. Usually, the patient begins to worry about returning to work and his usual life-style. For the surgical patient, it starts 2 or 3 days after transferring from the intensive care unit when his pain and lack of energy continue.

☑ **Intervention 2**

If the patient demonstrates signs of depression, use therapeutic communication techniques to help him put his feelings into words (see *Therapeutic communication techniques*, pages 17 to 19). Ask direct questions about what he is feeling.

Rationale and comments: By asking the patient to share his thoughts and feelings, the nurse can ease much of the tension associated with those thoughts. However, not all patients can express their feelings easily and some may need the nurse's assistance to do so. Asking direct questions may reveal more of what the patient is feeling than asking such general questions as "Would you like to tell me what you're thinking about?"

☑ **Intervention 3**

If the patient is not eating, see "Nutrition: Less Than Body Requirements" in this section for suggestions, and plan with the patient how much he will eat at each meal.

Rationale and comments: Lack of appetite, a common sign of depression, may be caused by dietary restrictions and the patient's anger over not being able to eat the foods he likes. Planning the patient's meals with him gives him a sense of control over the situation; feeling powerless is one of the causes of depression.

☑ **Intervention 4**

Establish a fluid plan with the patient (see "Bowel Elimination, Alteration in: Constipation" in this section for suggestions). Make sure the plan includes:
• giving the patient only one choice of fluid at a time. (Depressed patients have difficulty with making decisions, so their choices should be simple and concrete.)
• staying with the patient while he drinks the prescribed amount of fluid. (The patient will not be likely to drink the fluid on his own but may do so in the company of a nurse.)

• helping the patient to express anger constructively. (Being told that he must drink may make him angry, which can be therapeutic.)

Rationale and comments: Because depressed patients commonly do not drink as well as eat, they are at increased risk for insufficient fluid intake, leading to such complications as thickened pulmonary secretions, thicker blood (which can lead to blood clots), poor bowel elimination, and low urine output.

☑ Intervention 5

If the patient is unable to sleep, take the following measures:
• Make the patient as comfortable as possible by giving him a back rub, helping him with grooming, straightening the bed, adjusting him to a more comfortable position, turning down the lights, adjusting the room temperature, and making sure he has adequate pillows and blankets. (A deep, uninterrupted sleep may be all the patient needs to help lift his depression. Also, attention to his usual bedtime rituals may promote sleep.)
• Advise the patient to take a walk before settling down for the night, if his activity schedule permits. (Physical activity several hours before retiring helps the body achieve deep sleep.)
• Suggest that the patient take pain medication, if needed. If the patient is worried that he may be receiving too much pain medication, explain that his medication will be monitored carefully and that he will reduce his medication intake as the pain subsides. (Constant pain consumes much energy and can contribute to depression.)
• If the patient has had more than two nights of interrupted sleep, consider administering a hypnotic at the same time that pain medication is administered. (Pain medication may allow the patient to go to sleep and the hypnotic will help keep the patient asleep for several hours to provide the rest and refreshment he needs.)
• If at all possible, suspend monitoring the patient's nighttime vital signs. If a pulse check is required, take the pulse rate without waking the patient. If patient is on telemetry, disturb him only in the event of an abnormality.
• Use other means to help promote sleep, such as having the patient take a warm shower or giving him warm milk or some other protein if his condition and doctor's orders allow. (L-tryptophan, an amino acid present in milk and in various high-protein foods, reduces the length of time required to fall asleep.)

☑ Intervention 6

If the patient is sleeping most of the time, follow these procedures:
• Wake him up for meals, reminding him of his contract for eating and drinking.
• Tell him to bathe and assist him as needed. Allow him to rest between activities, as his condition requires.
• Avoid asking him direct questions concerning whether he wants to perform or participate in a specific activity, especially if he can answer with a "Yes" or "No" response. (Depressed patients usually do not wish to exert energy of any kind and are therefore more likely to answer "No" before thinking whether or not the request is something they want to do.)

• Tell him when to get out of bed (following his activity prescription), and walk with him as much as possible.

• If he expresses anger, accept it and use therapeutic communication techniques to help him channel the anger and to understand its source. (See *Therapeutic communication techniques*, pages 17 to 19.) However, remember to keep your own anger under control when responding to the patient's anger.

Rationale and comments: Anger is a normal response to being asked to do something that he may not wish to do. Depression is thought to occur when anger is directed toward the self, rather than outwardly toward others. Helping the patient direct his anger outwardly helps to lift his depression.

☑ Intervention 7
Ask the patient each day if he has had a bowel movement.

Rationale and comments: A depressed patient may not heed bodily sensations for bowel elimination. Also, his food and fluid intake will probably be low, contributing to the development of this condition.

☑ Intervention 8
Before discharge, discuss the following with patient and family:

• Explain that, like most patients (medical and surgical), he may experience fatigue after returning home; tell him that he should not let it frighten him. It usually diminishes as the patient increases his activities, not by staying in bed or in a chair all day.

• Ask the patient, family, and/or caregiver if they have thought about any of the following situations; help them talk about their concerns using therapeutic communication techniques.

—He won't be able to work anymore and will be condemned to a sickbed from now on.

—He can no longer enjoy sex. (He may have heard of others dying during orgasm and fears this may happen to him; see "Sexual Dysfunction" in this section.)

—He must avoid becoming excited. Talk with the patient about the difference between excitement and feeling upset. (Excitement can be an invigorating feeling, helping the patient overcome depression, whereas feeling upset drains the patient of energy and should be avoided when possible. Believing in this myth can cause the patient to think of all the things he might have to give up, thus contributing to his depression.)

—He will have another heart attack and die in his sleep. (Although the patient and family will eventually need to accept and get used to the thought that he may die of another attack, it is not likely helpful at this time to say so.)

—He will split open the sutures, or he knows that something is wrong because of the continuing pain. (Tell the patient and family that the incision will not open, and explain that it takes about 6 weeks for the sternum to heal, during which time the patient is likely to feel discomfort.)

• Ask them what methods they will use to overcome the patient's depression, and offer guidance if they request it. (The patient and family may have their own ways of solving personal problems; however, it may be possible to offer additional suggestions if they are having difficulty. See "Stress Management" in Section III for suggestions.)

• Tell the patient and family the following:

—Depression is usually self-limiting, usually subsiding in 3 months or less. (Knowing this, the patient and family can then spend their energy on moving ahead rather than wondering when the feeling is going to disappear.)

—An active exercise program and returning to work as soon as possible can help lift the depression. (Physical activity promotes well-being and provides a feeling of success and cardiovascular fitness. Work gives the patient a purpose for getting up each day and reminds him he is back to normal. Keep in mind that patients who were retired at the time of their MI will require a different stimulus to remind them they are getting better.)

—If the depression does not lift in 3 months, suggest they consider consulting a professional counselor. (Sometimes, having an MI creates other difficulties for the patient that are not overcome by the usual post-MI, postoperative recovery regimen; counseling may help.)

• Ask if the patient and family have any other concerns about the patient's returning home. (Verbalizing such concerns helps to reduce anxiety and can prompt suggestions for dealing with them before they become unmanageable. See "Family Processes, Alteration in" in this section for other suggestions for home teaching.)

Rationale and comments: Because the patient will have been on bed rest with limited activity during his hospitalization, he will be weak for at least 4 weeks after resuming activity. Warning the patient that this is likely to happen and that it has nothing to do with his heart may help prevent severe depression. Anticipating fears the patient or family may have after discharge gives them a chance to explore them now, thereby reducing their intensity later. If they encounter the fears later, they can recall the earlier discussion and may remember that talking about such fears reduced their intensity.

Diversional Activity Deficit

Diversional Activity Deficit related to prolonged hospitalization for prescribed medical therapy

SUPPORTING DATA
• Complaints of boredom
• Restlessness
• Anger over prolonged hospital stay

PLAN OF CARE
Outcome criteria
• Patient expresses feelings about prolonged hospitalization.
• Patient chooses strategies to decrease his diversional activity deficit.
• Patient engages in chosen activity.
• Patient reports decreased boredom and feelings of restlessness.

Interventions and rationales
☑ **Intervention 1**
Spend time talking to the patient about his emotional response to prolonged hospitalization. Explain that feelings of anger, frustration, fear, anxiety, and boredom are normal responses to prolonged hospitalization.

Rationale and comments: Patients may not recognize or understand the feelings that they are experiencing. A nurse's acknowledgment and acceptance of these feelings may help the patient accept and handle them.

☑ **Intervention 2**
Develop a plan with the patient to help decrease boredom using the following strategies:
• Allow the patient more control over daily routines.
• Have the patient ask family or friends to bring in books, tapes, or a radio.
• When his condition permits, suggest the patient spend time outside of his room. (A change in scenery and an opportunity to visit with other patients, family, or friends break up the monotony of the patient's day and make the time pass more quickly.)
• Enlist the use of patient support systems to provide visitors or other forms of diversion. Examples include church groups, social organizations, hospital volunteers, and other local volunteer groups.
• Ask the patient's family to bring in items from home to decorate his room. (Familiar objects from home decrease the antiseptic atmosphere of the patient's hospital room.)
• Suggest that the patient work on hobbies.

Rationale and comments: The patient plays a key role in decreasing a diversional activity deficit. The nurse can advise, recommend, and assist in obtaining resources; however, only the patient can determine which activities he enjoys.

☑ Intervention 3
Consult an occupational or recreational therapist, if indicated.

☑ Intervention 4
Assess for and reduce factors that limit the patient's ability to engage in diversional activities, including:
• pain
• fatigue
• anxiety
• depression
• financial concerns.

Rationale and comments: Multiple factors can contribute to the patient's diversional activity deficit. Reducing these factors can increase the patient's ability to engage in diversional activities.

Family Processes, Alteration in

Alteration in Family Processes related to anticipated or actual change in role or relationships or perceived or actual inadequate or absent support systems

SUPPORTING DATA
• Anticipated caregiver's lack of knowledge of home care
• Family members' concern about how they will continue present activities now that patient is ill
• Family members' or anticipated caregiver's fear or uncertainty about administering home care
• Spouse's concern about becoming the decision maker or about carrying out any other tasks the patient routinely performed
• Spouse's or significant other's feelings of loss of affection, emotional closeness, or sexual attention
• Spouse's or caregiver's lack of financial, emotional, or physical resources needed for anticipated home care

PLAN OF CARE
Outcome criteria
• Caregiver states plans for providing home care and comfort with those arrangements.
• Caregiver states resources to use if assistance is needed in areas identified as potentially problematic.

Interventions and rationales
☑ Intervention 1
Ask the patient, spouse, or significant other who the primary caregiver will be when the patient is discharged from the hospital. Consult the doctor, as needed, to determine the prognosis and anticipated date of discharge.

Rationale and comments: Discharge planning requires time and should begin as soon as possible. Discussing home care may be a source of hope to families and may help them through the crisis period; however, this should be individualized according to each family's needs.

☑ Intervention 2
Schedule time for discharge planning when you're least likely to be interrupted and when most of the family can be present.

Rationale and comments: Families find it difficult to maintain their concentration during interruptions for other care. Scheduling gives the activity the importance it deserves and allows more family members to attend than if teaching is done exclusively at the nurse's convenience.

☑ Intervention 3
Determine the amount and type of care the patient will need.

Rationale and comments: Care needs can range from seeing that a patient takes his own medications to administering total care to a bedridden patient.

☑ Intervention 4
Assess the patient's home situation according to the following criteria:
• Find out about the physical setup of the home, including:
—steps
—location of bathroom
—safety devices, including lights, handrails in tub, and a chair in the shower
—hazards, such as loose rugs, animals, or toys
—location of the patient's room in relation to the rest of the family's activities.
• Ask who the family decision maker is. (Patterns of family interaction are likely to be continued; however, if the patient was the decision maker and is now unable to make the decisions, this may be difficult on the rest of the family. This role shift can be frustrating to both the patient and the family, leading to other psychological effects, such as anger and isolation.)
• Collaborate with a social worker, if needed, for someone to visit the patient's home before discharge to gather data by observation rather than interview.

Rationale and comments: By gathering complete data on the home and assessing the patient's needs, the nurse can help the family better anticipate potential problem areas and can offer suggestions for adapting the environment to the patient's benefit.

☑ Intervention 5
Ask the patient's spouse or significant other and family members what resources are available for assistance in:
• lifting the patient or performing other physical tasks during the day or night, if needed
• obtaining groceries, medications, and other items (such as dressings) to care for the patient
• providing child care, if needed
• obtaining transportation
• paying for medications
• maintaining the house
• providing relief for the caregiver, as needed
• preparing meals
• getting the patient to the laboratory, doctor's office, or hospital.

Rationale and comments: By exploring all aspects of the patient's home life and anticipating both the patient's and family's needs, the nurse can help prepare the family to cope with maintaining usual routines while incorporating the additional care of a person with a chronic illness. Not all families will need the same amount of assistance.

✓ Intervention 6

Using role playing, review with the caregiver a typical day's sequence of events to see how the family will integrate the patient's care with daily routines.

Rationale and comments: By role playing, the caregiver and family can anticipate many of the difficulties that can arise during a typical day and can better plan how to deal with them.

✓ Intervention 7

Asking the caregiver's permission, refer the family to various resources, such as a visiting nurse, social worker, or clergy, if needed. First obtain the doctor's permission, per your institution's policy.

Rationale and comments: Families sometimes hesitate to accept help from outside sources; however, they may be more willing to do so if they are included in the decision process.

✓ Intervention 8

Discuss with the caregiver his feelings about caring for the patient at home. Pay particular attention to how much care he expects to provide as opposed to how much self-care he expects from the patient. (See *Therapeutic communication techniques,* pages 17 to 19.)

Rationale and comments: The patient's recovery depends on his ability to resume as much self-care as he can manage. Also, the more he does for himself, the less depressed he is likely to be.

✓ Intervention 9

Advise the caregiver to expect the patient to be depressed after returning home, explaining that it is a normal response after a serious illness or surgery.

Rationale and comments: Post-discharge depression is a common occurrence; the patient and family should be informed about this so that they aren't too worried and can take some measures to reduce its intensity and duration.

✓ Intervention 10

Review with the family which symptoms they should look for, depending on the patient's particular condition, and when to call the doctor.

Rationale and comments: Providing care is only one aspect of home care; monitoring the patient's condition is equally important and sometimes frightening. By being properly prepared, the family will feel more confident in their ability to care for the patient.

☑ **Intervention 11**
Review with the patient and family all the medications the patient will be taking.

Rationale and comments: Making sure the patient receives all his medications is one of the most important aspects of home care. Because administering numerous cardiovascular medications can be confusing, the patient and family should receive adequate instruction.

☑ **Intervention 12**
Ask the patient, family, and/or caregiver after each teaching session and before discharge if they have any questions or concerns about home care.

Rationale and comments: Questions or additional concerns can arise after the teaching session, but the patient, family, or caregiver may be hesitant to ask. Asking gives them the opportunity to talk about the subject further.

☑ **Intervention 13**
The day before the patient's discharge, ask the patient, family, and/or caregiver to state separately, in their own words, the prescribed regimen and their plans for carrying it out as well as their other home responsibilities. Correct any misconceptions and answer any remaining questions.

Rationale and comments: Asking those involved in caring for the patient after discharge to state their understanding of what they are expected to do is a more effective way of evaluating the teaching than just asking if they understood the explanations.

Alteration in Family Processes related to ill family member

SUPPORTING DATA
Family members may do any of the following:
• criticize the patient's nursing or medical care
• frequently request nursing care by using the patient's call light or making trips to the nurses' station
• use an insistent, demanding tone of voice
• provide total care for the patient, not allowing him to do things according to his physical or emotional ability or doctor's orders
• cry frequently, in and out of the patient's room, or refuse to go home for rest and relaxation despite the nurse's assurance that the patient will be all right
• ask questions about all aspects of the patient's nursing care while the nurse is attending the patient.

PLAN OF CARE
Outcome criteria
• Family members participate in the patient's care as directed, helping with what they can and are asked to do and allowing the patient to do what he can and should do for himself.

• Family members state that their home affairs are in order and satisfactory to them.
• Family members state they understand the care the patient is receiving.
• Family members state they feel confident with the nursing care the patient is receiving.

Interventions and rationales
☑ **Intervention 1**
Use therapeutic communication techniques to discuss the family's feelings about the patient's illness. (See *Therapeutic communication techniques,* pages 17 to 19.)

Rationale and comments: A serious illness to a family member is considered a crisis. Family members, like most individuals involved in a crisis, need the opportunity to talk about what has happened to them. Therapeutic communication techniques assist nurses in keeping the conversation focused on the family and their needs.

☑ **Intervention 2**
Ask the family to talk with you outside the room, preferably in a lounge or private room.

Rationale and comments: The family may be able to express themselves more fully outside the patient's hearing. Also, providing a private room and adequate seating promotes a feeling of importance to the activity as well as comfort. Developing a relationship with the family is as important as developing one with the patient.

☑ **Intervention 3**
Explain to the family the care plan for the patient. Inform them about:
• the patient's medical and nursing goals
• what interventions will be taking place
• what the patient will be expected to do for himself
• what the family can do to help the patient.

Rationale and comments: The family will be unable to participate unless they understand what is happening, what their role is, and what the patient is expected to do. They probably fear that the patient is going to die, regardless of whether they express this aloud, and want to do everything possible to prevent it from happening. However, they probably do not want to interfere with the care he is receiving. They have their own needs, which are affecting their behavior, and are probably unaware of how their behavior is affecting others involved in the patient's care.

☑ **Intervention 4**
Repeat the above information frequently, as needed, especially whenever a change in the care plan occurs.

Rationale and comments: Anxiety interferes with the family's ability to concentrate and hear clearly. Also, cardiovascular patients frequently have rapid changes in their condition; the family should be informed of these changes.

☑ Intervention 5

Ask the patient's family about the following:

• what arrangements they have made to ensure that they get adequate rest
• who may be available to help at home with such routine tasks as maintaining schedules, providing child care, and buying groceries
• concerns they have about themselves
• outside resources they can depend on for comfort while the patient is hospitalized, such as friends, church groups, and social organizations to which they belong.

Rationale and comments: Although the patient is hospitalized, the family needs to proceed with their own lives. However, the disruption caused by the patient's illness may be severe. Assisting the family with various arrangements eliminates one source of stress and allows them to concentrate on the patient. It also helps to maintain the family's overall health during the crisis.

☑ Intervention 6

Assist the family in making arrangements or contacting social services, depending on the above information.

Rationale and comments: Although discussing the situation is helpful, the family should proceed with definite plans as soon as possible. Nurses can usually provide the family the assistance they need; however, a social worker often has more readily available community information.

☑ Intervention 7

Ask the family periodically if the arrangements they made continue to be satisfactory. Frequency will depend on how difficult the problem was to solve in the first place.

Rationale and comments: Asking the family how their plans have fared shows that the nurse still cares about solving their problems. If the plans are not working, the family may be less hesitant to discuss them with someone who is sympathetic to their situation.

Fluid Volume Excess: Edema

Fluid Volume Excess: Edema related to complex neural, hormonal, and hemodynamic compensatory mechanisms that occur in response to the fall in cardiac output seen in congestive heart failure

SUPPORTING DATA
• Dyspnea on exertion
• Orthopnea
• Paroxysmal nocturnal dyspnea
• Rales and/or wheezes in lung fields
• Edema in dependent sites
• Weight gain of 2 lb or more per day
• Cough
• Nocturia, with oliguria during the day
• Increasing fatigue without increased activity
• Jugular vein distention
• Anorexia and nausea
• Abdominal distention

PLAN OF CARE
Outcome criteria
• Patient exhibits signs of decreased fluid volume excess, including:
—weight loss
—no additional weight gain
—decreased dyspnea
—improved arterial blood gas levels and chest X-rays
—decreased edema in dependent sites.

Interventions and rationales
☑ **Intervention 1**
Administer diuretics, as ordered.

Rationale and comments: Diuretics help reduce excessive water retention and relieve edema.

☑ **Intervention 2**
Limit the patient's sodium intake, as ordered, by:
• providing sodium-restricted meals
• advising him not to add salt to his meals
• providing low-sodium snacks between meals
• providing low-sodium fluids to drink
• explaining the need for restriction to the patient and family.

Rationale and comments: Restricting dietary sodium reduces the water retention in the body and helps relieve edema. Careful attention should be paid to the sodium content of snacks and fluids offered to the patient so that the total dietary intake of sodium does not exceed the amount prescribed.

☑ Intervention 3

Limit the patient's fluid intake, as ordered, using the following measures:
• Develop a fluid plan with the patient and family.
• Teach the patient and family how to monitor the patient's intake.

Rationale and comments: The doctor may order restricted fluid intake for some patients with congestive heart failure (CHF) to help decrease excessive water retention. The restriction may vary, usually ranging from 800 to 1,500 ml/day. Although patients should not exceed the prescribed fluid limit, they should try to drink all of the amount ordered over a 24-hour period to prevent such complications as constipation and fluid and electrolyte imbalances.

☑ Intervention 4

For patients who don't have a prescribed fluid limit, follow these measures:
• Monitor and record intake and output.
• Assess for signs of fluid volume excess (see "Supporting Data" above for details).
• Collaborate with the doctor about ordering a fluid limit if the patient's intake is consistently high and he shows signs of fluid volume excess.

Rationale and comments: By definition, all patients with CHF have some impairment in the heart's pumping action. Drinking large amounts of fluid may precipitate acute symptoms of CHF for some patients.

☑ Intervention 5

Assess and record data to evaluate the patient's fluid volume status. Follow these procedures:
• Maintain strict intake and output. (Intake and output records provide data about the patient's response to diuretics and a comparison of 24-hour intake to output).
• Obtain daily weights. (These provide the most consistently accurate information about the loss or gain of excessive fluid.)
• Auscultate the lungs for rales. (Decreased rales may indicate improvement; increased rales may indicate increased fluid volume excess and reflect a deterioration of the patient's condition.)
• Assess for edema in dependent sites, such as the sacrum in bedridden patients and the legs in ambulatory patients. (Decreased edema in these sites may indicate a decrease in fluid volume excess; increased edema may indicate increased retention of fluid and deterioration of the patient's condition.)
• Monitor pertinent laboratory and diagnostic studies, including:
—arterial blood gas levels
—chest X-ray reports
—serum electrolyte levels for imbalances that can develop as a result of diuretic therapy or sodium and fluid limits.

Gas Exchange: Impaired

Gas Exchange: Impaired, related to accumulation of fluid in the interstitial spaces and alveoli of the lungs secondary to congestive heart failure

SUPPORTING DATA
• Dyspnea on exertion
• Dyspnea at rest
• Orthopnea
• Paroxysmal nocturnal dyspnea
• Rales and/or wheezing in lung fields
• Cough (dry; hacking; or productive of frothy, sometimes blood-tinged, sputum)
• Arterial blood gas levels indicative of hypoxia and respiratory acidosis

PLAN OF CARE
Outcome criteria
• Patient demonstrates improved gas exchange as evidenced by:
—improved arterial blood gas levels
—improved chest X-rays
—decreased episodes of dyspnea
—decreased adventitious sounds in lung fields.

Interventions and rationales
☑ **Intervention 1**
Assist the patient to a position of comfort. Commonly used positions include:
• lying in bed, with head of bed elevated. (This position facilitates breathing.)
• sitting in a chair, with feet dependent. (This position facilitates venous pooling and decreases venous return to the heart. Unless contraindicated by unstable vital signs or other complications, chair rest is appropriate to decrease dyspnea.)
• sitting on side of the bed, with feet dependent and trunk and arms supported on overbed table. (Some patients prefer this position to relieve acute or severe episodes of dyspnea.)

☑ **Intervention 2**
Administer oxygen, as ordered.
Rationale and comments: Supplemental oxygen helps decrease hypoxia and relieve the subjective sensation of dyspnea.

☑ Intervention 3
If the patient requires continuous use of oxygen, take the following measures:
• Obtain a nasal cannula for him to use during meals.
• Connect extension tubing to the oxygen mask or cannula to permit the patient to move in the room with the oxygen running.
• Have the patient use a portable oxygen system whenever he leaves the room.

Rationale and comments: Patients who require continuous administration of oxygen can become acutely short of breath if oxygen is discontinued for even short periods of time.

☑ Intervention 4
Implement the measures outlined in "Fluid Volume Excess: Edema" in this section.

Rationale and comments: Impaired gas exchange in congestive heart failure (CHF) is directly related to the retention of excessive fluid, a result of complex neural, hormonal, and hemodynamic compensatory mechanisms that occur when the patient's cardiac output drops. Effective management of impaired gas exchange must include measures to reduce this excess fluid volume.

☑ Intervention 5
Implement measures to decrease the patient's anxiety as outlined in "Anxiety" in this section.

Rationale and comments: Anxiety adversely affects gas exchange by increasing the patient's respiratory rate and decreasing the depth of respiration. Relieving or reducing anxiety can facilitate the effectiveness of other measures employed to improve gas exchange.

☑ Intervention 6
Implement measures to limit the patient's activity as outlined in "Activity Intolerance related to decreased cardiac output" in this section.

Rationale and comments: Activity is a physiologic stress; in CHF the body's response to this stress may result in increased pulmonary vascular congestion and increased impairment of gas exchange in the alveoli. Rest decreases the body's demand for cardiac output and can facilitate the excretion of retained, excessive fluid, thus relieving pulmonary vascular congestion.

☑ Intervention 7
Assess the patient for changes in respiratory status, and notify the doctor when indicated. Follow these measures:
• Monitor the patient's respiratory status, including:
   —amount of dyspnea experienced
   —respiratory rate and rhythm
   —presence of rales on auscultation of lung fields.
• Check the patient's chest X-ray reports.
• Monitor the patient's arterial blood gas levels.

Grieving, Family

Grieving: Family related to actual loss of family member

SUPPORTING DATA
• Moaning, screaming, sobbing, pacing the floor, or wringing the hands
• Staring into space without saying anything and being unable to make decisions
• Thinking and acting logically and appropriately for the moment, but later being unable to remember what the decisions and actions were or how they were made

PLAN OF CARE
Outcome criteria
• Family shares feelings and concerns with the nursing staff.
• Family's anger is directed more at the nurse than at the patient.
• Deceased patient's family makes the necessary decisions before leaving the hospital.
• Deceased patient's family states they feel all right about leaving the hospital (after all arrangements have been made per institution's policy).

Interventions and rationales
☑ **Intervention 1**
Use therapeutic communication techniques during each interaction with the family (see *Therapeutic communication techniques,* pages 17 to 19).

Rationale and comments: Nurses can help family members to deal with the various emotions brought on by the patient's hospitalization and the realization that he might die. This is a particularly frightening time for both the patient and family.

☑ **Intervention 2**
If the patient is likely to die, listen to the family reminisce about the life they have shared.

Rationale and comments: Although nurses may feel helpless with a grieving family, their presence can be a source of comfort to the family.

☑ **Intervention 3**
See *Interventions to use with grievers* for suggested interventions that can be helpful to a bereaved person when death finally occurs.

Rationale and comments: The hospital nurse's role extends to the departure of the family and discharge of the body to the hospital morgue.

INTERVENTIONS TO USE WITH GRIEVERS

Interventions	Rationale and comments
• Stay with the griever as much as possible or send for another person to stay with him.	• Because death can leave a griever in a state of shock, the presence of a nurse or another person at this time is important.
• Sit in silence, looking for clues that the griever wishes to talk, including: —sighing —movement of the lips —movement of the body after sitting still for a while —looking at the nurse after a period of looking away.	• The griever may wish to talk about the deceased in an attempt to keep the person alive and to reduce the pain of the loss.
• Reflect the griever's cues as gently as possible with statements such as: —"You look as if you wished to say something." —"Was there something you wished to say?" —"You want to talk but are finding it difficult."	• The nurse's presence and gentle suggestions to talk may help the griever begin expressing his loss (an intellectual acknowledgment that a loss has occurred), which is the first step in the grieving process.
• Refrain from making comments that attempt to remove the pain or rationalize the loss or that try to make the griever focus on others who can fill the void in his life. Avoid such comments as: —"Think of your children, who need you now." —"It's God's will." —"Friends and family will help ease your pain."	• Although the nurse may wish to help the griever feel better, she cannot take away the pain of the loss; any comments or remarks that attempt to do so may reduce the griever's ability to express grief, a process that is, in itself, helpful and therapeutic.
• Expect outbursts of anger, and try to reflect them rather than react to them with such statements as: —"It just makes you furious that he died and left you alone like this." —"You're angry because I can't bring him back to you."	• Anger is a normal feeling in response to loss; if the nurse accepts it as such, the griever is more likely to accept it also.
• Touch the griever, as long as it is comfortable and appropriate to do so.	• Touch, when done in a comfortable manner, conveys caring, support, and a feeling that the griever is not alone. Nurses must be sensitive to the fact that some grievers may not allow themselves to be touched. Their unwillingness may be a reaction to anger, not a dislike of touch.

(continued)

INTERVENTIONS TO USE WITH GRIEVERS *(continued)*

Interventions	Rationale and comments
• Express your own feelings to the griever as long as they are honest and do not become the focus of the interaction. Expressions may include: —such statements as "I'm so sorry" —tears —quivering voice —spontaneous holding.	• The griever may find it comforting and therapeutic to know that the nurse cares enough to be touched by the loss also. However, it is not helpful for nurses to discuss their own needs at this time.
• Ask the griever to make any decisions only after the initial grieving has occurred; try to make the choices as simple as possible.	• In the period immediately after the patient's death, grievers experience many emotions and are unable to make decisions.

Grieving: Family related to anticipated loss of family member secondary to cardiovascular disease

SUPPORTING DATA
• Crying in response to news from the doctor about the patient
• Asking many questions of the intensive care unit staff or other personnel about the patient's condition
• Talking about how the patient and family used to be
• Finding it difficult to stay with the patient, even difficult to visit
• Refusing to leave the patient's bedside or the waiting room
• Questioning how family life will proceed after the anticipated death
• Being unable to sleep, eat, or engage in usual activities because of feelings of anxiety or depression
• Being unable to talk about the patient's condition or changing the subject if asked about his condition
• Showing irritability and even anger toward the patient or the staff
• Insisting on doing everything for the patient even though he is capable of doing things for himself
• Being unable to provide any care for the patient or calling the nurse for assistance every time the patient needs something
• Making statements about being unable to go on if the patient dies
• Calling all the relatives to come see the patient before it is too late
• Expressing disbelief of the situation and what is happening

---

PLAN OF CARE
Outcome criteria
• Patient and family share feelings and concerns with the nursing staff.
• Family's anger is directed more at the nurse than at the patient.

• Patient participates in his own care according to his abilities and doctor's orders.
• Family lets patient participate in his own care as above.
• Family provides care for things he is unable to do for himself.
• Family takes breaks from the patient's bedside.

Interventions and rationales

☑ Intervention 1

Use therapeutic communication techniques during each interaction with the family (see *Therapeutic communication techniques,* pages 17 to 19).

Rationale and comments: Nurses can help family members to deal with the various emotions brought on by the patient's hospitalization and the realization that he might die. This is a particularly frightening time for both the patient and family.

☑ Intervention 2

Explain to the family the plan of care for the patient and the care being administered to him.

Rationale and comments: Families find it easier to cope when they know what is happening.

☑ Intervention 3

Explain what care the family can give and show them how to do it.

Rationale and comments: Being able to participate in the care reduces feelings of helplessness and allows the family to express love and concern as well as to assist the nurse. It also prevents early separation from the patient.

☑ Intervention 4

Explain what care the patient can do for himself, and reinforce this each time you notice the family providing that care.

Rationale and comments: The family may feel that providing more care than what is required of them is helping the patient. However, explaining to them that they may be reinforcing the patient's helplessness, causing him to feel depressed, may help them refrain from giving such care.

☑ Intervention 5

Suggest that family members attend to their personal needs at least once a day. Explain that meeting their needs is just as important as meeting the patient's needs.

Rationale and comments: Often, family members feel that they need permission to leave. Avoid saying that nothing will happen to the patient while they are gone; his condition could change in the interim. If this occurs, the family may feel as though their leaving caused the change.

☑ Intervention 6

When alone with the patient, ask him how he feels about having someone with him all the time. Also ask whether he needs assistance with either bringing someone to be with him or giving him time alone. (*Note:* These interventions depend on your institution's policy and doctor's orders.)

Rationale and comments: Some patients want someone to be with them at all times and others want some time alone. Because some patients find it difficult to tell their family to leave, the nurse may need to intercede for the patient.

☑ Intervention 7

If the patient has been hospitalized previously, refer to his old chart for the following:
• clues as to what nursing behaviors or interventions may have helped the patient and family previously
• behaviors demonstrated or feelings expressed by the patient and family.

Rationale and comments: Family members, like most people, usually behave in a consistent manner. They're likely to repeat the same type of behavior with this hospitalization as they did in previous ones. Relying on documented notes from previous hospitalizations (the patient may have had several admissions because cardiovascular disease is a chronic condition) helps the present staff when planning care.

☑ Intervention 8

When contemplating the patient's discharge, work with family members to design a workable plan that encompasses and enhances the patient's abilities.

Rationale and comments: Although death may have been expected, the patient may not die and may go home. Planning ahead will help to avoid uncertainty when the patient returns home.

☑ Intervention 9

If the patient dies, see *Interventions to use with grievers,* pages 63 and 64.

Grieving, Individual Patient

Grieving related to actual loss secondary to amputation and diminishing activity tolerance

SUPPORTING DATA
• Feeling of being unable to lead a satisfying life after surgery
• Focusing only on things he will not be able to do
• Commenting about feeling less whole as a person
• Reviewing life in terms of what he has done wrong to deserve such an outcome
• Feeling unable to do any of his previous activities
• Feeling irritable and using sarcasm
• Refusing to participate in activities of which he is capable
• Turning his back on the nurse or family
• Being unable or unwilling to talk about feelings
• Expressing depression directly or indirectly by:
  —sadness
  —psychomotor retardation
  —apathy
  —crying
  —agitation
  —restlessness
• Expressing anger or hostility directly or indirectly by:
  —negative verbalizations
  —aggressive behavior
  —passive aggressiveness (withholding, withdrawal, or jealousy)
(See also "Supporting Data" for "Depression, Reactive: Situational" in this section.)

PLAN OF CARE
Outcome criteria
• Patient states he has one or more methods to try when he has uncomfortable thoughts about his losses.
• Patient performs self-care voluntarily to the limit of his abilities.

Interventions and rationales
☑ Intervention 1
If not already known from admission data base, find out how the patient usually discharges feelings of tension and anger.

Rationale and comments: Patients react in similar ways to stress. By knowing what these ways are, nurses can recognize the behavior when it occurs, especially if the behavior is indirect.

☑ **Intervention 2**

Use therapeutic communication techniques whenever the patient displays or alludes to any of the feelings and behaviors described earlier in "Supporting Data" (see *Therapeutic communication techniques*, pages 17 to 19).

Rationale and comments: Patients facing loss of a limb or other functional abilities experience considerable tension that is often difficult to express directly. Nurses can help them sort out their feelings.

☑ **Intervention 3**

Determine whether the patient is using coping mechanisms to deal with his loss (see *Coping mechanisms*).

Rationale and comments: Like most people, the patient uses coping mechanisms to maintain personal integrity and reduce the degree of threat when under a great deal of stress. Learning that he may lose a limb or that he may need to give up some of his favorite activities requires much energy. Nurses can help by understanding that the patient may not wish to think about his illness for a while and by assisting him to conserve his energy.

COPING MECHANISMS

Mechanism	Definition	Example
Regression	Ego defense mechanism in which the patient retreats to using less mature responses in an attempt to cope with stress and to maintain ego integrity. With this mechanism, the patient may cry or whine instead of asking for what he desires.	"Will you hand me the glass? I don't think I can reach it."
Repression, suppression, or denial	Unconscious or conscious attempts to remove intolerable thoughts of death or anxious feelings from the mind to maintain an emotional equilibrium. Although these processes consume energy and alter reality, they make life bearable for the moment. With any of these mechanisms, the patient may disregard doctor's orders and get out of bed or engage in numerous activities while trying to keep busy all day. Some use of these mechanisms is normal to reduce the intensity of feelings produced by crisis.	"No, I'm not upset that I had a heart attack. Things like that don't bother me." "I had only a mild heart attack."

COPING MECHANISMS *(continued)*

Mechanism	Definition	Example
Rationalization	A form of reasoning in which the patient fails to recognize true causal relationships and emphasizes the minor aspects or minimizes the major aspects of a situation to hide his true feelings and thoughts or to devalue the importance of a nonattainable object or situation	"It's not that important that I can't play golf anymore." (Said by a patient who played golf every day before his heart attack)
Depersonalization	Mechanism by which the patient loses his sense of identity and feels less human or less important; results from severe stress	"I can't believe this is happening to me."
Projection	Mechanism by which the patient externalizes his own undesirable condition, thoughts, or feelings by ascribing them to others	"My wife is more upset that I'm going to lose my leg than I am."
Intellectualization	Mechanism by which the patient focuses on the facts of his illness to give him a sense of predictability, control, and hope. With this mechanism, he can isolate feelings from thoughts, which leads to a feeling of detachment from the illness (he may refuse to deal with the notion of living with the condition).	The patient may learn the intricate details of his condition and treatment and use the technical terminology in conversation.
Obsessive-compulsive behavior	Mechanism based on intellectualization and isolation of feelings from thoughts by which the patient orders his world to reduce anxiety and to give him a feeling of control. The patient may blindly follow a regimen, such as exercising regardless of how tired he is.	"I never take my medication until after I've had my juice."

(continued)

COPING MECHANISMS *(continued)*

Mechanism	Definition	Example
Counterphobic behavior	Self-destructive, cavalier, or uncaring behaviors in which the patient engages to demonstrate his mastery over the threat of illness. Such counterphobic behaviors may be difficult to distinguish from denial; they may even be a combination of both.	The patient gets out of bed despite doctor's orders to the contrary. The patient eats a regular diet instead of the prescribed low-salt diet.
Sublimation	Mechanism by which the patient channels unacceptable thoughts and feelings into socially acceptable ones; activities may be as vigorous as the patient's condition permits.	Pacing the floor Meditation

☑ Intervention 4

Assess the patient and family for the particular stage of grief each may be experiencing as a reaction to the loss. Stages include the following:
• avoidance phase
—disbelief
—dejection
—shock
—numbness
—somatic distress
• confrontation phase
—anger
—yearning
—bargaining
—depression
• reestablishment phase
—acceptance
—looking at alternatives
—acceptance of new identity.

Rationale and comments: Patients and families must first absorb the idea of the loss, then accept it, and then develop a way of living with the loss. This takes time and energy. Because these phases are not discrete and one phase is not necessarily complete before another phase starts, you'll need to assess patients and families at each contact.

☑ Intervention 5

Use the following suggested interventions for the three stages listed above.
• Avoidance phase
—Stay with the patient as long as possible after he receives the news of his loss, even though he may not wish to discuss it.

—Discuss the news with the patient if he wishes to talk about it. (He may not wish to discuss how he feels about the news at this time, as it is a normal initial reaction to separate facts from feelings.) Answer his questions honestly, then leave if he dismisses you verbally or nonverbally. He may turn away, turn on the television, reach for the phone to call someone, talk only to his spouse or a visitor (thus excluding you), or focus conversation on you instead. (The patient will use various behaviors to maintain his own integrity and sense of control, allowing him to absorb the news a little at a time.)

• Confrontation phase
—Listen for and respond to expressions of feeling with therapeutic communication techniques (see *Therapeutic communication techniques,* pages 17 to 19). (During this phase, the patient's feelings may be intense and can be frightening. Helping him to clarify what is happening can assist him through this difficult time.)
—Provide as many opportunities as possible for the patient to express anger. Let him talk about it or expend the energy of anger in walking or performing other physical activities. Do not take his anger personally. (Anger, the main feeling of this phase, is difficult for the nurse to treat and the patient to experience.)

• Reestablishment phase
—Using therapeutic communication techniques, respond to the patient's expressions about envisioning his life without the limb or the particular role he is struggling to relinquish (see *Therapeutic communication techniques,* pages 17 to 19). (This phase may not be seen in the hospital, depending on the length of time the patient is hospitalized and on the severity of the loss. However, these phases are not absolute or discrete, and the patient may move in and out of them. Therefore, you need to be prepared to assist the patient when he is in this phase.)
—Answer honestly any questions the patient has, consulting other sources as necessary. (Knowledge of what the patient can expect after the loss or what alternatives there are for role change help him regain a feeling of control.)
—If another patient in the hospital is experiencing the same loss and is available to talk with the patient, try to arrange for the two to meet. (This helps the patient see how others are coping with the loss and can assist him in the grieving process.) After the meeting, give the patient an opportunity to discuss his feelings.

☑ **Intervention 6**

Ask the patient what methods or techniques he is using to relieve his uncomfortable feelings and whether they are working.

Rationale and comments: If other methods have proved effective in the past, the nurse can suggest them to the patient.

☑ **Intervention 7**

Use the interventions in "Stress Management" in Section III to teach the patient methods of relaxing and of stopping uncomfortable thoughts. This teaching is best accomplished when the patient is in a relatively calm state.

Rationale and comments: By practicing his own methods, the patient will have a feeling of mastery and reduce his dependence on the nurse or family for emotional care. Keep in mind that any immediate crisis will have to pass before the patient is able to listen to any new ways of managing his feelings.

☑ Intervention 8
Ask the patient daily if he needs additional help applying any of the suggestions.

Rationale and comments: Asking ensures that the patient knows the nurse is interested in his progress. It also gives an indication of how the patient is progressing and whether he needs additional assistance.
Note: Remember that you cannot eliminate the patient's source of grief; however, you may be able to help reduce his fear by listening; by helping to clarify what is happening to him; and by your actions, presence, calm manner, use of therapeutic communication techniques, appropriate physical care (including back rubbing, positioning, and offering of food and fluids), and referral when you have used all of your resources. When the patient's fear is reduced, he feels better able to manage his life and has less stress on his heart.

Grieving related to anticipated loss (death) secondary to failing myocardial function

SUPPORTING DATA
• Asks "Why me?" and reviews life in terms of what he has done wrong to deserve such an outcome
• States inability to do any of his previous activities
• Displays irritability and uses sarcasm
• Refuses to participate in activities of which he is capable
• Turns his back on the nurse or family
• Is unable or unwilling to talk about feelings
• Expresses depression directly or indirectly by:
  —sadness
  —psychomotor retardation
  —apathy
  —crying
  —agitation
  —restlessness
• Expresses anger or hostility directly or indirectly by:
  —negative verbalizations
  —aggressive behavior
  —passive aggressiveness (withholding, withdrawal, or jealousy)
• May state the following specific fears:
  —fear of the unknown
  —fear of loneliness
  —fear of loss of family and friends

—fear of loss of self-control
—fear of disability
—fear of suffering and pain
—fear of loss of identity
—fear of sorrow
—fear of regression
—fear of mutilation, decomposition, and premature burial
• Expresses guilt and shame with such statements as:
— "I'm costing my family so much money."
— "I'm afraid my wife will get sick spending so much time on me."
— "I'm sorry I got mad at you; I can't seem to help myself."
— "I'm sorry you have to clean me up like this; I used to be able to do it myself."

PLAN OF CARE
Outcome criteria
• Patient states he has one or more methods to try when he has uncomfortable thoughts about dying and his losses.
• Patient performs self-care voluntarily, according to his abilities.
• Patient is active to the limits of his abilities.

Interventions and rationales
☑ Intervention 1
If not already known from admission data base, find out how the patient usually discharges feelings of tension and anger.

Rationale and comments: Patients react in similar ways to stress. By knowing what these ways are, nurses can recognize the behavior when it occurs, especially if the behavior is indirect.

☑ Intervention 2
Use therapeutic communication techniques whenever the patient displays or alludes to any of the feelings and behaviors described above in "Supporting Data" (see *Therapeutic communication techniques,* pages 17 to 19).

Rationale and comments: Patients facing impending death experience considerable tension that is often difficult to express directly. Nurses can help them sort out such feelings.

☑ Intervention 3
If the patient demonstrates specific coping mechanisms, consider the following interventions (see *Coping mechanisms,* pages 68 to 70):
• Regression
—Meet the patient's dependency needs by doing more of his physical care than usual, telling him more often and very specifically when you will return, answering his call light as soon as possible, and offering help rather than waiting for him to ask for it. (It takes much energy to assimilate the news that no further treatment is available at this time. Anticipating and meeting dependency needs helps to conserve energy.

His initial reaction to the stress may be to want to retreat. Usually most patients soon regain their usual ways of caring for themselves after being allowed to retreat for a while.)

—Set limits that are reasonable, not arbitrary; explain them to the patient and family, and maintain them firmly when or if his regression becomes a problem to the staff, family, or himself. (Problems can arise when the regression defense mechanism is disproportionate to the disabling effects of the illness. Setting limits helps the patient feel secure and lets him know you are looking out for his best interest.)

—Within the patient's capacity, help him plan to accomplish something each day. He will feel better if he can see gradual progress or, if that is impossible, if he can maintain as much functioning as possible. (Dwelling on his impending death provokes anxiety; by living day to day, he can help control the anxiety.)

• Repression

—Talk about the things the patient wants to discuss in a friendly, casual way, letting him guide the conversation. (If you bring up thoughts of his illness and potential or actual losses and he has succeeded in blocking them out of his mind, he will not know what you are talking about.)

• Suppression

—Look for excessive talking, sleeping, or activity of any kind. (These activities help him keep anxious thoughts at a distance and may keep others from talking about stressful matters.)

—If the patient is awake at night, ask if he would like to talk about what is on his mind. (The lack of distractions and his horizontal positioning during the night may make him especially prone to anxious thoughts. He may need just a gentle invitation to speak about his thoughts.)

—If the patient declines to talk, you may offer him a back rub or food or fluids (as allowed and available); ask if the room temperature is comfortable, whether he has adequate covers, or if he needs to void; readjust his position; or find out if you can do anything else for him. (All these activities demonstrate to the patient that you are concerned and willing to comfort him and let him control the content of any interaction. He may not want to think about his illness for a while.)

—See "Sleep-Pattern Disturbance" in this section for additional suggestions if the patient persistently has difficulty sleeping. (Lack of sleep or the inability to sleep at night contributes to ongoing feelings of anxiety and depression.)

• Denial

—Let the patient determine the content of the conversation, including the desire not to talk. (Denial allows the patient time to collect himself and mobilize other, less radical defenses.)

—Avoid repeatedly explaining the patient's condition to him if he does not seem interested in hearing about it, but be ready to explain whenever he is ready to relinquish some of his denial. (A general principle of nursing care is to never remove the defense of denial unless something else is available to put in its place.)

- Rationalization
  —Neither agree nor disagree with the patient's explanations, but always give accurate explanations if asked a direct question. (Remember, each of these mechanisms is a way the patient has of protecting himself from stress; the nurse tries not to participate in any of the patient's distortions. Answering accurately helps maintain the nurse-patient relationship and may assist the patient to assess his situation more realistically.)
- Depersonalization
  —Stay with the patient as long as possible if he is experiencing a sensation of unreality. (Because this can be frightening to the patient, your calm presence and willingness to listen can be reassuring.)
  —If the feeling persists, you may need to call a family member to stay with the patient or suggest psychiatric consultation. (This defense is maladaptive as well as uncomfortable and frightening to the patient. Having another person in the room at all times may be necessary, not only for his comfort but also for his safety. A psychiatrist may be needed to suggest other care methods and medications to help him through this form of adaptation.)
- Projection
  —Avoid opposing or siding with the misconceptions shown in projection. (Anger and hostility are normal reactions to distressing news, and projection is one way the patient has of managing those strong feelings.)
  —Offer the patient the opportunity to express his anger and hostility. This can be done by reflecting the apparent feelings or by mentioning ways in which he can express anger, such as pounding a pillow or screaming. (Acknowledging the feeling sometimes makes it easier for the patient to accept it. If he cannot discuss the feeling directly, indirect methods will at least reduce the energy created by the feeling and assist the patient to feel more comfortable.)
  —In a nonjudgmental way, question why he thinks and feels as he does, and ask what he would need to correct the problem. (Remember that "why" questions are difficult to answer, so your tone must be gentle and wondering for the patient not to feel attacked and accused.)
- Intellectualization
  —Ask the patient what he is feeling when he discusses an issue factually. (Focusing on feelings gives the patient permission to talk about them if he can or will.)
  —Answer the patient's questions honestly and accurately, even if you suspect he's using the questioning as a defense. (Failure to answer would increase the patient's anger. He needs to use whatever defense he thinks will help him through this experience.)
- Obsessive-compulsive behavior
  —Abide by the patient's desires as much as possible. (As long as his rigidity does not interfere with his care, it makes him feel better.)
  —If you find it impossible to accept a particular behavior, explain why, ask how the patient will feel if he is unable to carry out the behavior, and seek a mutually agreeable substitute. (This lets the patient know the nurse is concerned and not arbitrary. Given the opportunity, the patient may be able to substitute one behavior for another.)

• Counterphobic behavior
—Respond to rebellious behavior with a gentle question, such as "I wonder why you persist in this behavior when your doctor has asked you not to?" (This may help the patient to assess his behavior; however, this kind of behavior may be the only way the patient can feel in control, manage the stress, and maintain his integrity. Remember that "why" questions are difficult to answer; he may not even know the answer but may know only that he can't stop the behavior.)
—Find as many ways as possible for the patient to make choices. Help him to develop a morning schedule that is within doctor's orders, or select the menu and determine when he can eat between-meal snacks, if ordered and allowed. (If the patient can feel some control in his life, he may have less need to act in more destructive ways.)
• Sublimation
—Suggest various ways, compatible with the patient's usual methods of discharging feelings, for him to express anger and tension, such as tearing up paper, going for a walk, breathing deeply, tensing and relaxing all muscle groups, or pounding a pillow. (Any means of getting rid of uncomfortable feelings must be acceptable to the patient; use of familiar techniques adds to the stress-releasing value of the technique. Sometimes, feelings have to be discharged rather than understood. Healthy use of this mechanism is harmless, may be beneficial to society if the patient's energies are directed toward volunteer work, and promotes patient well-being.)

⊠ Intervention 4
Assess the patient and family for their particular stage of grief as a reaction to the news that no further medical treatment is available. Stages include:
• avoidance phase
—disbelief
—dejection
—shock
—numbness
—somatic distress
• confrontation phase
—anger
—yearning
—bargaining
—depression
• reestablishment phase
—acceptance
—looking at alternatives
—accepting a new identity.

Rationale and comments: Patients and families undergoing losses of any kind must first absorb the idea of the loss, then accept it, and then develop a way of living despite the loss or impending death of the patient. All of this takes time and energy. Because these phases are not discrete and one phase is not necessarily complete before another one starts, you'll need to assess them with each contact.

☑ Intervention 5

Consider these suggested interventions for the three stages of grief listed on the opposite page.

• Avoidance phase

—Stay with the patient as long as possible after he receives the news, even though he may not wish to discuss it or may discuss it but not the feelings associated with the news. (Your presence can serve as an anchor during this time of turmoil. He may want to separate facts from feelings, which is a normal initial reaction.)

—Answer his questions honestly if the patient asks any.

—If the patient dismisses you verbally or nonverbally, leave the room. He may turn away, turn on the television, reach for the phone to call someone, talk only to his spouse or a visitor (thereby excluding you), or focus the conversation on you. (He may use these various behaviors to maintain his own integrity and a sense of control, enabling him to absorb the news a little at a time.)

• Confrontation phase

—Listen for and respond to expressions of feeling with therapeutic communication techniques (see *Therapeutic communication techniques,* pages 17 to 19). (During this phase, the patient's feelings may be intense and can be frightening. Your presence and help in clarifying what is happening can assist the patient through this difficult time.)

—Provide as many opportunities as possible for the patient to express anger, such as by talking about it or expending energy by walking. Remember not to take his anger personally or to return anger. (Anger, the main feeling of this phase, is a difficult emotion for the nurse to treat and the patient and family to feel.)

• Reestablishment phase

—Respond to the patient's expressions relating to how he thinks he can live with the idea of a limited future using therapeutic communication techniques (see *Therapeutic communication techniques,* pages 17 to 19). (This phase may not be seen in the hospital, depending on the length of time the patient is hospitalized and the severity of the loss. However, the phases are not absolute and the patient may switch from one phase to another; you'll need to be prepared to encounter this phase if it occurs.)

—Answer the patient's questions honestly about what he can expect, consulting other sources as necessary. (Knowing what to expect in his future allows the patient to make plans for the rest of his life and helps him regain a feeling of control and energy. Although you may not always have the information the patient needs, try to help the patient find the answers to his questions.)

☑ Intervention 6

Ask the patient what methods or techniques he is using to relieve his uncomfortable feelings and whether they are working.

Rationale and comments: If certain methods have proven effective in the past, they can be suggested to the patient.

☑ Intervention 7

Use the interventions in "Stress Management" in Section III to teach the patient methods of relaxing and of stopping uncomfortable thoughts. This teaching can best be done when the patient is in a relatively calm state.

Rationale and comments: By using his own methods, the patient will have a feeling of mastery and reduce his dependence on the nurse or his family for emotional care. However, any immediate crisis will have to pass before the patient is able to listen to any new ways of managing his feelings.

☑ Intervention 8

Ask the patient daily if he needs additional help applying any of the suggestions.

Rationale and comments: Asking if he needs help lets the patient know the nurse is interested in his progress. It also indicates whether he needs additional assistance.

Note: Remember that you cannot remove the patient's source of grief; however, you may be able to help reduce his fear by listening; helping to clarify what is happening to him; and by your presence, calm manner, use of therapeutic communication techniques, appropriate physical care (including back rubbing, positioning, and offering of food and fluids), and referral when you have used all of your resources. When the patient's fear is reduced, he feels better able to manage his life and has less stress on his heart.

Noncompliance

Noncompliance related to difficult regimen; lack of knowledge; lack of resources, such as money or care assistance; denial of illness; or difference in value system with health care workers

SUPPORTING DATA
• Stated inability by patient or family to carry out what is ordered because it:
—is too difficult
—is too confusing to follow the procedure
—costs too much money
—takes too much time
—doesn't help the patient
—bothers the patient to swallow all those pills each day
—inhibits their life-style
• Agreeing to follow prescriptions when in hospital, but failing to comply (obvious at follow-up visit from patient's weight gain, continued blood pressure elevation, or other parameters)
• Expressed feelings that the patient isn't sick and thus doesn't need medication
• Fear that weight loss will result in loss of strength
• Fear of being labeled a sissy if he agrees to take medications and to adhere to other medical requests
• Family's indication that the patient will not comply with doctor's orders
• Patient's feeling that family is smothering him

PLAN OF CARE
Outcome criteria
• Patient and family state the prescribed regimen.
• Patient and family state plans for following the prescribed regimen.
• Patient states reasons for not following the regimen, if he is, in fact, not following it.
• Patient and family state consequences of not following regimen if that is the choice they have made.

Interventions and rationales
☑ Intervention 1
Plan an uninterrupted period to sit down and talk with the patient.

Rationale and comments: Spending time with the patient to identify factors contributing to noncompliance is just as important as spending time with him to change a dressing or adjust an I.V. line.

☑ Intervention 2

Plan a separate time to talk with the patient's family.

Rationale and comments: For the initial investigation, nurses should probably see the family separately from the patient so that each has a chance to discuss the situation from his own viewpoint.

☑ Intervention 3

Assess the patient or family for reasons for noncompliance. Use therapeutic communication techniques (see *Therapeutic communication techniques,* pages 17 to 19). Follow these procedures:
• Assess the patient's feelings about the regimen to get a clear picture of his point of view. (You'll need to clarify how he feels emotionally before you can begin to deal with the more cognitive or intellectual aspects of the situation.)
• Assess what the regimen means to the patient. This may or may not be the same as his feelings for the regimen. (If his self-concept is diminished in some way by having to adhere to certain behaviors, regardless of the behaviors' values, he may not follow the regimen.)
• Assess what interferes with his following the prescribed regimen. If the patient is having difficulty expressing himself, try to elicit responses to the following. Ask if he feels the regimen:
—is too difficult
—is too time consuming
—causes discomfort or pain
—takes too much energy
—causes uncomfortable side effects
—is dangerous or risky in some way
—is too much trouble
—makes him feel embarrassed or conspicuous in some way
—is too expensive
—does not help him
—isolates him from his friends.
Before changing the subject, ask him if he has any other reasons for not being able to carry out the regimen. (Despite your best effort, you may have failed to ask about the one thing the patient considers to be the most important reason.)
• Assess the patient's family, asking the same questions about feelings, meaning, and problems. (You may discover that their feelings and meanings differ considerably from those of the patient's, which could explain his difficulty in carrying out the regimen. Or you may find that the patient and family see the situation the same way, which may make the problem easier to solve.)
• Review the patient's home situation in relation to how it affects the regimen (see "Family Processes, Alteration in" in this section).

☑ Intervention 4

Ask the patient what he thinks the best solution to the problem would be.

Rationale and comments: Including the patient in finding a solution to the problem may assist him to comply with a new program.

☑ **Intervention 5**

Ask the family members what they think the best solution to the problem would be.

Rationale and comments: Including the family may help the patient to comply. Also, the family is more likely to carry out something they helped to prepare.

☑ **Intervention 6**

Plan to spend an uninterrupted period with the patient and family to discuss the results of the assessment and the proposed solutions; you may need to schedule more than one session.

Rationale and comments: Providing the patient and family with feedback allows each person to hear each other's viewpoints on the subject. This has to be handled objectively to avoid creating any feelings of defensiveness in either the patient or family that might hinder further problem solving.

☑ **Intervention 7**

Carry out the nursing responsibilities resulting from the proposed solution. Follow these procedures:
• Teach and demonstrate. Remember that lack of knowledge is often a reason for noncompliance.
• Make appropriate referrals as needed:
—Refer the patient and family to the appropriate social services. (Lack of money, transportation, or assistance in the home may be the problem.)
—Refer the patient to a doctor. (By changing the patient's medication, the doctor may eliminate some of the uncomfortable side effects the patient may be experiencing, thereby resulting in greater compliance.)
—Refer the patient to a nutritionist or clinical dietitian. (Adjusting the patient's diet or suggesting new ideas for food preparation may increase compliance in this area.)
—Refer the patient to a cardiac rehabilitation program or physical therapist according to your institution's policy. (The patient and family may not be aware of the resources available or of the benefits of exercise in promoting a feeling of well-being and cardiovascular fitness.)
• Write down plans and discuss how to implement them with the patient and family. (Written plans reinforce the regimen, provide a source of reference when the patient and family are away from the nurse, and ensure that the patient and family are following the same information.)
• Use contracting, setting various specific goals, or reward systems to motivate the patient to adhere to the regimen. (Keep in mind that all patients do not respond to the same reward system.)
• Ask the patient and family what problems they anticipate with the plan, and problem-solve with them to think of ways of overcoming these difficulties.

• Discuss the patient's feelings about the regimen if this seems helpful. (The patient or family has to accept responsibility for care, if possible, despite how they actually feel about it. However, the feelings of anger that come with change need to be expressed; the nurse can help them with these feelings.)

• Suggest that the patient or family seek professional help, according to your institution's policy, if their problems extend beyond the scope of your nursing responsibility. (Severe anxiety and depression can drastically interfere with compliance and require professional help, for example.)

Rationale and comments: Identifying the problems and concerns of the patient and family and establishing a plan of care may be the nurse's primary duties; however, the nurse then has a responsibility to assist the patient and family to overcome the problems as much as she can.

Nutrition, Alteration in: Less Than Body Requirements

Alteration in Nutrition: Less Than Body Requirements related to anorexia, inability to eat sufficient amounts secondary to dyspnea, fatigue, patient's dislike of prescribed diet, or increased metabolic demands

SUPPORTING DATA
• Anorexia
• Consistently refusing meals
• Consistently eating less than half of meals supplied

PLAN OF CARE
Outcome criteria
• Patient increases amount eaten during each meal and snack.
• Patient increases calorie intake per day (as measured by calorie count).

Interventions and rationales
☑ Intervention 1
Assess and reduce the factors contributing to the patient's inadequate nutrition. Such factors may include:
• pain
—Administer pain medication before meals, timing the administration so that the patient is comfortable but not excessively sedated at mealtimes.
—Implement other pain-relief measures as indicated by the patient's condition.
• the patient's emotional response to diagnosis, surgery, and prognosis. (Some patients react to a diagnosis of cardiovascular disease with anger, grief, or depression, which can cause anorexia and result in inadequate nutrition.)
• dyspnea and fatigue. (These conditions often decrease a patient's ability to eat sufficient amounts of food to meet the body's metabolic demands.)
—Watch for signs that the patient is becoming dyspneic or fatigued, including statements by the patient that he is too tired or too short of breath to eat and obvious signs that he is significantly short of breath when eating.
—Provide rest periods immediately before and after meals.
—If the patient is receiving oxygen by face mask, provide a nasal cannula for him to use during meals.

(See "Activity Intolerance," "Gas Exchange, Impaired," and "Fluid Volume Excess: Edema" in this section for additional interventions.)
• the patient's dislike of the prescribed diet or foods supplied on meal trays.
—Listen for statements by the patient that the food is tasteless or that he does not like certain foods. (Cardiac patients are often placed on restricted diets that represent a significant and unappealing change from typical home meals. If the prescribed meals are too unappealing to him, he may refuse to eat sufficient amounts to meet the body's metabolic demands.)
—Assess the patient's usual dietary habits and preferences compared with his current diet. (This can assist the dietitian in developing a diet more palatable to the patient.)
—In collaboration with the dietitian, include foods that are more palatable to the patient on his meal tray. (Including such foods and avoiding those foods he especially dislikes gives him a sense of control and may increase his nutritional intake.)
—With the dietitian's assistance, ask for the patient's family to bring in foods from home that are more appealing to the patient.

☑ Intervention 2
Implement the following general measures to facilitate increased nutritional intake:
• Offer the patient small, frequent meals (four to six per day). (Smaller meals are easier for the patient to eat and digest and cause less stress on the heart.)
• In collaboration with the dietitian, provide the patient with appropriate snacks between meals.
• Assist the patient with selecting foods from the menu, setting up his meal trays, and eating, as needed.
• Suggest that family members or friends visit during meals. (Having company may divert the patient and increase the amount of food he eats.)

☑ Intervention 3
Assess the interventions' effect on the patient's nutritional intake by the following measures:
• recording the amount of each meal or snack eaten
• recording the amount and type of fluids drunk
• consulting with the doctor or dietitian about obtaining a calorie count for several days
• obtaining daily weights.

Rationale and comments: Body weight alone may be a misleading measure of nutritional status because the edema seen in various cardiovascular diseases can increase overall body weight and mask continued inadequate nutrition.

Physical Mobility: Impaired

Impaired Physical Mobility related to amputation of one or both legs secondary to vascular disease

SUPPORTING DATA
• Below the knee amputation of one or both legs
• Above the knee amputation of one or both legs
• Needing assistance or aids to ambulate safely
• Needing assistance or aids to transfer from bed to chair or bedside commode
• Needing assistance or aids to perform self-care activities
• Needing assistance or aids to move or turn in bed

PLAN OF CARE
Outcome criteria
• Patient performs prescribed exercises to increase upper body strength and muscle strength of both legs and to maintain normal function of the remaining intact limb.
• Patient develops no contractures.
• Patient increases mobility as evidenced by transferring himself from the bed to a chair, wheelchair, and bedside commode, then back to the bed.

Interventions and rationales
☑ Intervention 1
Use proper patient positioning to decrease the risk of contractures. Follow these procedures:
• Keep the patient's residual limb extended when he is lying in bed or sitting in a chair.
• Avoid using a pillow under the residual limb when he is lying in bed or sitting in a chair. (Some surgeons permit a pillow under the residual limb for no more than 48 hours after surgery to decrease stump edema.)
• Keep the residual limb adducted (never abducted) when the patient is lying in bed.
• If his respiratory and cardiovascular status permit, position the patient prone for 30 minutes several times a day.
• Have the patient avoid prolonged sitting.

Rationale and comments: Developing contractures will further decrease a patient's mobility and significantly interfere with rehabilitation and fitting of a prosthesis.

☑ Intervention 2
In collaboration with the doctor and physical therapist, implement an exercise program with the patient.

• Have the patient perform prescribed exercises to increase the upper body strength he will need to perform bed-to-chair transfers. Take the following measures:

—Install an over-the-bed trapeze for the patient to use to move himself in bed.

—Have the patient perform active range-of-motion (ROM) exercises for the arms four times a day.

—With the patient sitting in bed, have him lift his hips off the bed by pushing down with arms three or four times a day. (This exercise strengthens his triceps muscles, which are necessary for self-transfer).

• Have the patient perform prescribed exercises to strengthen muscles for ambulation with assistive devices or a prosthesis as directed by a physical therapist. Prescribed exercises will vary depending on the level of amputation, the patient's condition, and the rehabilitation goals. Common exercises may include the following:

—Have the patient squeeze his buttocks together, then release them.

—For a patient with a below-the-knee amputation, have him tighten his kneecap for 10 seconds, then release it (quadriceps setting).

—With the patient lying supine in bed, have him bend his unaffected leg at the knee and place his foot flat on the bed. Then have him raise his shoulders and head off the bed. (This strengthens the abdominal muscles.)

☑ Intervention 3

Maintain the dressings as prescribed to decrease edema and promote healing (see "Amputation, Leg [for Vascular Disease]" in Section II).

Rationale and comments: Postoperative edema can interfere with healing and thus delay prosthetic fitting and increased mobility.

☑ Intervention 4

Implement the following measures to prevent damage to the nonamputated leg:

• Have the patient perform active ROM exercises with the nonamputated leg, including dorsal flexion/plantar flexion, ankle rotation, and knee bending (with assistance).

• Provide meticulous skin and foot care.

Rationale and comments: Since the patient's mobility is already impaired because of the amputation, damage to the other limb could further reduce his mobility and impede rehabilitation. The patient may tend to use the heel of the remaining foot to push himself up in bed, thereby increasing the risk of skin breakdown on the heel.

☑ Intervention 5

In collaboration with the doctor and physical therapist, have the patient increase mobility by:

• using a trapeze or side rails to move or turn himself in bed

• learning to transfer from the bed to a chair, wheelchair, or bedside commode

• ambulating under the direction of a physical therapist.

Respiratory Function, Alteration in

Alteration in Respiratory Function related to incisional pain and decreased mobility after surgery

SUPPORTING DATA
• Shallow respirations
• Rapid respirations
• Diminished breath sounds in lung fields evidenced on auscultation
• Arterial blood gas levels indicative of hypoxia
• Chest X-ray report noting atelectasis

PLAN OF CARE
Outcome criteria*
• Patient's respiratory status returns to normal as evidenced by normal chest X-ray, arterial blood gas levels, and breath sounds on auscultation of lung fields.

Interventions and rationales
☑ **Intervention 1**
Implement the interventions listed in "Respiratory Function, Potential Alteration in" in this section.

Rationale and comments: Deep-breathing exercises, use of an incentive spirometer, coughing, and increasing physical activity are appropriate interventions to use in preventing and treating atelectasis.

☑ **Intervention 2**
Administer supplemental oxygen, as prescribed, to relieve hypoxia and dyspnea.

☑ **Intervention 3**
In collaboration with the doctor and respiratory therapist, administer nebulization treatments to deliver medications or moisture directly into the upper and lower airways, facilitating the mobilization of retained secretions.
• During treatment, instruct the patient to breathe in slowly through the mouth; then have him hold his breath briefly at the end of inhalation and exhale slowly.

*For patients with no underlying chronic respiratory conditions, such as chronic obstructive pulmonary disease; if chronic respiratory disease is present, these criteria need to be modified according to the patient's condition.

• Have the patient repeat the deep-breathing sequence every few breaths during the treatment.
• Instruct the patient to cough, as necessary, to clear the airway during treatment.

☑ Intervention 4
In collaboration with the doctor and respiratory therapist, implement chest physiotherapy (PT).
• Before beginning chest PT, determine which lung segments to treat by auscultating lung fields and reviewing chest X-ray reports.
• Closely monitor the patient's respirations and pulse rate and rhythm during treatment; stop chest PT if these vital signs indicate that the patient is not tolerating treatment.
• Chest PT may include the following:
   —postural drainage (standard positions for postural drainage may need to be modified for patients with cardiovascular disease)
   —cupping and clapping
   —vibration
   —nasotracheal suction (for patients who are unable to cough effectively enough to remove secretions from the respiratory tract).
Note: For details on how to perform postural drainage, cupping and clapping, and vibration, consult a medical-surgical nursing or respiratory therapy text.

☑ Intervention 5
Assess the patient's response to interventions. Follow these measures:
• Assess his respiratory status, including auscultating breath sounds.
• Monitor chest X-ray reports.
• Monitor arterial blood gas levels.

Respiratory Function, Potential Alteration in

Potential Alteration in Respiratory Function related to pain and decreased activity after surgery

SUPPORTING DATA
• Patient is in postoperative period after coronary artery bypass surgery, valve replacement surgery, amputation, or peripheral vascular bypass surgery

PLAN OF CARE
Outcome criteria*
• Patient's respiratory rate and rhythm are normal.
• Patient has no adventitious sounds during lung auscultation.
• Patient's chest X-ray and arterial blood gas levels are within normal limits.

Interventions and rationales
☑ Intervention 1
Ask the patient to breathe deeply and cough every 1 to 2 hours while awake and every 2 to 4 hours at night after transferring from the intensive care unit. Follow these measures:
• Ask the patient to use his incentive spirometer. Instruct him to:
—take a slow, deep breath
—sustain the breath for at least 3 seconds
—exhale slowly
—repeat the exercise 5 to 10 times, pausing in between to breathe normally.
• Ask the patient to deep breathe 5 to 10 times per hour, pausing in between to breathe normally. Instruct him to use one of the following techniques:
—Tell him to inhale slowly through the nose until he feels his abdomen rise with the breath. Then have him exhale slowly through the mouth while contracting abdominal muscles.
—Instruct him to lie on his back with knees bent and feet flat; then have him place one hand on his chest and one on his abdomen. Tell him to push his abdomen against his hand while inhaling and to pull the abdomen in while exhaling. (Note that this exercise may also be done with the patient in a sitting position.)

*For patients with no underlying chronic respiratory conditions, such as chronic obstructive pulmonary disease; if chronic respiratory disease is present, these criteria need to be modified according to the patient's condition.

• Ask the patient to cough after performing deep-breathing exercises. Follow these measures:
—Assist him to splint the incision, as needed.
—Have him sit up straight or lean forward slightly.
—Instruct him to take a deep breath slowly and to hold it, count to three, then cough deeply and forcefully.
• If the patient does not cough effectively, use the following strategies:
—Administer pain medication before having the patient cough and deep breathe as indicated (the pain from a chest incision can interfere with the patient's ability to deep breathe and cough).
—Have the patient take a deep breath and cough two times while exhaling that breath (often the second cough from a single breath is more effective).
—Have the patient take a small breath and cough slightly on exhalation; then have him take a deeper breath and cough harder on exhalation. Finally, have him take an extremely deep breath and cough very forcefully on exhalation.

Rationale and comments: Deep breathing helps to prevent atelectasis and improve ventilation. Coughing helps to promote lung expansion and facilitates removal of any retained secretions. The exercises should be done on an around-the-clock basis. Some patients, especially those who have undergone chest surgery, tend to cheat—consciously or unconsciously—when taking deep breaths. They may use the accessory muscles of the neck and take a seemingly deep breath, or they may take a number of rapid, shallow breaths. In either case, these breaths are ineffective in preventing atelectasis.

☑ Intervention 2
Have the patient turn from his side to back to side every 2 hours while in bed.

Rationale and comments: Turning helps to facilitate alveolar inflation and prevent stasis of secretions.

☑ Intervention 3
Implement pain-relief measures.

Rationale and comments: Pain is a major cause of the patient's inability to cough, breathe deeply, or move after surgery.

☑ Intervention 4
Progress the patient's activity level out of bed when appropriate.

Rationale and comments: Having the patient get out of bed to move to a chair or ambulate helps improve ventilation and prevent atelectasis. Movement may dislodge mucus in the tracheobronchial tree and facilitate effective coughing.

☑ Intervention 5

Assess the patient for the following indications that he is developing atelectasis (if present, implement measures outlined in "Respiratory Function, Alteration in" in this section):
• arterial blood gas levels that indicate continued or increased hypoxia
• chest X-ray report noting development of atelectasis
• clinical signs of hypoxia, including:
—irregular pulse because of premature ventricular beats (changes in pulse rate and rhythm can be an early indication of hypoxia)
—tachycardia
—increased respiratory rate
—confusion and disorientation
—elevated temperature
—diminished breath sounds or rhonchi present on auscultation of lungs
—dry, hacking, shallow, ineffective cough that tires the patient.

☑ Intervention 6

Assess for factors that increase the patient's risk for developing atelectasis, and intervene appropriately. Factors include:
• inadequate pain relief
• excessive sedation from use of prescribed analgesics. If this occurs, reduce the medication's dosage or frequency of administration (if permitted by doctor's orders). Consult the doctor about changing medications, if indicated.
• inadequate sleep at night
• inadequate rest during the day
• refusal to breathe deeply, cough, or move. Determine the patient's reasons for the refusal, and intervene as indicated. (Frequently, a patient's refusal is related to pain or fatigue; relieving these conditions can promote compliance with respiratory care measures.)
• inadequate nutrition. (If the patient's nutritional intake is insufficient to meet the body's metabolic demands, he may have insufficient energy to participate in respiratory care measures.)

Self-Concept, Alteration in

Alteration in Self-Concept: Disturbance in Body Image related to feelings of powerlessness or loss of control secondary to loss of limb, insertion of pacemaker, or change in cardiovascular status after myocardial infarction or coronary artery bypass surgery

SUPPORTING DATA
• Refusal to look at residual limb
• Refusal to look at pacemaker insertion site
• Refusal to touch surgical incision sites
• Comments about being less than a whole person, disliking body appearance, or not being able to trust the body in the usual way
• Sexually oriented comments or advances by the male patient to enhance his feelings about himself or his attractiveness to others
• Lack of attention to personal grooming
• Signs of depression, including:
—weeping
—loss of appetite
—excessive sleeping
—lack of energy
—refusal to participate in self-care, recreational, or diversional activities
—anger toward family and staff
• Refusal to see family and friends
• Refusal to adhere to prescribed medical regimen
• Exhibition of demanding behavior toward family and staff
• Pain that continues beyond healing of surgical incisions
• Signs of anxiety, including:
—sleeplessness
—fear of moving
—fear of heart or pacemaker failure
• Refusal to discuss amputation, pacemaker insertion, or myocardial infarction; or changing the subject whenever it is discussed
• Expressions of loss, including:
—sadness
—anger
—disbelief

PLAN OF CARE
Outcome criteria
• Patient and family share their thoughts and concerns with the nurse.
• Patient and family state resources to which they can turn if feelings are too strong to manage alone.

• Patient engages in self-care to the best of his abilities.
• Family assists patient in self-care and allows him to do as much as possible.

Interventions and rationales

☑ **Intervention 1**

Using therapeutic communication techniques, try to elicit the patient's feelings about his illness or surgery (see *Therapeutic communication techniques*, pages 17 to 19).

Rationale and comments: The patient may feel threatened by his altered body appearance and may find it difficult to discuss. Part of the nurse's responsibility is to assist the patient to clarify his feelings to himself.

☑ **Intervention 2**

If the patient is showing signs of anxiety, see "Anxiety" in this section.

☑ **Intervention 3**

If the patient is showing signs of depression, see "Depression, Reactive: Situational" in this section.

☑ **Intervention 4**

If the patient is showing signs of grieving, see "Grieving, Individual Patient" in this section.

☑ **Intervention 5**

If the patient is showing signs of sleeplessness or excessive sleeping, see "Sleep-Pattern Disturbance" in this section.

☑ **Intervention 6**

If the patient's family is having difficulty listening to the patient's concerns, see "Family Processes, Alteration in" in this section.

☑ **Intervention 7**

If the patient is showing signs of noncompliance, see "Noncompliance" in this section.

Rationale and comments: Patients sometimes do the opposite of what is best for them to prove there is nothing wrong with them and that they are still in control.

☑ **Intervention 8**

Consult the doctor about referring the patient and family to other health care professionals if their feelings are interfering with the patient's expected recovery.

Rationale and comments: Helping the patient to overcome an altered self-concept may be impossible to achieve before he is discharged from the hospital. (Depression, in particular, can interfere with recovery from surgery.) Referring the patient and family for additional professional help may be necessary.

☑ Intervention 9

If the male patient makes sexually oriented comments or advances, respond with therapeutic communication techniques rather than value judgments. If he persists despite your firm but gentle refusals, refer him to the appropriate health care professional.

Rationale and comments: A male patient may use sex to confirm his self-concept. Using therapeutic communication techniques may assist him to discuss his deeper feelings, whereas responding with value judgments stops the exploration of these feelings. A patient's persistence in continuing to focus on sexual matters despite the nurse's offer to explore the feelings prompting such actions may require the help of another professional. Although a nurse is not expected to accept a patient's sexual overture, she has a responsibility to respond to the patient in a therapeutic way as far as she is able.

☑ Intervention 10

Speak with the patient's family alone on at least one occasion to find out if they can share any information about the patient's feelings that you don't already know.

Rationale and comments: The patient may be more willing to share such information with his family than with a nurse; however, he may be willing to discuss the information if the nurse brings up the subject.

☑ Intervention 11

When speaking with the patient's family about their knowledge of the patient's feelings, take the opportunity to focus on any concerns the family may have about the patient.

Rationale and comments: The family needs an opportunity to discuss the patient when not in his presence. Knowing that the nurse is concerned about their feelings may help them to care for him when circumstances may make that difficult.

Alteration in Self-Concept: Disturbance in Self-Esteem related to alteration in body image, activity intolerance, feelings of powerlessness, change in family role, loss of or change in employment status secondary to cardiac and peripheral vascular disease

SUPPORTING DATA

• Comments denoting feelings of inadequacy, such as:
  —"I'm not worth anything to anybody anymore."
  —"There's no use trying; I can't do it."
  —"There's no reason to go on when I feel so awful about myself."
  —"I never can do anything right."
• Refusal to participate in self-care activities
• Making no references to the future

• Signs of depression, including:
—weeping
—lack of appetite
—excessive sleeping
—comments about lack of energy
—irritability or anger toward staff and family
—expressions of loss
• Frequent, repeated stories about past accomplishments
• Boastful comments about future dreams that may be unrealistic based on the patient's condition
• Refusal to adhere to prescribed medical orders

PLAN OF CARE
Outcome criteria
• Patient and family share their thoughts and concerns with the nurse.
• Patient and family state resources to which they can turn if feelings of low self-esteem continue.
• Patient participates in self-care to the best of his abilities.
• Patient adheres to the prescribed medical regimen.

Interventions and rationales
☑ **Intervention 1**
Use therapeutic communication techniques whenever the patient makes a self-derogatory remark (see *Therapeutic communication techniques,* pages 17 to 19). Also, avoid using false or inappropriate reassurance (see *Blocks to communication,* page 22).

Rationale and comments: Using therapeutic communication techniques helps the patient hear what he said and gives him a chance to reevaluate its validity. Using false or inappropriate reassurance blocks the exploration of feelings.

☑ **Intervention 2**
If the patient shows signs of depression, see "Depression, Reactive: Situational" in this section.

Rationale and comments: Depression can lead to feelings of low self-esteem and, conversely, feelings of low self-esteem can lead to depression.

☑ **Intervention 3**
If the patient shows signs of noncompliance, see "Noncompliance" in this section.

Rationale and comments: The patient may use noncompliance as a way to bolster his self-esteem and to give him a feeling of control.

☑ **Intervention 4**
Discuss with the patient's family away from the patient their knowledge of his feelings about the illness. Also, try to elicit their reactions to these feelings.

Rationale and comments: The patient's family is often aware of feelings that have not been expressed to the nurse. They need an opportunity to express their own feelings to continue caring for the patient physically and psychologically.

☑ Intervention 5

Consult the doctor about referring the patient to other health care professionals if the depth of his low self-esteem is beyond the scope of your nursing responsibilities and the family's ability to cope with it.

Rationale and comments: Because nurses and the patient's family are not always able to treat all the patient's concerns, consultation with a doctor and referral to other professionals may be needed.

☑ Intervention 6

Refer to "Stress Management" in Section III for post-hospital care suggestions for both the patient and family.

Rationale and comments: Raising the patient's low self-esteem completely during his hospitalization may be impossible. However, as the patient's physical ability improves after discharge, his self-esteem may also rise.

Sexual Dysfunction

Sexual Dysfunction related to fear and lack of knowledge of effects of cardiovascular disease on sexual activity

SUPPORTING DATA
• Diagnosis of angina or myocardial infarction
• Current hospitalization for coronary artery bypass surgery
• Indirectly expressed concerns by patient or partner about resuming sexual activity
• Requests by patient or partner for information about resuming sexual activity

PLAN OF CARE
Outcome criteria
• Patient and partner state measures to take to limit the patient's myocardial oxygen demand during sexual activity.
• Patient and partner report no further concerns regarding the resumption of sexual activity.

Interventions and rationales
☑ **Intervention 1**
Collect baseline data from the patient and his partner, including:
• concerns about resuming sexual activity
• knowledge about how to resume sexual activity safely
• previous patterns of sexual activity, such as:
—partner's availability
—usual time of day and frequency of intercourse
—average duration of intercourse
• past experience with chest pain during sexual stimulation or intercourse. (The patient's previous experience with chest pain may increase his or his partner's fear of resuming activity and may discourage the patient from even attempting to resume activity. Fear also triggers a physiologic response that increases stress on the heart.)
• history of sexual difficulty 1 to 3 months before the patient's cardiac problems developed. Some patients may have sexual difficulties unrelated to their heart disease and may need referral to an appropriate professional.
• medications the patient is currently taking. (Some cardiac medications have side effects that interfere with sexual activity [see *Effects of selected cardiovascular medications on sexual function*, page 98].)
• the patient's response to activity progression. A patient's exercise tolerance is often a good indication of his physiologic readiness for sexual activity.

EFFECTS OF SELECTED CARDIOVASCULAR MEDICATIONS ON SEXUAL FUNCTION

Medication	Effect
thiazide diuretics	• Possible decreased vaginal lubrication and libido
spironolactone (Aldactone)	• Impotence • Irregular menstrual periods • Possible decreased libido
rauwolfia alkaloids (Reserpine)	• Impotence • Decreased libido • Ejaculation disorders
methyldopa (Aldomet)	• Impotence • Decreased libido • Ejaculation disorders
clonidine (Catapres)	• Impotence
propranolol (Inderal)	• Impotence • Decreased libido • Increased fatigue

---

• the patient's emotional response to diagnosis of cardiovascular disease. (Responses include depression, anxiety, and feelings of powerlessness, which can interfere with the resumption of satisfying sexual activity.)
• the patient's and his partner's willingness to discuss the topic.

Rationale and comments: This topic often needs to be initiated by the nurse; mentioning sexual activity as one of a list of energy-consuming activities the patient will be able to resume is a comfortable way to introduce the topic. Keep in mind that timing and sensitivity are important. Other topics, such as finances, returning to work, and the patient's prognosis, may have more immediate concern and should be addressed first.

☑ **Intervention 2**
Assist the patient and his partner to resume some sexual activity in the hospital setting.
• Ensure that they have ample time to visit privately and without interruption.
• Suggest that the patient wear his own clothes rather than a hospital gown.
• Suggest that the female patient resume wearing cosmetics and jewelry, if she desires.
• Tell the patient and his partner that hugging, kissing, caressing, and holding are not stressful on the heart and may be resumed in the hospital if desired.

Rationale and comments: These activities help to promote sexual identity and intimacy without increasing stress on the heart. They can also help facilitate a satisfying resumption of full sexual activity when the patient is physically ready.

☑ Intervention 3

Collaborate with the doctor about when the patient may resume sexual activity. Common indications for resumption of full sexual activity include the patient's ability to:
• climb 20 steps in 10 seconds without showing signs of activity intolerance
• walk several blocks at a brisk pace without showing signs of activity intolerance
• increase his pulse rate to a specified level without showing signs of activity intolerance.

Rationale and comments: These activities use about the same amount of energy that is involved in sexual intercourse with one's usual partner.

☑ Intervention 4

Provide specific instruction about the safe resumption of sexual intercourse following these procedures:
• Instruct the patient and his partner about when they may resume sexual intercourse.
• Instruct the patient to:
  —use a familiar, comfortable setting with his usual partner. (An unfamiliar setting, a new partner, or a room that is too hot or too cold may increase stress on the heart during intercourse.)
  —use positions that are familiar and comfortable. (This decreases stress on the heart. Patients who have undergone coronary artery bypass grafting may need to modify positions slightly to decrease incisional discomfort.)
  —rest before and after intercourse. (Attempting sexual activity when fatigued increases stress on the heart and decreases the likelihood of a satisfying experience. Rest after intercourse helps to limit stress on the heart.)
  —wait at least 3 hours after drinking alcoholic beverages or eating a large meal before having intercourse. (Engaging in intercourse after ingesting alcohol or a large meal is extremely stressful on the heart.)
  —avoid anal intercourse; it increases the risk of parasympathetic stimulation and bradycardia.
  —consider using foreplay to allow the heart rate and blood pressure to rise gradually, which is less stressful on the heart.
• If sexual activity elicits anginal pain:
  —instruct the patient to take one sublingual nitroglycerin tablet before having intercourse. (This helps to decrease chest pain during intercourse.)
  —suggest that the patient consider extending the amount of time spent in foreplay.
• Instruct the patient and his partner that the following warning signs indicate an intolerance for sexual activity:
  —chest pain that occurs during or after intercourse
  —marked shortness of breath that exceeds normal tachypnea experienced during intercourse and that persists for 5 to 10 minutes after orgasm
  —rapid heart rate or palpitations that persist for 10 minutes after orgasm
  —marked fatigue the day after intercourse
  —sleeplessness after the sexual experience.

• Instruct the patient to refrain from further intercourse and to notify the doctor if any of these signs occur. (The doctor may be able to alter the patient's medical regimen to increase activity tolerance.)

☑ Intervention 5
Explain to the patient the relationship between emotional response to cardiovascular disease and sexual functioning.

Rationale and comments: Such emotions as fear, anxiety, and depression can interfere with sexual performance and satisfaction with sexual activity. Feelings of personal failure and sexual inadequacy can result when a patient cannot perform at his previous sexual level. These feelings may further interfere with achieving satisfying sexual activity. Helping the patient and his partner understand the emotional and pharmacologic reasons for possible difficulties may limit the feelings of guilt and failure.

☑ Intervention 6
Explain to the patient the possible side effects his medication may be having on sexual functioning (see *Effects of selected cardiovascular medications on sexual function,* page 98).

☑ Intervention 7
Provide appropriate written materials for the patient and his partner. (These materials reinforce verbal teaching and provide a source of information after discharge from the hospital.)

☑ Intervention 8
Suggest the services of outside resources, as needed, including the following:
• participation in an outpatient cardiac rehabilitation program. (Participation in such a program may help increase activity tolerance.)
• sexual counseling. (Illness and hospitalization may aggravate long-standing sexual difficulties between partners. Resolution of these or other persistent problems that develop as a result of the patient's illness may require the expertise of a counselor.)
• urologic examination. (Impotence in the male patient may be related to atherosclerosis in the arteries supplying the penis.)

Skin Integrity: Impaired

Impaired Skin Integrity related to tissue ischemia in lower extremities caused by reduced blood flow to the tissue secondary to the presence of one or more atherosclerotic lesions in peripheral circulation

SUPPORTING DATA
• Presence of injury on leg or foot (such as a blister, cut, or an area of breakdown)

PLAN OF CARE
Outcome criteria
• Existing areas of impaired skin integrity heal without incident.

Interventions and rationales
☑ **Intervention 1**
Continue routine skin care measures outlined in "Skin Integrity: Potential for Impairment" in this section.

☑ **Intervention 2**
Implement the prescribed care for the injured area; common measures may include:
• dressing changes
• use of whirlpool treatments
• surgical debridement by the doctor.

Rationale and comments: Wet-to-dry dressings are frequently prescribed initially to debride the wound mechanically. If granulation occurs, wet-to-wet dressings may be used to promote tissue growth and repair. Whirlpool treatments may also help to debride injured areas. Surgical debridement may be necessary to remove necrotic tissue and promote healing.

☑ **Intervention 3**
Implement the following measures to control diabetes mellitus when applicable:
• Monitor the patient's blood glucose levels and report abnormal results.
• Administer prescribed hypoglycemic agents.
• Provide a calorie-restricted diet, as ordered.
Note: For a complete discussion on care of the patient with diabetes mellitus, consult a medical-surgical textbook.

Rationale and comments: Many patients with occlusive arterial disease are also diabetic. Uncontrolled diabetes can interfere with healing. Patients who take oral antidiabetic agents at home may require insulin during hospitalization to maintain blood glucose levels within the desired range. The patient may be discharged on insulin or may be returned to oral agents.

☑ Intervention 4
Assess the patient for signs of infection in the injured area, and intervene if they are present.
• Signs include:
—redness, warmth, and edema at site
—change in drainage to purulent
—fever
—elevated white blood cell count
—failure of ulcer to begin to heal.
• If signs of infection are present:
—notify the doctor
—obtain a culture of the wound (may require a doctor's order)
—administer prescribed antibiotics
—continue prescribed measures for treatment of injury.

Rationale and comments: The presence of continued or increased infection may indicate the need for more aggressive measures, including surgical debridement or amputation.

☑ Intervention 5
Assess and report the patient's response to treatment including:
• change in characteristics of injury
• results of repeat wound cultures.

Rationale and comments: Indications of healing include the presence of granulation tissue, decreasing purulent drainage, or decreasing size of wound.

Skin Integrity: Potential for Impairment

Potential for Impaired Skin Integrity related to edema, impaired tissue perfusion, decreased mobility, and anorexia associated with congestive heart failure

SUPPORTING DATA
• Edema in dependent body sites
• Activity limited by doctor's orders or patient condition
• Diagnosis of acute congestive heart failure (CHF)
• Decreased intake (eats less than half of food served at each meal)

PLAN OF CARE
Outcome criteria
• Patient shows no evidence of impaired skin integrity.

Interventions and rationales
☑ **Intervention 1**
Implement routine skin care measures, including:
• daily inspection of skin for evidence of impaired skin integrity.
• massage of patient's back, sacrum, buttocks, and heels with lotion at least once during a shift.
• use of a turning sheet to move patient up in bed. (Use of a turning sheet eliminates shearing forces that can damage the patient's already fragile skin.)
• changing the patient's position every 2 hours, keeping in mind the following:
—Position him to facilitate breathing. (Patients with CHF will not tolerate positions that increase their difficulty in breathing.)
—Turn the patient from side to back to side while he is in bed.
—May also get the patient out of bed and into a chair (unless contraindicated).
• assisting the patient from the bedpan or bedside commode as soon as toileting is complete. (Allowing the patient to sit for long periods on a bedpan or bedside commode can put prolonged pressure on his buttocks.)

☑ **Intervention 2**
Handle edematous areas carefully. Follow these suggestions:
• Avoid shearing forces on these tissues when moving patient.
• Avoid the use of tape on edematous areas.
• Position the patient to decrease pressure on edematous areas.
• Use such aids as heel protectors, as needed.

Rationale and comments: Edematous areas are at high risk of developing impaired skin integrity because the circulation is already compromised.

☑ **Intervention 3**
Reduce the patient's specific risk factors for impaired skin integrity as indicated:
• For edema and impaired tissue perfusion, see "Fluid Volume Excess: Edema" and "Gas Exchange: Impaired" in this section.
• For anorexia and inadequate nutritional intake, see "Nutrition, Alteration in: Less than Body Requirements" in this section.
• For decreased activity, see "Activity Intolerance" in this section.

Potential for Impaired Skin Integrity related to tissue ischemia in lower extremities caused by reduced blood flow to the tissue secondary to the presence of one or more atherosclerotic lesions in peripheral arterial circulation

SUPPORTING DATA
• Atherosclerotic obstruction in peripheral arterial circulation documented by angiography, Doppler ultrasound, or plethysmography
• Absent or diminished peripheral pulse(s) in leg
• Intermittent claudication
• Foot or toe pain at rest
• Current hospitalization for peripheral arterial bypass surgery or past history of such surgery
• Current hospitalization for amputation secondary to complications from occlusive arterial disease

---

PLAN OF CARE
Outcome criteria
• Patient shows no evidence of impaired skin integrity.

Interventions and rationales
☑ **Intervention 1**
Inspect the patient's legs and feet daily for signs of injury, redness, or irritation or for other signs of impaired skin integrity.

Rationale and comments: Many patients with occlusive arterial disease may have some neuropathy that decreases their perception of pain; daily inspection is the only reliable means of identifying injury or other impairment of skin integrity.

☑ **Intervention 2**
Wash the patient's feet daily, following these guidelines:
• Use warm (not hot) water. Immersing feet in water that is too hot may result in ischemic damage.

• Use mild soap.
• Gently pat feet dry, making sure to dry well between the toes.
• Apply mild lotion to dry areas of the foot. Do not apply lotion to the area between the toes, as this is susceptible to infection and breakdown.
• Dust the feet gently with cornstarch if sweating is a problem.

☑ Intervention 3
Implement the following measures to decrease risk of injury:
• Ask the patient to wear shoes or slippers and socks when walking in the room or hall. (Appropriate footwear should provide good support, protect the heel and toe, be flat, and fit correctly.)
• Promote increased circulation to the legs. Follow these procedures:
—Position the patient with the head of the bed elevated 30 degrees. (This position facilitates blood flow to the legs and may help to decrease ischemia.)
—Keep the patient's legs and feet warm by having him wear cotton or wool socks and by keeping the room temperature comfortably warm. (Cold causes vasoconstriction, which decreases blood flow and can increase ischemia.)
—Do not apply any form of heat directly to the legs or feet. (Direct heat increases tissue metabolism and oxygen demands, possibly resulting in increased tissue ischemia.)
—Instruct the patient to refrain from smoking.
• Have the patient use heel protectors or a bed cradle. (These aids can decrease pressure on susceptible areas.)

Rationale and comments: Injuries heal slowly with occlusive arterial disease; therefore, prevention is vital.

☑ Intervention 4
Teach the patient how to care for feet properly at home.

Sleep-Pattern Disturbance

Sleep-Pattern Disturbance related to dyspnea, anxiety, medication side effects, pain, noise, treatment disruptions, lack of exercise, nightmares

SUPPORTING DATA
• Fatigue and sleepiness during daytime hours
• Sleeplessness during the night, observed or reported
• Patient's request to not be awakened at night for vital signs and other treatments
• Frequent calls to the nurse during the night to request fluids or pain medication, to get assistance with going to the bathroom or fixing blankets, to make room temperature adjustments, or to turn off the light or close the door
• Complaints that nurses make too much noise during the night
• Taking a long time to fall asleep or awakening after 2 to 4 hours and being unable to return to sleep
• Requests for sleep medication every night
• Complaints of pain during the night
• Decreases in activity tolerance

PLAN OF CARE
Outcome criteria
• Patient states he slept well.
• Patient states he feels refreshed.
• Patient remains oriented and alert during the day and does not complain of drowsiness.
• If patient desires, he is able to reduce intake of sleep medication.

Interventions and rationales
☑ Intervention 1
Assess the patient for the following, if not already in the data base:
• usual time for retiring and awakening
• usual ways to promote sleep, including reading, watching television, eating, sexual activity, listening to music, meditation, or taking a bath or shower
• usual measures the patient takes to counteract insomnia and their effectiveness
• frequency of difficulty with sleeping before his hospitalization. (Keep in mind that a patient who normally has frequent difficulty with sleeping is more likely to experience difficulty in the hospital than a patient who rarely experiences difficulty with sleeping.)

Rationale and comments: Understanding the patient's present difficulty requires knowing his usual sleep pattern. Methods to promote sleep are usually developed over many years; patients feel more comfortable if they can follow their usual routines in strange surroundings or when problems arise.

☑ Intervention 2
Implement a schedule for bedtime activities that most closely resembles the patient's usual pattern and make sure it is compatible with hospital policy and doctor's orders. For example, a schedule might include the following:
• mild exercise. (Keep in mind that vigorous exercise is stimulating, rather than relaxing. Also, afternoon exercise has been found to promote slow-wave sleep more than evening exercise.)
• shower or bath. (Warm water can be relaxing as well as refreshing.)
• brushing teeth
• straightening the bed
• adjusting the room temperature or covers
• administering medications (those regularly scheduled or those for pain). (Because pain is frequently an impediment to sleep, avoid having to arouse the patient to take medications after he is relaxed and ready for sleep.)
• back rub. (Giving the patient a back rub not only relaxes his muscles but also shows you care for him and provides a time for conversation if the patient so desires.)
• adjusting lights and closing the door
• administering sleep medications. Only do this if the patient is used to taking them on a routine basis. (If sleeping pills are part of patient's ritual, elimination of them will be more disruptive than helpful.)

Rationale and comments: The closer the activities resemble a familiar pattern, the greater their effect is likely to be.

☑ Intervention 3
Check the patient 1 hour after administering care to see if he is asleep.

Rationale and comments: The patient is the true judge of the effectiveness of nursing actions.

☑ Intervention 4
If the patient is still awake, take the following measures:
• Ask him if he has a specific reason—physical or psychological—for being awake; often, the patient knows what is keeping him awake.
• Try to make the patient as comfortable as possible.
• Listen to the patient, using therapeutic communication techniques (see *Therapeutic communication techniques,* pages 17 to 19), if reasons are more psychological in nature. (Because anxieties often arise at night, thereby interfering with sleep, assisting the patient to express them may help him to sleep.)
• Offer sleep medication if sleeplessness occurs early in the night. (Sleep medication given too late causes the patient to feel groggy during the day; this may result in his sleeping during the day, then remaining awake during the next night. You'll need to decide if the patient's need for sleep is more important than reducing his sleep medication.)

• Discuss with the patient any plans to reduce the use of sleeping pills. (When frequent use of sleeping pills is discontinued, disrupted sleep patterns occur for several days. The patient may wish to postpone this disruption until after discharge from the hospital.)

☑ **Intervention 5**

Try any of these other suggestions to help the patient sleep:
• Administer pain and sleep medications together. (As the pain medication relieves pain, the sleep medication takes over and provides a prolonged sleep.)
• Suggest that the patient drink a glass of warm milk or eat some other food within his dietary restrictions. (High-protein foods contain L-tryptophan, which is helpful in inducing sleep. Also, if the patient is in the habit of snacking before bedtime, absence of a snack will interfere with sleep.)
• Tell him to try meditation, deep-breathing exercises, listening to music, or watching television (if he's in a private room). (If the patient knows meditation, he is likely to use it on his own; he can be taught deep-breathing exercises in a few minutes.)
• Have him concentrate on staying awake. (This seems to have the opposite effect of inducing sleep.)

☑ **Intervention 6**

Ask the patient to try staying awake during the day except for taking one or two brief naps if he has had a myocardial infarction (MI) or heart surgery.

Rationale and comments: Sleeping during the day turns the sleep cycle around; however, if the patient is seriously ill, he probably will not be able to stay awake all day, nor should he. Naps are recommended for patients who have had an MI or surgery. As recovery from these events occurs, the patient will be able to spend more time awake during the day; also, he'll be able to establish a new sleep pattern that incorporates the naps into the schedule.

☑ **Intervention 7**

Try to schedule the patient's treatments, vital signs measurements, and medications to occur at one given time to avoid waking the patient frequently during the night.

Rationale and comments: Rapid-eye-movement sleep, the most refreshing sleep, generally occurs in the later portion of an uninterrupted sleep period. If the patient is wakened frequently, he will never experience this sleep and, consequently, will not feel rested.

☑ **Intervention 8**

Discuss with the doctor whether all the procedures currently done during the night are necessary (not all nursing procedures have to be done during the night even if presently scheduled).

Rationale and comments: The patient's failure to complete 90-minute cycles of sleep can lead to serious complications, such as myocardial irritability and ventricular dysrhythmias, because of the rapid, alternating bursts of sympathetic and parasympathetic autonomic stimulation.

SECTION II: STANDARD CARE PLANS

Amputation, Leg
(for Vascular Disease)

ASSOCIATED NURSING DIAGNOSES
Anxiety
Bowel Elimination, Alteration in: Constipation
Comfort, Alteration in: Acute Pain
Depression, Reactive: Situational
Family Processes, Alteration in
Grieving, Family
Grieving, Individual Patient
Nutrition, Alteration in: Less Than Body Requirements
Physical Mobility, Impaired
Respiratory Function, Alteration in
Respiratory Function, Potential Alteration in
Self-Concept, Alteration in
Skin Integrity, Impaired
Skin Integrity, Potential for Impairment
Sleep-Pattern Disturbance

ASSOCIATED TEACHING PLANS
Amputation, Leg: Home Care
Atherosclerosis: Disease Process and Risk Factors
Cardiovascular Disease Risk Factors: Cigarette Smoking
Cardiovascular Disease Risk Factors: Diabetes Mellitus and Atherosclerosis
Cardiovascular Disease Risk Factors: Dietary Measures to Control
    Hyperlipidemia
Hypertension, Essential: Disease Process and Risk Factors
Occlusive Arterial Disease: Disease Process and Home Care

Interventions and rationales
☑ Intervention 1
Collect data on the patient preoperatively, including the following:
• presence and status of any concurrent medical problems
• presence of infection in the leg to be amputated
• the patient's fluid and electrolyte status
• the patient's nutritional status
• the patient's and family's knowledge about the proposed surgery, post-operative care, and rehabilitation measures
• the patient's and family's anxiety and other emotional responses to the upcoming amputation
• financial concerns, including loss of job or income secondary to amputation as well as the cost of medical care, rehabilitation, and prosthesis.

Rationale and comments: Many patients who undergo amputation have one or more concurrent medical problems that may affect their postoperative recovery. Careful preoperative assessment provides baseline data that can assist the nurse in recognizing significant postoperative changes.

☑ Intervention 2
Assist with any scheduled diagnostic tests. Tests may include:
• arterial blood pressure measurements in the thigh and ankle of the affected leg
• skin temperature measurements
• radioisotope scanning to determine cutaneous, local blood flow
• arteriography (see *Tests used to diagnose occlusive arterial disease in the legs*, pages 199 to 200).

Rationale and comments: Diagnostic tests may be used to determine the approximate or planned level of amputation. However, the final decision about the exact level is made in the operating room by the surgeon on the basis of the degree of bleeding of the skin edges.

☑ Intervention 3
Assist with measures to improve the patient's overall status preoperatively, including:
• performing dressing changes and administering antibiotics, as prescribed, to treat infection
• implementing measures to facilitate blood flow to the involved leg as outlined in the nursing diagnosis care plan for "Skin Integrity, Potential for Impairment related to tissue ischemia" in Section I
• implementing measures to improve nutritional status as outlined in "Nutrition, Alteration in: Less Than Body Requirements" in Section I
• implementing measures to control diabetes when applicable. (Consult a medical-surgical nursing textbook for a complete discussion of care of diabetic patients.)
—Monitor blood glucose levels and report abnormal results.
—Administer prescribed hypoglycemic agents.
—Provide a calorie-restricted diet, as ordered.

Rationale and comments: Many patients with vascular disease resulting in lower limb amputation are also diabetic; uncontrolled diabetes can interfere with healing. Patients who take oral antidiabetic agents at home may require insulin during hospitalization to maintain blood glucose levels within the desired range. Patients may be discharged on insulin or may be switched back to oral agents.

☑ Intervention 4
In collaboration with the doctor, physical therapist, and prosthetist, implement preoperative teaching. Be sure to include the following points in your discussion with the patient:
• the surgical procedure planned. Advise the patient that the level of amputation will be determined by the doctor on the basis of diagnostic tests and the patient's clinical condition.

• type of dressing planned postoperatively (see *Types of dressings used after amputation* for information about commonly used dressings).
• rehabilitation measures planned, including exercises and prosthesis.

☑ Intervention 5
Assess the patient upon his return from surgery. Include the following data:
• the level of amputation performed
• intraoperative and postoperative complications
• the type of dressing on the residual limb
• the amount and type of drainage present from the operative site.

☑ Intervention 6
Implement the prescribed medical orders, which may include the following:
• taking vital sign measurements every 15 minutes until the patient is stable, then every 4 hours
• maintaining the patient on bed rest with the foot of the bed elevated for the first 24 to 48 hours (to decrease edema in the residual limb)
• advancing the patient's activity to getting out of bed and sitting in a chair with assistance for short periods (Sitting for long periods can result in hip flexion contractures and impede rehabilitation.)
• implementing an exercise program directed by the physical therapist
• administering prescribed medications, including:
  —analgesics to control postoperative pain
  —antibiotics to prevent a wound infection
  —stool softeners and laxatives
• not allowing the patient to smoke. (Smoking promotes vasoconstriction, which can interfere with postoperative healing and can compromise circulation to the remaining leg.)

☑ Intervention 7
Assess the patient for signs of postoperative hemorrhage and notify the doctor if such signs are present. Observe for:
• character and the amount of drainage from the wound drain every 4 to 8 hours, as indicated
• changes in vital signs indicative of hemorrhage
• signs of excessive bleeding on the residual limb dressing.

Rationale and comments: Hemorrhage from the surgical site can be a serious complication after amputation.

☑ Intervention 8
Assess patient for such signs of wound infection as:
• elevated temperature
• elevated white blood cell count
• purulent drainage from the incision site
• failure of the incision site to heal
• increased pain in the incision site.

Rationale and comments: Infection after amputation is a serious complication. It not only can interfere with normal healing but also can delay prosthetic fitting and may result in additional surgery to revise the stump.

TYPES OF DRESSINGS USED AFTER AMPUTATION

Molded rigid dressing

Description
- Made of plaster of paris
- Applied in operating room at close of surgery to conform to the shape of the residual limb

Purpose
- Limits the development of postoperative edema in the residual limb
- Facilitates earlier prosthesis fitting by decreasing the time needed to shrink the residual limb
- Facilitates healing of the surgical incision by limiting edema, which can interfere with capillary circulation in wound edges
- May be used with a temporary prosthesis

Concerns
- Requires application by specially trained personnel
- Does not permit daily inspection of wound or surgical incision for evidence of infection or impaired healing
- Increases risk of impaired circulation

Controlled environment therapy

Description
- Consists of a sterile bag encasing the residual limb and a console by which to control settings

Purpose
- Decreases postoperative edema in the residual limb
- Decreases pain caused by increased edema
- Increases circulation to wound to facilitate healing
- Permits easy, continuous wound inspection

Concerns
- Limits the patient to his hospital room and decreases overall activity because of the size of the console
- Prohibits the patient from lying prone
- Increases the risk of hip flexion contractures
- Increases the amount of time the patient spends in bed, thus increasing the need for skin care measures and other measures to decrease the risk of other complications associated with bed rest

Elastic or Ace wraps

Description
- Lightweight, inexpensive means of wrapping residual limb
- Consists of 4″ or 6″ elastic wraps that are applied to the residual limb smoothly, without wrinkles, using a figure-eight configuration and angular turns

Purpose
- Used to control postoperative edema in the residual limb
- Permits frequent wound inspection
- Permits frequent dressing changes, as needed.

Concerns
- Least effective in controlling edema
- Requires skill in applying; incorrect application can result in misformed stump or delayed prosthetic fitting.
- Part of dressing can slip and form a tourniquet around the residual limb, thus interfering with circulation and impairing healing.
- Requires frequent observation for dressing status and reapplication as needed

(continued)

TYPES OF DRESSINGS USED AFTER AMPUTATION *(continued)*

Shrinkers

Description	• Tubular dressing made of rubber and reinforced cotton • Available in various sizes and worn suspended from the patient's waist, belt or garter, or shoulder harness
Purpose	• Controls postoperative edema in the residual limb
Concerns	• Possible interference with circulation to distal part of residual limb because of incorrect fit • Can be expensive because the patient must purchase additional shrinkers in smaller sizes as residual limb shrinks • Because the dressing may slip or roll after application, it must be observed frequently and reapplied as necessary.

☑ Intervention 9

If signs and symptoms of infection develop, take the following measures:
• Notify the doctor.
• Obtain a wound culture (this may require a doctor's order in some institutions).
• Administer prescribed antibiotics.
• Implement any prescribed dressing changes. (Dressing changes may include sterile dry dressings or wet-to-dry dressings using normal saline solution, povidone-iodine, or another prescribed solution.)
• Assess for signs of healing. Decreased drainage, warmth, and redness indicate improvement.
• Continue measures to promote good nutrition.
• Continue measures to promote circulation to the residual limb.
• Continue to implement measures to control blood glucose levels.
• Prepare the patient for additional surgical procedures, if ordered. (Incision and drainage of the wound or revision of the stump may be necessary in severe infection.)

Rationale and comments: Control of diabetes becomes more difficult when infection is present. A vicious cycle can develop: infection causes increased blood glucoses levels; with increased blood glucose levels, infection is hard to resolve and the wound fails to heal. Maintaining blood glucose levels within the desired range will help combat infection and promote healing.

☑ Intervention 10

Implement measures to manage these common postoperative problems:
• pain (see "Comfort, Alteration in: Acute Pain" in Section I)
• atelectasis (see "Respiratory Function, Alteration in" and "Respiratory Function, Potential Alteration in" in Section I)
• deep vein thrombosis (see "Deep Vein Thrombosis, Prevention of" in this section)

• impaired skin integrity (see "Skin Integrity, Impaired" and "Skin Integrity, Potential for Impairment"in Section I)
• constipation (see "Bowel Elimination, Alteration in: Constipation" in Section I)
• postoperative depression (see "Depression, Reactive: Situational" in Section I).

☑ **Intervention 11**
Implement measures to promote optimal rehabilitation (see the measures outlined in "Physical Mobility, Impaired" in Section I).

Angina Pectoris

ASSOCIATED NURSING DIAGNOSES
Activity Intolerance
Activity Intolerance, Potential for
Anxiety
Bowel Elimination, Alteration in: Constipation
Depression, Reactive: Situational
Family Processes, Alteration in
Grieving, Family
Grieving, Individual Patient
Noncompliance
Self-Concept, Alteration in
Sexual Dysfunction
Sleep-Pattern Disturbance

ASSOCIATED TEACHING PLANS
Angina Pectoris: Disease Process and Home Care
Atherosclerosis: Disease Process and Risk Factors
Cardiac Anatomy and Physiology: Heart and Blood Vessels
Cardiovascular Disease Risk Factors: Cigarette Smoking
Cardiovascular Disease Risk Factors: Diabetes Mellitus and Atherosclerosis
Cardiovascular Disease Risk Factors: Dietary Measures to Control Hyperlipidemia
Hypertension, Essential: Disease Process and Risk Factors
Medication Guidelines
Stress Management

☑ Interventions and rationales
Intervention 1
Obtain a history of the patient's angina pain on admission, including the following data:
• the patient's description of the pain
• location of the pain
• duration of the pain
• radiation of the pain to other areas
• frequency of the attacks
• pattern to the attacks
• factors that aggravate the pain
• factors that relieve the pain.

Rationale and comments: Because symptoms of angina may vary from patient to patient, this information will provide baseline data about the patient's individual signs and symptoms and will aid the nurse in recognizing and treating acute attacks.

☑ Intervention 2

Monitor the patient for any signs of acute attacks during the hospital stay. Signs may include:
- chest pain
  - —often described as tightness, discomfort, sensation of pressure, or a feeling of constriction
  - —often located substernally or retrosternally
  - —may radiate to the neck, jaw, teeth, back, shoulders, arms, elbows, or wrists (radiates to left side more frequently than to right side)
  - —unaffected by changes in position or by respirations
  - —usually subsides within 15 minutes with rest or after administration of nitroglycerin
  - —may be accompanied by nausea and vomiting, dyspnea, diaphoresis, pallor, or anxiety
- changes in vital signs
- ischemic changes on EKG
- less common signs and symptoms, including:
  - —chest pain that begins as a dull ache in the wrist or elbow and that moves to a substernal or retrosternal area
  - —complaint of numbness in an extremity
  - —pain that is located in only the neck, jaw, throat, or teeth
  - —shortness of breath and fatigue without pain.

Rationale and comments: Angina pectoris occurs when an imbalance between myocardial oxygen supply and demand develops, resulting in myocardial ischemia. Although the most common symptom of angina is chest pain, symptoms may be variable. Some patients may experience only mild chest pain with few accompanying symptoms; mild chest pain still represents myocardial ischemia and should be treated. In other patients, sensations of pain may be masked by beta-adrenergic blocker therapy and the neuropathies associated with diabetes mellitus.

☑ Intervention 3

Treat acute attacks of angina pectoris, following these procedures:
- Have the patient stop all activity and sit down.
- Administer sublingual nitroglycerin.
  - —Place one tablet under the patient's tongue; instruct him to let the tablet dissolve.
  - —Monitor the patient's response to the nitroglycerin. Ask if the pain is lessening, then check his pulse and blood pressure.
  - —If pain is not relieved and the patient's systolic blood pressure drops significantly, withhold further administration of nitroglycerin and notify the doctor.
  - —If pain is not relieved by one nitroglycerin tablet and blood pressure has not dropped significantly, continue to administer one nitroglycerin tablet every 5 minutes until pain is relieved or a maximum of three tablets have been given. (The number may vary according to doctor's orders.)

• If sublingual nitroglycerin is ineffective in relieving the patient's chest pain, implement the following measures:

—Administer morphine sulfate (or other medications) if prescribed for the relief of acute attacks, evaluate the patient's response after a few minutes, and notify the doctor.

—If no additional medications are prescribed to treat acute attacks, notify the doctor immediately.

• Administer oxygen by nasal cannula, as ordered.

• Take measures to decrease the patient's anxiety.

• If the patient is on continuous EKG monitoring, obtain a rhythm strip to check for evidence of ischemia and/or dysrhythmias.

Rationale and comments: Treatment centers on prompt action.

• Stopping activity decreases myocardial oxygen consumption and lessens myocardial oxygen demand.

• Sublingual nitroglycerin, the drug of choice to treat acute angina attacks, decreases myocardial oxygen demand and increases oxygen supply through collateral vessels to the ischemic area. Because this drug is a vasodilator, it can cause hypotension.

• Chest pain unrelieved by nitroglycerin is a strong indication that the patient may be experiencing a myocardial infarction. Additional prompt treatment is needed to limit damage to the myocardium.

• Morphine sulfate is often the drug of choice to treat chest pain unrelieved by sublingual nitroglycerin.

• Administration of supplemental oxygen helps to decrease hypoxia, which can increase myocardial work load and oxygen demand, thereby increasing myocardial ischemia.

• Anxiety increases myocardial oxygen consumption and can increase myocardial ischemia.

☑ **Intervention 4**

Implement the following frequently prescribed medical orders, as ordered:

• Administer prescribed medications, which commonly include:

—sublingual nitroglycerin to treat acute attacks

—long-acting antianginals, such as long-acting nitrates (see *Nitrates*), calcium channel blockers (see *Calcium channel blockers*, page 120), and beta-adrenergic blockers (see *Beta-adrenergic blocking agents*, page 191) to decrease the frequency of episodes of myocardial ischemia

—laxatives or stool softeners to prevent straining with defecation. (Straining increases myocardial oxygen demand and may precipitate an acute episode of myocardial ischemia.)

—antianxiety medications. (Anxiety increases myocardial oxygen demand and the risk that the patient will have an acute episode of myocardial ischemia.)

• Administer oxygen, as ordered or needed, to help prevent hypoxia, which can increase myocardial work load and oxygen consumption. (Keep in mind that the prescribed FIO_2 or liter flow will vary, depending on the patient's arterial blood gas levels and respiratory status.)

COMMONLY PRESCRIBED MEDICATIONS

NITRATES

Examples	• Erythrityl tetranitrate (Cardilate) • Isosorbide dinitrate (Isordil, Sorbitrate) • Nitroglycerin ointment (Nitro-Bid ointment, Nitrol ointment) • Nitroglycerin, sustained-release (Nitro-Bid) • Nitroglycerin, transdermal patches (Nitro-Dur, Transderm-Nitro, Nitrodisc) • Pentaerythritol tetranitrate (Peritrate)
Actions	• Systemic vasodilator • In the presence of coronary artery disease, increases oxygen supply to ischemic areas of myocardium by causing dilatation of collateral vessels • Decreases myocardial oxygen demand
Uses	• Prevents or reduces the number of acute ischemic attacks in patients with coronary artery disease
Side effects	• Flushing • Headache • Hypotension • Tachycardia
Nursing responsibilities	• Monitor the patient's vital signs carefully, especially for signs of hypotension. • Note and report any change in the pattern of angina attacks. • Assess and report any medication side effects.

• Limit the patient's activity to decrease myocardial work load and oxygen consumption. Depending on the patient's status, restrictions may include:
—room rest
—bed rest with bathroom privileges
—strict bed rest.
• Restrict the patient's diet, as ordered. Common restrictions include:
—no caffeine or stimulants. (Caffeine, a central nervous system stimulant, can increase myocardial oxygen consumption by increasing blood pressure and heart rate, thereby provoking an acute episode of myocardial ischemia.)
—low saturated fat and low cholesterol diets.
• Maintain continuous EKG monitoring, as ordered.
• Maintain a heparin lock or a keep-vein-open I.V. line, as ordered.

Rationale and comments: Different types of angina have been identified; treatment and prognosis of the patient's condition may vary depending on his specific type of angina (see *Classification of angina,* page 121, for a brief description of each type).

CALCIUM CHANNEL BLOCKERS

Examples	• Diltiazem (Cardizem) • Nifedipine (Procardia) • Verapamil (Calan, Isoptin)
Actions	• Dilates coronary arteries • Prevents coronary artery spasms • Slows conduction through the sinoatrial and atrioventricular nodes
Uses	• Reduces or prevents myocardial ischemia by increasing myocardial oxygen supply • Prevents myocardial ischemia caused by coronary artery vasospasm • Treats and controls supraventricular tachydysrhythmias (I.V. verapamil) • Under investigation for use in controlling hypertension
Side effects	*Note:* These vary with each drug. • Verapamil: constipation, headache, heart block, flushing, peripheral edema • Nifedipine: hypotension, reflex tachycardia, flushing, tremor, nervousness, peripheral edema • Diltiazem: heart block, dry mouth
Cautions	• Verapamil is contraindicated for use in patients with congestive heart failure. • Diltiazem should be used cautiously in patients with heart block or hypotension.
Nursing responsibilities	• Monitor the patient's vital signs carefully for hypotension and changes in pulse rate or rhythm. • Notify the doctor if vital signs don't fall within preset parameters.

☑ **Intervention 5**

Monitor the patient for development of acute MI (see "Myocardial Infarction, Acute" in this section for signs and symptoms).

Rationale and comments: Because patients with angina may progress to MI, prompt recognition and treatment can limit complications and death.

☑ **Intervention 6**

Assist with evaluating the patient's progress and response to therapy.
• Monitor the patient for any changes in the pattern of attacks, and notify the doctor accordingly.
• Assess the patient's response to increasing activity.

Rationale and comments: Angina attacks that increase in frequency, duration, or severity are a warning that the patient is at high risk for developing an MI in the near future. Conversely, angina attacks that decrease in severity and frequency are an indication that medical and nursing measures are effective in limiting episodes of myocardial ischemia.

CLASSIFICATION OF ANGINA

Stable angina	• Predictably precipitated by some type or degree of exertion or stress (stress may be physical or emotional) • Produces certain characteristics that are similar with each attack • Responds to rest or nitroglycerin • Frequently caused by atherosclerotic lesions that develop in coronary arteries and partially obstruct the lumen of the artery. During times of increased myocardial oxygen demand (such as with exertion), the heart is unable to sufficiently increase blood flow through the diseased arteries to meet this demand. As a result, an imbalance between myocardial oxygen supply and demand occurs and the patient experiences myocardial ischemia. • May be managed with long-acting antianginal medications and reduction of risk factors
Unstable angina	• Includes four subgroups: —recent-onset angina (occurring within 6 weeks); attacks occur frequently and interfere significantly with patient's usual activities —angina that occurs at rest —chronic stable angina that increases in frequency, intensity, or duration —angina that develops within days to weeks after myocardial infarction • Frequently indicates critical atherosclerotic lesions in one or more coronary arteries • Indicates increased risk for the development of an acute myocardial infarction or sudden death • Extent of coronary artery disease determined by cardiac catheterization • May be treated with medications, coronary artery bypass grafting, or percutaneous transluminal coronary angioplasty
Variant angina	• May occur at rest or with activity • May be precipitated by smoking or alcohol consumption • Caused by coronary artery spasm. The spasm interferes with blood flow through the artery and creates an imbalance between myocardial oxygen supply and demand. It may occur in the presence or absence of atherosclerotic lesions in the coronary arteries. • Treated with calcium channel blockers to control the coronary artery spasms

☑ Intervention 7

Assist with procedures to assess the extent of coronary artery disease. Common procedures include:

- Holter monitoring
- exercise stress test
- exercise stress test with radionuclide imaging
- cardiac catheterization.

(For specific details on these procedures, see *Diagnostic tests: Coronary artery disease, angina, myocardial infarction, congestive heart failure.*)

Rationale and comments: Long-term medical management depends, in part, on the extent of atherosclerosis in the coronary arteries.

DIAGNOSTIC TESTS: CORONARY ARTERY DISEASE, ANGINA, MYOCARDIAL INFARCTION, CONGESTIVE HEART FAILURE

Holter monitor	
Purpose	• Detects episodes of myocardial ischemia that are asymptomatic except for ST wave changes • Evaluates myocardial response to activity after myocardial infarction (MI) • Assesses for presence of potentially dangerous dysrhythmias • Monitors effectiveness of medications prescribed to restore balance between oxygen supply and demand
Procedure	• Noninvasive procedure with minimal risks involved • May be done on an inpatient or outpatient basis • Involves continuous ambulatory recording of patient's EKG • Requires a recording device to be worn by patient for a prescribed period (usually 24 to 48 hours) • Requires that patient follow usual daily routine; the patient or a family member keeps a record of activities performed during the recording period
Preparation	• Instruct the patient or family member on how to keep a diary to record activities during the recording period. • Instruct the patient to avoid disconnecting the monitor leads for any reason and to avoid wetting the leads or recording device during the recording period.
Postprocedure	• None
Exercise stress test	
Purpose	• General diagnostic screening for coronary artery disease (CAD); can indicate the presence of CAD but does not give specific information about the number or precise location of occlusions

DIAGNOSTIC TESTS: CORONARY ARTERY DISEASE, ANGINA, MYOCARDIAL INFARCTION, CONGESTIVE HEART FAILURE
(continued)

Exercise stress test *(continued)*

Purpose *(continued)*	• Provides guidelines for physical activity for healthy adults as well as for MI patients or those who have undergone coronary artery bypass grafting (CABG) surgery • Identifies pathologic responses to exercise, including myocardial ischemia and dysrhythmias • Assists in identifying patients at high risk for experiencing a second cardiac event • Provides objective data on exercise capacity of patients with valvular heart disease
Procedure	• Noninvasive procedure involving low risk to the patient • Requires patient to perform some type of exercise while being monitored for changes in vital signs and EKG pattern or for development of other symptoms of myocardial ischemia; patient exercises until set parameters are reached. • Exercise performed may include walking on a treadmill or riding a stationary bicycle. • Involves two major types of exercise tests: symptom-limited and graded (also called submaximal). In the symptom-limited test, the patient exercises until he complains of exhaustion or develops angina, dyspnea, local muscle fatigue, ischemic ST wave changes, hypotension, or ventricular dysrhythmias. The test is structured to try to elicit these symptoms within 6 to 15 minutes. In the graded test, the patient exercises until he achieves a predetermined work load or a preset pulse rate for a specific period of time.
Preparation	• Patient should avoid smoking for at least 2 hours before the test. • Depending on institutional policy, patient may be allowed a light meal or nothing by mouth before the test. • Patient should avoid hot showers or strenuous activity before the test. • Have the patient wear good walking shoes and comfortable clothes. (Female patients may prefer slacks; provide pajama bottoms for male and female patients in the hospital.)
Postprocedure	• None

Thallium 201 myocardial imaging or scintigraphy: Resting

Purpose	• Provides estimate of area at risk during evolution of MI • Differentiates ischemia or infarct from normal, healthy tissue • Differentiates ischemia from an infarct • Does not differentiate between old and acute MI • Assists in assessing the effectiveness of thrombolytic therapy

(continued)

DIAGNOSTIC TESTS: CORONARY ARTERY DISEASE, ANGINA, MYOCARDIAL INFARCTION, CONGESTIVE HEART FAILURE
(continued)

Thallium 201 myocardial imaging or scintigraphy: Resting *(continued)*

Procedure	• Involves minimal risk to the patient • Requires I.V. injection of thallium 201, a radioisotope; then, patient is scanned using a special camera. Normal myocardial tissue takes up the radioisotope; areas of infarct or ischemia do not. On scan, infarcted or ischemic areas show up as a "cold spot." If a cold spot appears on the initial scan, a repeat scan will be done several hours later. If the cold spot persists, the area is infarcted; if the cold spot has disappeared, the area was ischemic.
Preparation	• Explain to the patient that he may feel uncomfortable lying still on the table. • No special preparation is necessary.
Postprocedure	• None

Thallium 201 myocardial imaging or scintigraphy: Exercise

Purpose	• Differentiates ischemia or infarct from normal, healthy tissue • Differentiates ischemia from an infarct • For other specific purposes, see *Exercise stress test.*
Procedure	• Involves few risks to the patient • Requires patient to perform a set amount of exercise while being monitored for signs and symptoms of myocardial ischemia (protocol similar to that of *Exercise stress test*). Before patient stops exercising, he is injected with thallium 201 I.V., then he continues to exercise for 45 to 60 seconds more. Within 10 minutes after receiving the injection, the patient is scanned with a special camera. • For a brief description of findings, see *Thallium 201 myocardial imaging or scintigraphy: Resting.*
Preparation	• Same as for *Exercise stress test*
Postprocedure	• None

Technetium pyrophosphate scanning

Purpose	• Identifies location or extent of infarct • Confirms MI when it cannot be diagnosed by enzyme studies or EKG changes • Confirms extension of MI
Procedure	• Involves minimal risks to the patient • Requires I.V. injection of a radioisotope; then, patient is scanned 1 to 2 hours after injection using a special camera. Areas of MI take up the radioisotope (shown on scan as a "hot spot"); normal myocardial tissue does not • Optimal time period for this scan: 48 to 72 hours after onset of symptoms; scans done earlier than 12 hours or later than 6 to 7 days after onset of symptoms may appear negative.

DIAGNOSTIC TESTS: CORONARY ARTERY DISEASE, ANGINA, MYOCARDIAL INFARCTION, CONGESTIVE HEART FAILURE
(continued)

Technetium pyrophosphate scanning *(continued)*

Preparation	• Explain that patient may be uncomfortable lying flat and still during the scanning. • No special patient preparation is necessary.
Postprocedure	• None

Echocardiography, two-dimensional

Purpose	• Assesses left ventricular function • Identifies apical mural thrombus • Estimates damage from MI and risk for subsequent complications • May give indication of multivessel CAD • Assesses valvular function • Confirms diagnosis of pericardial effusion
Procedure	• Noninvasive procedure with little risk to the patient • May be done at patient's bedside • Uses ultrasound scanning techniques to provide a cross-sectional view of the heart and its structures
Preparation	• Tell patient that he may be asked to turn in bed or to hold his breath at specific points during the test. • No special preparation is required.
Postprocedure	• None

Multiple-gated acquisition cardiac blood pool imaging (MUGA)

Purpose	• Assesses for presence of CAD • Evaluates left ventricular function or provides an estimate of ejection fraction • Assesses amount of damage from MI • Provides estimate of risk second cardiac event • Assists in diagnosis of right ventricular infarct • Assists in diagnosis of ventricular aneurysm
Procedure	• Involves minimal risks to the patient • Requires 5 to 10 ml of the patient's blood to be labeled with a radioactive tracer; the blood is injected I.V. The patient is scanned as blood passes through the heart; scans are computer-analyzed. • May be done as a resting or an exercise study
Preparation	• No special preparations are needed for the resting study. • For the exercise study, see *Exercise stress test* for information about an exercise protocol.
Postprocedure	• None

(continued)

DIAGNOSTIC TESTS: CORONARY ARTERY DISEASE, ANGINA, MYOCARDIAL INFARCTION, CONGESTIVE HEART FAILURE
(continued)

Cardiac catheterization

Purpose	• Identifies the specific location of atherosclerotic lesions in coronary arteries • Evaluates left ventricular function and provides an estimate of ejection fraction • Identifies the presence and type of valvular disease • Provides data to determine patient suitability for CABG surgery • Assists in determining type of medical care indicated after MI • Evaluates patient suitability for angioplasty and thrombolytic therapy • Assesses patency of grafts after CABG surgery • Assesses effectiveness of angioplasty and thrombolytic therapy
Procedure	• Requires a catheter to be inserted, under fluoroscopy, through the skin and into the arterial or venous circulation (usual sites include the brachial or femoral vessels). The catheter is threaded through the vascular system and positioned in the heart. Contrast medium is injected and serial X-rays are taken. • May cause the patient to feel a sensation of warmth or flushing when the contrast medium is injected • Involves evaluation of coronary circulation, pressures in the heart chambers, and valvular functioning • Patient is awake for procedure but may be mildly sedated. • Involves the following risks to the patient: allergic reaction to the contrast medium, hemorrhage, dysrhythmias, formation of thrombus at insertion site, and cerebrovascular accident
Preparation	• Obtain the patient's informed consent, as per institutional policy. • Assess the patient for allergy to shellfish, iodine, or other contrast media. Notify the doctor if the patient is allergic. • Scrub and shave the insertion site according to institutional policy. • Make sure the patient receives nothing by mouth for 6 to 8 hours before the test. • Premedicate the patient with a mild sedative, as ordered. • Start an I.V. line or heparin lock, as ordered. • Assess the patient's vital signs and peripheral pulses for baseline comparison after the procedure. • Complete other preprocedural routines per institutional policy.

DIAGNOSTIC TESTS: CORONARY ARTERY DISEASE, ANGINA, MYOCARDIAL INFARCTION, CONGESTIVE HEART FAILURE
(continued)

Cardiac catheterization (continued)

Postprocedure
- Maintain a pressure dressing at the insertion site.
- Check the patient's vital signs every 15 minutes until he is stable.
- Keep the patient on bed rest for 4 to 8 hours, as ordered, with the head of the bed elevated less than or equal to 30 degrees.
- Check the pulse distal to the insertion site; evaluate for changes in quality from preprocedural findings.
- Check the extremity for changes in warmth and color from preprocedural findings; notify the doctor about any changes.
- Check the insertion site for bleeding or hematoma formation; if significant bleeding occurs, notify the doctor and apply direct pressure sufficient to control the bleeding but not to occlude distal pulses.
- Unless contraindicated, instruct the patient to drink increased amounts of fluids.
- Medicate the patient for pain, as indicated and as ordered.

Congestive Heart Failure

ASSOCIATED NURSING DIAGNOSES
Activity Intolerance
Anxiety
Bowel Elimination, Alteration in: Constipation
Depression, Reactive: Situational
Family Processes, Alteration in
Fluid Volume Excess: Edema
Gas Exchange, Impaired
Grieving, Family
Grieving, Individual Patient
Noncompliance
Nutrition, Alteration in: Less Than Body Requirements
Self-Concept, Alteration in
Skin Integrity, Potential for Impairment
Sleep-Pattern Disturbance

ASSOCIATED TEACHING PLANS
Cardiac Anatomy and Physiology: Heart and Blood Vessels
Congestive Heart Failure: Disease Process and Home Care
Deep Vein Thrombosis: Disease Process and Prevention
Fluid Plan
Medication Guidelines
Oxygen Use at Home
Radial Pulse Measurement
Sodium-Restricted Diet

Interventions and rationales
☑ Intervention 1
Obtain an appropriate patient history on admission, including data on:
• dyspnea that occurs:
   —with activity (have the patient specify the amount of activity)
   —when the patient is lying flat and that is relieved or lessened when the patient sits up with feet in a dependent position (orthopnea)
   —while the patient is sleeping, awakening him 2 to 3 hours after retiring, and is relieved or lessened when the patient stands up out of bed (paroxysmal nocturnal dyspnea).
• coughing. Assess whether the cough is:
   —dry, hacking, and nonproductive
   —productive of frothy pink sputum.

• fatigue. Ask whether the fatigue:
—occurs with exertion
—occurs gradually, increasing over time without a corresponding increase
 in activity
—interferes with the patient's ability to perform activities of daily living
• peripheral edema. Find out whether the edema occurs as:
—swelling in feet or hands
—a weight gain of 2 lb or more over 24 hours.
• changes in voiding patterns, including:
—oliguria during the day
—nocturia.
• GI symptoms. Assess for:
—anorexia and nausea
—abdominal distention.
• other signs and symptoms resulting from decreased cerebral circulation
secondary to decreased cardiac output, including:
—insomnia
—dizziness
—confusion
—anxiety
—lethargy.

☑ **Intervention 2**
Perform a physical assessment on admission, collecting the following data:
• appearance of acute distress
• changes in vital signs, including:
—tachycardia
—faint or irregular pulse
—hypotension
—tachypnea
• abnormal respiratory findings, including:
—rales and wheezing on auscultation (usually first heard in lung bases,
 often the right base before the left)
—cyanosis in severe heart failure
• abnormal cardiac findings, including:
—edema in dependent sites (frequently seen in the sacrum of patients
 confined to bed and in the legs of ambulatory patients)
—distention of external jugular veins noted with the head of the bed
 elevated more than 15 degrees
—point of maximal impulse (PMI) that is displaced down and laterally
• abnormal GI findings, including:
—enlarged liver or spleen
—abdominal tenderness or distention.

Rationale and comments: Congestive heart failure (CHF) is a clinical
syndrome that results when the heart is unable to pump enough blood to
meet the body's metabolic demands at rest or with activity. Each patient
can present with a variable set of symptoms; several factors influence what
symptoms a patient experiences (see *Bases of symptoms seen in congestive
heart failure*, page 130, for more information).

BASES OF SYMPTOMS SEEN IN CONGESTIVE HEART FAILURE

Symptoms of congestive heart failure (CHF) develop when the heart is unable to pump enough blood to meet the body's metabolic demands at rest or with activity. Some symptoms are directly related to the drop in cardiac output; their severity depends on the degree of failure present. Other symptoms develop as a result of the body's compensatory mechanisms.

When the cardiac output falls, complex neural, hormonal, and hemodynamic mechanisms begin to operate in an attempt to increase cardiac output to meet the body's needs. These mechanisms result in fluid retention, vasoconstriction, and the redistribution of blood flow from the periphery to the heart and other vital organs. If the patient has CHF, these changes fail to increase cardiac output and instead cause pulmonary and systemic vascular congestion, which results in many of the signs and symptoms commonly seen in CHF.

Dyspnea, one of the earliest and most common signs of CHF, occurs because of the accumulation of fluid in the interstitial spaces and alveoli of the lungs. The degree of activity needed to induce dyspnea gives an indication of the severity of heart failure present. Orthopnea, another respiratory symptom, occurs in part because of the increased venous return to the heart from the abdomen and legs when the patient assumes a recumbent position. Paroxysmal nocturnal dyspnea results from the increased venous return to the heart that occurs with recumbency and the suppression of the respiratory center during sleep.

Fatigue, another common symptom in CHF, results from the decrease in cardiac output seen in CHF as well as from decreased blood flow to the skeletal muscles that occurs as the body tries to compensate for the reduced cardiac output.

Peripheral or systemic edema occurs because of accumulation of fluid in the extravascular spaces.

Oliguria occurs from decreased cardiac output and subsequent decreased kidney perfusion. Nocturia occurs because the demand for cardiac output may decrease at night, thereby increasing renal perfusion and the subsequent formation of urine.

Vascular congestion of abdominal organs can result in enlargement of the liver and spleen, abdominal tenderness or distention, and subjective complaints of nausea and vomiting.

☑ **Intervention 3**

Implement the prescribed medical care, which may include the following:
• Administer prescribed medications. Some commonly prescribed cardiac medications include:
—cardiac glycosides (see *Cardiac glycosides*)
—diuretics (see *Diuretics*, page 132)
—vasodilators (see *Vasodilators*, page 133)
—angiotensin-converting enzyme inhibitors (see *Angiotensin-converting enzyme inhibitors*, page 134).
• Administer oxygen, as ordered, to help reduce dyspnea.
• Limit the patient's activity; common restrictions include:
—bed rest with bathroom privileges
—chair rest
—strict bed rest.
• Provide a sodium- and/or fluid-restricted diet, as ordered.

COMMONLY PRESCRIBED MEDICATIONS

CARDIAC GLYCOSIDES

Examples	• Digoxin (Lanoxin) • Digitoxin (Crystodigin)
Actions	• Increases force of myocardial contraction, resulting in more complete emptying of ventricles • Slows conduction through the atrioventricular node by increasing the refractory period of the node
Uses	• Relieves symptoms of congestive heart failure • Improves oxygen delivery to tissues • Slows heart rate in presence of certain dysrhythmias
Toxic effects	• Anorexia, nausea, and vomiting • Visual disturbances, including green- or yellow-tinted vision, double vision, blurred vision, white dots appearing in the visual field; cardiac dysrhythmias, including heart block and premature ventricular contractions
Cautions	• Has a narrow therapeutic range (0.8 to 2.4 ng/ml); toxicity can develop rapidly. Factors increasing the risk of toxicity include renal or hepatic dysfunction, rapid I.V. administration, and hypokalemia; elderly patients are also more at risk. • Aluminum-containing antacids and kaolin-pectin interfere with absorption.
Nursing responsibilities	• Check the apical pulse rate before administering the drug. If the pulse rate is less than 60 beats/minute (or as specified by the doctor), hold the dose and notify the doctor. • Monitor the patient closely for signs of digitalis toxicity. • Monitor potassium levels (especially if the patient is taking potassium-wasting diuretics concurrently). • Do not administer aluminum-containing antacids or kaolin-pectin within 2 hours before or after administering digitalis glycosides.

Rationale and comments: Various medications are prescribed to improve the heart's effectiveness as a pump. As the heart's pumping action improves, the patient experiences fewer signs and symptoms of heart failure.

Limiting activity decreases myocardial work load by decreasing the demand for cardiac output; decreased demand for cardiac output lessens the need for redistribution of blood flow and can result in effective diuresis and improvement in the patient's clinical condition. Unless the CHF is severe, patients usually are not placed on strict bed rest because of the complications associated with immobility.

☑ **Intervention 4**

Implement measures to manage edema, including:
• using the measures outlined in "Fluid Volume Excess: Edema" in Section I
• administering diuretics, as ordered
• providing a sodium- or fluid-restricted diet, as ordered.

COMMONLY PRESCRIBED MEDICATIONS

DIURETICS

Potassium-wasting diuretics	• Chlorothiazide (Diuril) • Furosemide (Lasix) • Hydrochlorothiazide (Esidrix) • Methyclothiazide (Enduron) • Polythiazide (Renese)
Potassium-sparing diuretics	• Spironolactone (Aldactone)
Actions	• Prevents the reabsorption of sodium and water, thereby increasing sodium excretion and the reduction of edema • Site of action in kidney depends on specific drug used
Uses	• Decreases congestive heart failure symptoms by decreasing edema (systemic and/or pulmonary) • Controls hypertension
Side effects	• Fluid and electrolyte imbalances
Nursing responsibilities	• For patients receiving potassium-wasting diuretics: —Assess serum potassium levels closely. —Assist the patient to include potassium-rich foods in the diet. —Consult the doctor about potassium supplements if indicated. • For all patients: —Monitor electrolyte levels, intake and output, and daily weight.

Rationale and comments: Edema is a common problem associated with CHF. The measures listed in this intervention help to decrease fluid retention and alleviate edema and its associated symptoms.

☑ **Intervention 5**

Implement the following measures to manage the patient's dyspnea:
• Use the interventions outlined in "Gas Exchange, Impaired" in Section I.
• Administer diuretics, as ordered.
• Provide a sodium- or fluid-restricted diet, as ordered.
• Administer supplemental oxygen, as ordered.

Rationale and comments: Caused by accumulation of fluid in the interstitial spaces and alveoli of the lungs, dyspnea can be one of the most troublesome and frightening symptoms of CHF for a patient.

☑ **Intervention 6**

Implement measures to decrease the patient's risk of developing deep vein thrombosis (see "Deep Vein Thrombosis, Prevention of" in this section for details).

COMMONLY PRESCRIBED MEDICATIONS

VASODILATORS

The vasodilators listed below include arterial vasodilators and selective nitrates commonly prescribed to control congestive heart failure (CHF). Although nitrates are also used to treat angina pectoris (see *Nitrates,* page 119), they may be prescribed to control CHF as discussed below.

Arterial vasodilators

Examples	• Hydralazine hydrochloride (Apresoline) • Minoxidil (Loniten)—for hypertension only
Action	• Directly dilates arteries, resulting in decreased blood pressure and decreased systemic vascular resistance
Uses	• Increases cardiac output in CHF • Controls hypertension
Side effects	• Headache • Anorexia and nausea • Sweating
Cautions	• May cause hypotension in patients with CHF: often used in combination with nitrates
Nursing responsibilities	• Monitor the patient's blood pressure before administering medication; consult doctor about the lowest acceptable limit for systolic blood pressure (maybe as low as 90 mm Hg in patients with CHF).

Nitrates

Examples	• Isosorbide dinitrate (Isordil, Sorbitrate) • Nitroglycerin ointment (Nitro-Bid ointment, Nitrol ointment) • Nitroglycerin, sustained-release (Nitro-Bid)
Actions	• Systemic vasodilator • Decreases ventricular filling pressures by increasing venous pooling
Uses	• Decreases symptoms caused by the complex compensatory mechanisms that occur in CHF
Cautions	• May cause hypotension • Is often combined with an arterial vasodilator for optimal control of CHF
Side effects	• Flushing • Headache • Hypotension • Tachycardia
Nursing responsibilities	• Monitor the patient's blood pressure before administering medication; consult doctor about the lowest acceptable limit for systolic blood pressure (may be as low as 90 mm Hg in patients with CHF). • See *Nitrates*, page 119, for other nursing responsibilities.

COMMONLY PRESCRIBED MEDICATIONS	
ANGIOTENSIN-CONVERTING ENZYME INHIBITORS	
Example	• Captopril (Capoten)
Actions	• Thought to interfere with the synthesis of angiotensin I to angiotensin II, resulting in decreased peripheral vascular resistance and decreased secretion of aldosterone
Uses	• Improves cardiac output in congestive heart failure • Controls hypertension (particularly when other agents are ineffective or cause unacceptable side effects); usually combined with thiazide diuretic for blood pressure control
Side effects	• Proteinuria • Neutropenia • Agranulocytosis • Rash with pruritus and fever • Flushing and pallor • Hypotension • Tachycardia • Chest pain
Caution	• Should be used cautiously in patients with renal disease or autoimmune disorders
Nursing responsibilities	• Monitor the patient's blood pressure before giving medication; consult doctor about lowest acceptable limit for systolic blood pressure (may be as low as 90 mm Hg in patients with CHF).

☑ Intervention 7

Monitor the patient for worsening CHF.

• Assess for signs of increasing CHF; notify the doctor if any of the following signs are present:

—increased edema in dependent sites
—weight gain of 2 lb (0.9 kg) or more over 24 hours
—increasing dyspnea with activity
—increasing fatigue with activity
—increasing rales or wheezing in lung fields
—worsening arterial blood gas levels
—chest X-ray report noting increased congestion
—nonspecific anxiety
—insomnia
—development of a cough.

• Assess the patient for factors that may cause signs of increased heart failure, including:

—electrolyte imbalances (may predispose the patient to dysrhythmias)
—digitalis toxicity (This effect can develop easily, especially in elderly patients and those with decreased renal function, and can result in dysrhythmias.)

—infection (Infection, with its accompanying fever and increased metabolic demands, increases the demand for cardiac output and may result in more acute symptoms of failure.)

—dysrhythmias. (Dysrhythmias can cause decreased cardiac output that may aggravate existing CHF. Also, rapid dysrhythmias increase the work load of the heart and can aggravate CHF.)

Rationale and comments: Initial signs of increasing CHF can be very subtle and easily overlooked. Because deterioration can occur rapidly, frequent assessment is vital.

☑ Intervention 8

Monitor the patient for development of pulmonary edema.

• Assess the patient for symptoms of pulmonary edema, including:

—complaint of feeling suffocated

—complaint of anxiety, agitation, or pallor

—diaphoresis

—cold, clammy, cyanotic skin

—respiratory rate greater than 30 to 40 breaths/minute

—use of accessory muscles with respiration

—cough producing profuse amounts of frothy, pink, or blood-tinged mucus

—rales, rhonchi, or wheezing in lung fields

—hypotension

—tachycardia.

• Notify the doctor immediately of the patient's condition.

• While waiting for further instructions from the doctor, implement the following measures:

—Position the patient with his head elevated and legs dependent to facilitate breathing and promote venous pooling.

—Administer oxygen by nasal cannula or face mask to decrease hypoxia.

—Stay with the patient to help reduce fear, which can increase respiratory distress.

• Implement the prescribed orders, which may include the following:

—Start an I.V. line or heparin lock.

—Administer the prescribed I.V. medications, such as morphine sulfate, digitalis, furosemide or another potent diuretic, aminophylline, nitroglycerin, or nitroprusside. (These medications reduce congestion, improve the heart's pumping ability, and decrease anxiety and respiratory distress.)

—Assist with transferring the patient to the ICU.

Rationale and comments: Pulmonary edema may occur abruptly in patients with CHF. Because this is a clinical emergency, prompt recognition and treatment are vital. Patients with acute pulmonary edema are frequently transferred to the ICU. However, staff nurses may be involved in implementing initial measures before the actual transfer.

☑ Intervention 9
Assist with diagnostic procedures. Commonly used diagnostic tests include the following (see *Diagnostic tests: coronary artery disease, angina, myocardial infarction, congestive heart failure,* pages 122 to 127):
• multiple-gated acquisition study (MUGA)
• two-dimensional echocardiography
• low-level exercise stress test
• cardiac catheterization.

Rationale and comments: Diagnostic tests are used to identify underlying causes of CHF and to evaluate left ventricular function.

☑ Intervention 10
Evaluate the patient's progress by:
• auscultating lung fields for changes in rales, rhonchi, and wheezing
• obtaining daily weights and recording the patient's daily intake and output
• assessing the status of edema in dependent sites
• assessing the patient's response to increased activity.

Coronary Artery Bypass Surgery (Post ICU)

ASSOCIATED NURSING DIAGNOSES
Activity Intolerance
Activity Intolerance, Potential for
Anxiety
Bowel Elimination, Alteration in: Constipation
Comfort, Alteration in: Acute Pain
Depression, Reactive: Situational
Family Processes, Alteration in
Grieving, Family
Grieving, Individual Patient
Noncompliance
Nutrition, Alteration in: Less Than Body Requirements
Respiratory Function, Alteration in
Respiratory Function, Potential Alteration in
Self-Concept, Alteration in
Sexual Dysfunction
Sleep-Pattern Disturbance

ASSOCIATED TEACHING PLANS
Atherosclerosis: Disease Process and Risk Factors
Cardiac Anatomy and Physiology: Heart and Blood Vessels
Cardiovascular Disease Risk Factors: Cigarette Smoking
Cardiovascular Disease Risk Factors: Diabetes Mellitus and Atherosclerosis
Cardiovascular Disease Risk Factors: Dietary Measures to Control
  Hyperlipidemia
Coronary Artery Bypass Grafting Surgery: Home Care
Exercising after Myocardial Infarction or Heart Surgery
Hypertension, Essential: Disease Process and Risk Factors
Medication Guidelines
Sexual Activity and Heart Disease
Stress Management

Interventions and rationales
☑ Intervention 1
Obtain baseline data upon receiving the patient from the intensive care unit (ICU). Data should include the following information:
• complications during or after surgery, including:
  —low cardiac output

—dysrhythmias (For more information about commonly seen dysrhythmias, see *Common dysrhythmias seen in patients with cardiovascular disease.*)
—respiratory complications
—reoperation for excessive bleeding
—cerebrovascular accident (CVA)
—myocardial infarction (MI)
• pattern of vital signs
• presence of invasive lines, including:
—patent venous access line (may be a peripheral or central line heparin lock or an I.V. line)
—pacemaker wires
—chest tubes (rarely present after transfer from the ICU
• status of incision line(s)
• fluid and electrolyte status, including:
—recent electrolyte values
—urine output
—current weight.

Rationale and comments: Complications that occur during or after surgery can influence the patient's later postoperative course. For example, low cardiac output that occurs in the immediate postoperative period can cause later complications, such as renal failure and myocardial ischemia. Reoperation increases the patient's risk of developing a wound infection. CVA, although considered a relatively rare complication after surgery, will significantly alter the medical and nursing management of the patient.

Temporary pacemaker wires may be inserted during surgery. The wires may not be connected to an external pacemaker, but carefully protected in some type of dressing. If the patient develops rhythm disturbances requiring the use of a pacemaker, the wires may be rapidly and easily attached to an external pacemaker. In some institutions, these wires are removed before the patient is transferred from the ICU; in others, the patient is transferred with the wires in place.

✓ Intervention 2
Implement the prescribed medical care regarding the patient's:
• activity. Patients may:
—sit in a chair and ambulate to the bathroom on the day of transfer
—increase their activity according to the exercise plan.
• diet. Common restrictions include:
—low cholesterol or low saturated fat diet
—calorie restrictions if weight loss is indicated
—sodium- or fluid-restricted diet if the patient has congestive heart failure (CHF).
• continuous EKG monitoring, as ordered.
• respiratory care, including administration of oxygen, as indicated by patient condition.

(Text continues on page 142.)

COMMON DYSRHYTHMIAS SEEN IN PATIENTS WITH CARDIOVASCULAR DISEASE

This chart presents a brief overview of common dysrhythmias along with their clinical signs and symptoms and common management procedures. A discussion of how to recognize characteristic EKG tracings for these dysrhythmias exceeds the scope of this text.

Sinus tachycardia

Description	• Regular rhythm • Rate exceeding 100 beats/minute • Impulse initiated by sinoatrial (SA) node at rate faster than normal • Normal conduction of impulse through heart
Signs and symptoms	• May be accompanied by dyspnea • Other signs and symptoms often dependent on underlying cause
Common causes	• Pain • Activity or exercise • Anxiety • Hypoxia (multiple causes, including congestive heart failure [CHF], atelectasis, and pulmonary embolism)
Comments or concerns	• Sinus tachycardia is a clinical symptom. The patient should always be carefully assessed for the underlying cause. • Sinus tachycardia increases stress on the heart by increasing the cardiac work load.
Management	• Treat the underlying cause.

Atrial fibrillation

Description	• Rhythm is irregularly irregular. • Rate is variable; ventricular rate in untreated atrial fibrillation may go as high as 180 beats/minute. • On palpation, peripheral pulses will have variable force. Some beats will feel strong; others will be barely palpable. • Impulses are initiated in atria. • Fibrillation is characterized by chaotic and irregular atrial impulses that result in ineffective atrial contractions. • Impulses travel irregularly to the atrioventricular (AV) node; ventricles respond irregularly to the atrial impulses, resulting in the characteristic irregularly irregular rhythm seen in atrial fibrillation.
Signs and symptoms	• Feeling of palpitations • Signs and symptoms of decreased cardiac output, including hypotension, decreased activity tolerance, dizziness, and fatigue
Common causes	• Frequently seen chronically in patients with history of mitral valve disease • Pericarditis that occurs after coronary artery bypass grafting or valve replacement surgery • Associated with atherosclerotic coronary heart disease

(continued)

**COMMON DYSRHYTHMIAS SEEN IN PATIENTS
WITH CARDIOVASCULAR DISEASE** (continued)

Atrial fibrillation (continued)

Comments or concerns	• May easily result in decreased cardiac output • Increases risk of thrombus and subsequent emboli formation • May trigger acute CHF in patient with compromised myocardial (especially left ventricular) function • Rapid ventricular rates increase stress on heart
Management	• Digitalis is usually the drug of choice to slow the ventricular rate. • If digitalis is ineffective, other antiarrhythmic medications may be prescribed, including propranolol and quinidine (see *Antiarrhythmic medications*, pages 144 and 145). • Treat the underlying cause.

Premature ventricular contractions

Description	• An abnormal beat is initiated in the ventricle, resulting in an irregularity in the pulse rhythm; amount of irregularity depends on number of premature ventricular contractions (PVCs). • On palpation of the pulse, PVC often feels like a "missed" or a "skipped" beat. • Impulses are initiated in ventricles by cells that normally do not act as pacemakers for the heart. • Conduction through the ventricles is abnormal; this results in compromised ventricular contraction and decreased cardiac output. • PVCs may occur in isolation or in groups of two or three or more.
Signs and symptoms	• Signs and symptoms are often associated with number of PVCs occurring per minute. • Isolated or infrequent PVCs are often unaccompanied by any other signs or symptoms. • Symptoms seen with increased PVCs are related to decreased cardiac output and may include hypotension and dizziness. • Apical-radial pulse deficit may be present.
Common causes	• Hypoxia • Digitalis toxicity • Hypokalemia • Myocardial ischemia
Comments or concerns	• PVCs may precipitate additional serious dysrhythmias, such as ventricular tachycardia and ventricular fibrillation. PVCs that occur in pairs, in groups of three or more, or arise from a variety of places in the ventricle are warning signs that serious dysrhythmias may be developing; these types of PVCs should be treated.
Management	• I.V. lidocaine, administered as a bolus, is the drug of choice for immediate treatment.

COMMON DYSRHYTHMIAS SEEN IN PATIENTS WITH CARDIOVASCULAR DISEASE *(continued)*

Premature ventricular contractions *(continued)*

Management *(continued)*	• Treat any underlying cause. • Oral antiarrhythmic medications may be indicated (see *Antiarrhythmic medications*, pages 144 and 145, for additional information).

Ventricular tachycardia

Description	• Life-threatening dysrhythmia characterized by three or more PVCs in a row • Results in ineffective ventricular contraction and diminished cardiac output
Signs and symptoms	• Hypotension • Loss of consciousness • Can lead to cardiopulmonary arrest
Common causes	• Untreated or uncontrolled PVCs • Other causes under *Premature ventricular contractions*
Comments or concerns	• May lead to ventricular fibrillation and cardiopulmonary arrest
Management	• Immediate intervention is necessary. • I.V. lidocaine, administered as a bolus, is the initial drug of choice; may be followed by continuous lidocaine drip, if needed. • Electric countershock (defibrillation) may be necessary. • Cardiopulmonary resuscitation (CPR) may be required if indicated by patient status. • Treat the underlying cause. • To prevent recurrent episodes, oral antiarrhythmic medications may be prescribed when the patient's condition permits.

Ventricular fibrillation

Description	• Chaotic ventricular rhythm that results in completely ineffective ventricular contraction • Results quickly in cardiopulmonary arrest
Signs and symptoms	• Loss of consciousness • Loss of palpable pulse and blood pressure • Respiratory arrest
Common causes	See *Premature ventricular contractions* and *Ventricular tachycardia* above.
Comments or concerns	• Life-threatening dysrhythmia that requires immediate, aggressive treatment
Management	• Immediate electric countershock (defibrillation) is required. • CPR, as necessary. • Treat the underlying cause. • To prevent recurrent episodes, oral antiarrhythmic medications may be prescribed when the patient's condition permits.

(continued)

**COMMON DYSRHYTHMIAS SEEN IN PATIENTS
WITH CARDIOVASCULAR DISEASE** *(continued)*

Heart block	
Description	• Heart block includes a group of dysrhythmias in which normal conduction of the impulse from the SA node through the AV node to the ventricles does not occur. • In first-degree heart block, the least serious type, the impulses are conducted more slowly than usual; however, all impulses reach the ventricles. • In second-degree heart block, some impulses are blocked and do not reach the ventricles. • In third-degree heart block, all impulses from the atria are blocked and do not reach the ventricles.
Signs and symptoms	• Depends on type of heart block present • First-degree heart block: usually asymptomatic • Third-degree heart block: heart rate drops to 40 beats/minute or less; often accompanied by signs of decreased cardiac output, such as syncope
Common causes	• Often associated with history of valvular heart disease • May be caused by damage to electrical conducting system of heart secondary to myocardial infarction • May be caused by digitalis toxicity
Management	• First-degree heart block rarely requires treatment. • With second-degree heart block, if the patient is asymptomatic, treatment is rarely indicated. • For symptomatic second-degree heart block and third-degree heart block, I.V. atropine sulfate may be given for severe bradycardia. • Heart block may require insertion of a pacemaker (may be temporary or permanent).

☑ **Intervention 3**

Administer medications as prescribed; commonly prescribed medications may include:

• antiplatelet medications (see *Antiplatelet medications*)
• cardiovascular medications, such as:
  —antiarrhythmic medications (see *Antiarrhythmic medications*, pages 144 and 145)
  —cardiac glycosides (see *Cardiac glycosides*, page 131)
  —diuretics (see *Diuretics*, page 132)
  —antihypertensive medications (see *Beta-adrenergic blocking agents*, page 191; *Adrenergic antagonists*, page 175; and *Angiotensin-converting enzyme inhibitors*, page 134)
  —analgesics
  —prophylactic antibiotics
  —stool softeners and laxatives.

Rationale and comments: Patients who have undergone CABG may also have other concurrent cardiovascular problems, such as dysrhythmias, hypertension, and CHF. Prophylactic antibiotics are often limited to the

COMMONLY PRESCRIBED MEDICATIONS	

ANTIPLATELET MEDICATIONS

Example	• Dipyridamole (Persantine)
Actions	• Decreases risk of formation of platelet thrombi by inhibiting platelet aggregation • Increases coronary blood flow by selectively dilating coronary arteries
Uses	• Considered possibly effective in the long-term management of angina pectoris • Often combined with another antiplatelet medication to maintain grafts after vascular bypass surgery (not an approved use; currently under investigation) • May be used in combination with an anticoagulant or another antiplatelet medication to decrease the risk of coronary thrombosis (under investigation)
Side effects	• Skin rashes • Flushing • Headache • Dizziness • Nausea and vomiting • GI bleeding • Hypotension
Nursing responsibilities	• Assess for side effects. • Observe for bleeding, especially when drug is combined with anticoagulant therapy.

first 48 hours postoperatively. However, some doctors may prescribe them for a longer period. Use of stool softeners and laxatives prevents straining with defecation, thus decreasing stress on the heart.

☑ Intervention 4
Implement measures to prevent or treat the following common postoperative problems:
• pain (see "Comfort, Alteration in: Acute Pain" in Section I)
• depression (see "Depression, Reactive: Situational" in Section I)
• postoperative atelectasis (see "Respiratory Function, Potential Alteration in" in Section I)
• constipation (see "Bowel Elimination, Alteration in: Constipation" in Section I)
• postoperative infection of incision lines
—Perform routine incision line care.
—Instruct the patient to avoid using lotions, creams, or powders on incision lines.
—Assess the incision for signs of inflammation.
• edema in the donor leg
—Have the patient wear elastic hose (antiembolism stockings), as ordered.
—Have the patient use elastic (Ace) wraps, as ordered.
—Tell the patient to elevate his leg when sitting.
—Tell the patient to avoid crossing his legs at all times.

ANTIARRHYTHMIC MEDICATIONS

Type 1$_a$ Antiarrhythmic agents

Examples	• Disopyramide (Norpace) • Procainamide (Pronestyl, Procan SR) • Quinidine sulfate (Quinidex); quinidine gluconate (Quinaglute)
Actions	• Decreases automaticity and prolongs the effective refractory period
Uses	• Effective in treating dysrhythmias caused by disturbances in automaticity or reentry, such as atrial fibrillation, premature ventricular contractions (PVCs), and ventricular tachycardia
Side effects	• GI distress • Dysrhythmias • Heart block • Quinidine: hypersensitivity, thrombocytopenia, hypotension • Procainamide: thrombocytopenia, weakness, and systemic lupus erythematosus-like syndrome • Disopyramide: dry mouth, urine retention, and increased glaucoma
Cautions	• Use cautiously if the patient has dysrhythmias (other than those above), heart block, or hepatic or renal disease. • Other cautions vary with specific medications.
Nursing responsibilites	• Monitor the patient's vital signs. • Assess pulse rate and rhythm. • Monitor serum drug levels, as ordered. • Administer quinidine with food at evenly spaced intervals. • Assess the patient for side effects.

Local anesthetic agents and anticonvulsant agents

Examples	• Lidocaine (Xylocaine): I.V. use only • Phenytoin (Dilantin): I.V. or oral use
Actions	• Decreases automaticity and prolongs the effectiveness of the refractory period
Uses	• Suppresses and controls ventricular dysrhythmias, such as premature ventricular beats and ventricular tachycardia
Side effects	• Vary with agent prescribed • Lidocaine: dizziness, hypotension, confusion, nausea, and respiratory depression • Phenytoin: drowsiness and gum hyperplasia
Cautions	• For treatment of dysrhythmias, use only lidocaine labeled for cardiac use (contains no preservatives or epinephrine).
Nursing responsibilities	• Monitor the patient's vital signs. • Monitor for side effects. • Administer phenytoin at evenly spaced intervals. • Consult institutional policy on administration of I.V. phenytoin (medication precipitates in many diluents).

ANTIARRHYTHMIC MEDICATIONS *(continued)*

Beta-adrenergic blocking agents

See *Beta-adrenergic blocking agents,* page 191, for details.

Cardiac glycosides

See *Cardiac glycosides,* page 131, for details.

Calcium channel blockers

See *Calcium channel blockers,* page 120, for details.

Bretylium

Examples	• Bretylium (Bretylol)
Actions	• Suppresses dysrhythmias by antiadrenergic action and by increasing the threshold for ventricular fibrillation
Uses	• Treatment and control of life-threatening ventricular dysrhythmias that have not responded to lidocaine or procainamide
Side effects	• Hypotension • Nausea and vomiting
Cautions	• None
Nursing responsibilities	• Infuse I.V. dose over 8 to 10 minutes if permitted by patient status. • If continuous infusion used, monitor blood pressure carefully.

Rationale and comments: Removal of the saphenous vein initially reduces venous return and causes edema in the donor leg.

☑ **Intervention 5**
Monitor the patient and implement measures to control dysrhythmias.
• Check the patient's vital signs every 4 hours or as indicated by the patient's condition.
• Maintain continuous EKG monitoring for rate or rhythm changes.
• Assess the patient for the following signs and symptoms of decreased cardiac output:
—dizziness
—excessive fatigue
—hypotension
—confusion
—malaise or weakness.

Rationale and comments: Commonly seen dysrhythmias include atrial fibrillation and premature ventricular contractions (*see Common dysrhythmias seen in patients with cardiovascular disease,* pages 139 to 142, for additional information on these dysrhythmias). Signs of decreased cardiac output may be the initial clinical clue that the patient is experiencing a dysrhythmia.

☑ Intervention 6

If significant dysrhythmias occur, take the following measures:
• Have the patient stop and rest if he is engaged in an activity, as dysrhythmias can be an indication of activity intolerance.
• Assess the patient for signs of decreased cardiac output (see Intervention 5 above).
• Administer oxygen, as ordered, if it is available. (Hypoxia can precipitate dysrhythmias; also, some patients experience dyspnea with dysrhythmias.)
• Notify the doctor immediately.
• Administer antiarrhythmic medications as ordered. (see *Antiarrhythmic medications*, pages 144 and 145, for information).
• Assess the patient closely for response to antiarrhythmic medications, including:
—checking pulse rate and rhythm
—assessing for signs of decreased cardiac output
—monitoring serum drug levels as ordered
—monitoring for side effects and symptoms of drug toxicity.
• Assess the patient's vital signs for indications of deterioration in cardiovascular condition, because the cardiovascular status of patients with dysrhythmias can change rapidly.
• Provide explanations to the patient or his family, and assist them in coping with their anxiety.
• If long-term antiarrhythmic therapy is ordered, implement the following measures:
—Administer prescribed medications.
—Assess the patient's vital signs and EKG rhythm for changes.
—Continue to explain to the patient and family about the patient's progress and prescribed treatment.

Rationale and comments: Significant dysrhythmias are those which greatly increase the oxygen demand of the heart by increasing myocardial work load, reduce cardiac output to the point at which the patient experiences symptoms, or are early indications that more serious rhythm disturbances may be developing.

Dysrhythmias can be anxiety-provoking for the patient and his family. The nursing activity that occurs when a dysrhythmia develops (such as checking vital signs and giving medications) may give the patient the idea that something serious is wrong with his heart; careful and repeated explanations of what is occurring and how the patient is doing can help to decrease anxiety.

Some patients will require antiarrhythmic medications on a long-term or permanent basis to control their heart rhythm. Because individual response varies, each patient's medication regimen will be different. Initially, the doctor may need to alter the patient's prescribed medications frequently to achieve a regimen with maximum benefit and minimum side effects. This process can be quite confusing and tedious to the patient and his family; frequent explanation of which medications are prescribed, how they work, and why changes were made can help them cope more effectively.

☑ Intervention 7

Monitor the patient and implement measures to control pericarditis.

• Assess the patient for symptoms (see *Characteristics of noncardiac chest pain*, pages 184 and 185).
• Administer prescribed medications, including:
—mild analgesics
—nonsteroidal anti-inflammatory medications
—steroids prescribed for severe pericarditis that does not respond to nonsteroidal anti-inflammatory agents.
• Explain the cause and treatment of pericarditis to the patient and his family.

Rationale and comments: Pericarditis, an inflammation of the pericardial sac surrounding the heart, is a common complication after cardiac surgery. A classic symptom of pericarditis is chest pain.

✓ Intervention 8
Monitor the patient and implement the following measures to control the complication of pulmonary vascular congestion:
• Note common signs and symptoms, including:
—X-ray reports noting interstitial or alveolar edema
—decreasing PO_2 on arterial blood gas measurements
—complaints of dyspnea or orthopnea
—weight gain of 2 lb (0.9 kg) or more over 24 hours.
• Implement the prescribed medical care, including:
—administering prescribed diuretics (see *Diuretics*, page 132)
—administering oxygen, as ordered
—implementing fluid restrictions, as ordered
—obtaining repeat arterial blood gas levels and chest X-rays, as ordered
—continuing to monitor daily weights and intake and output.

Rationale and comments: Pulmonary vascular congestion can occur in the interstitial or alveolar spaces of the lung as a result of CHF or noncardiac causes, including fluid and colloid shifts that occur in response to the loss of total serum protein during surgery. Some patients may be asymptomatic; the only indication may be the presence of interstitial or alveolar edema on X-ray. Frequently, the use of diuretics and oxygen therapy is sufficient to treat this complication; however, sometimes fluid intake may need to be restricted temporarily for some patients. Improvement is indicated by fluid weight loss, improved arterial blood gas levels, and decreased edema as noted on X-ray reports.

✓ Intervention 9
Monitor the patient and implement measures to control the complication of CHF. (See "Congestive Heart Failure" in this section for more information.)

Rationale and comments: Some patients develop CHF after coronary artery bypass surgery because of dysrhythmias or damage to the myocardium that occurs before, during, or after surgery.

✓ Intervention 10
Monitor the patient and implement measures to control the complication of postoperative wound infection.

• If signs and symptoms of infection develop:
—Notify the doctor.
—Obtain a wound culture, as ordered.
—Administer prescribed antibiotics.
—Implement prescribed dressing changes.
—Assess for signs of healing.
—Notify the doctor if wound edges separate, drainage increases, or wound dehiscence occurs. (Continued infection may result in mild separation of incision edges or wound dehiscence.)

☑ **Intervention 11**

For patients with chest tubes in place after transfer from ICU, implement the following measures:
• Determine the type and location of chest tubes.
• Assess and record the type and amount of drainage at least once per shift.
• Maintain a sterile chest tube system.
• Set the suction at the prescribed level. (A commonly used system is the Pleur-evac.)
—Orders may call for chest tubes for straight drainage only.
—Check the amount of water in the suction control chamber; make sure the amount is correct for the amount of suction prescribed. (The amount of water in the suction control chamber determines the amount of suction applied.)
—If the fluid level is below the prescribed amount, add additional fluid according to the manufacturer's or institution's policy.
• Make sure the system is correctly set up and functioning appropriately.
—Make sure the water-seal chamber is filled to the correct level.
—Check that the suction control chamber is bubbling gently. (Vigorous bubbling is unnecessary; it will not increase the amount or effectiveness of the suction.)
—Check the tubing and connections to make sure there is no air leak.
• Maintain a dry, intact dressing around the insertion site.
• Assist the patient to manage chest tubes correctly when ambulating.
—Maintain a closed system.
—Avoid elevating the tubes above the level of the chest to prevent reflux of fluid back into the chest.
—Handle the tubes gently to avoid drainage from spilling from one collection chamber to the next and to facilitate accurate measurement of drainage.

Rationale and comments: At the end of the surgical procedure, one or more chest tubes are routinely placed for drainage; they are brought outside the body through stab wounds. Chest tubes may be pleural or mediastinal; although care measures for both types of tubes are about the same, the system for a pleural tube must remain airtight to prevent serious respiratory complications, such as tension pneumothorax.

These tubes are usually removed before the patient is transferred from the ICU; however, an isolated patient may be transferred with these tubes still in place.

Deep Vein Thrombosis

ASSOCIATED NURSING DIAGNOSES
Anxiety
Bowel Elimination, Alteration in: Constipation
Comfort, Alteration in: Acute Pain
Noncompliance

ASSOCIATED TEACHING PLANS
Cardiac Anatomy and Physiology: Heart and Blood Vessels
Deep Vein Thrombosis: Disease Process and Prevention
Medication Guidelines

Interventions and rationales
☑ **Intervention 1**
Assess the patient for clinical indications of deep vein thrombosis, including:
• edema in one extremity evidenced by:
  —asymmetrical ankle edema
  —increased diameter of one calf, ankle, or thigh in relation to the other
  —pitting edema in one leg only
  —loss of concavity of the malleolar space in one leg
• complaint of heavy, dull, aching pain unaffected by exercise
• tenderness with direct palpation over the affected vein
• positive Homan's sign (pain in the calf on dorsiflexion of the foot)
• dilatation of superficial veins
• mottled or cyanotic skin
• affected extremity warmer to touch than the unaffected extremity
• signs and symptoms of pulmonary embolism (see Intervention 8 below
for details).

Rationale and comments: Patients with deep vein thrombosis may have
variable signs and symptoms, most commonly those related to venous
congestion caused by the occlusion of a vein by the thrombus. Edema in
only one extremity is one of the most reliable clinical indications (except
in patients who have undergone saphenous vein grafting to one or more
coronary arteries; they may have edema in the donor leg that is unrelated
to deep vein thrombosis). A positive Homan's sign occurs in only a minority
of patients with deep vein thrombosis. In some patients, deep vein thrombosis may be asymptomatic; the first clinical indication may be development
of a pulmonary embolus.

☑ **Intervention 2**
Assess the patient for risk factors associated with deep vein thrombosis
(see "Deep Vein Thrombosis, Prevention of" in this section).

Rationale and comments: Because many of the clinical signs and symptoms seen in deep vein thrombosis are nonspecific and may be caused by other problems, such as muscle injury or infection, diagnosis on the basis of clinical signs and symptoms alone is insufficient. Determining the presence of risk factors can provide additional information needed to evaluate the patient's condition.

☑ Intervention 3
Assist in preparing the patient for prescribed diagnostic measures, including the following:
• venography
• Doppler ultrasound
• radioiodinated fibrinogen uptake
• impedance plethysmography.
(See *Tests used to diagnose deep vein thrombosis.*)

Rationale and comments: Diagnostic tests are used to establish a definitive diagnosis of deep vein thrombosis.

☑ Intervention 4
Implement the prescribed medical care regarding the following:
• activity
—Maintain the patient on bed rest with the foot of the bed elevated 30 degrees (unless contraindicated) until the acute episode has resolved.
—After the acute episode, advance the patient's activity level; this should be done on an individual basis.
• application of warm, moist heat to the affected extremity, as ordered
—Follow institutional or manufacturer's guidelines when applying moist heat.
• administration of analgesics, as prescribed
• application of Ace wraps or elastic stockings, as prescribed (usually after the episode has resolved).

Rationale and comments: Limiting activity to bed rest with the foot of the bed elevated 30 degrees facilitates venous return to the heart and decreases venous stasis.
   The acute episode of deep vein thrombosis usually resolves within 5 to 10 days. Warm, moist heat applied to the affected extremity helps to relieve vasospasm and edema. Mild analgesics are usually sufficient to control the discomfort associated with deep vein thrombosis. Ace wraps or elastic stockings decrease venous stasis by compressing the superficial veins and increasing blood flow through the deep veins. They are most commonly prescribed after the acute episode has resolved.

☑ Intervention 5
Implement the prescribed anticoagulant therapy, including:
• administration of heparin, as prescribed
—Note that heparin is usually given by continuous I.V. drip or intermittent I.V. bolus.

TESTS USED TO DIAGNOSE DEEP VEIN THROMBOSIS

Venography

Purpose
- Visualizes the venous system directly; used to detect or rule out the presence of clots in venous circulation
- Because of associated risks, should only be used when risk factors or clinical signs and symptoms strongly indicate the presence of a deep vein thrombosis

Procedure
- This is an invasive procedure.
- The patient is placed on a tilted X-ray table, with no weight bearing permitted on the affected extremity.
- An I.V. line is started in the foot of the affected extremity; contrast medium is injected into venous circulation and is observed under fluoroscopy as it fills the venous system. This enables areas of occlusion caused by deep vein thrombosis to be precisely identified.
- Side effects of the procedure include a warm, flushed sensation, nausea, vomiting, and a slight metallic taste in the mouth. Other side effects may include pain, swelling, and edema in the affected extremity.
- Risks include allergic reaction to the contrast medium and development of a venous thrombus in reaction to the medium.

Preparation
- Assess the patient for allergies to iodine or shellfish and for previous reaction to any contrast media; if allergy is suspected, notify the radiologist when scheduling the test.
- On the day of the test, restrict the patient's oral intake, as directed. (Depending on institutional policy, the patient may be allowed liquids or nothing by mouth.)
- Administer the patient's routine prescribed medications, as ordered or according to institutional policy.
- Obtain an informed consent per institutional policy.
- Explain the procedure to the patient. Tell him that he may be asked to plantar-flex his foot or perform Valsalva's maneuver to facilitate filling of the venous system with contrast medium. Have the patient practice both.
- Premedicate the patient with a mild sedative before the procedure, if ordered.

Postprocedure
- Monitor the patient's vital signs every 15 minutes until he is stable; then, follow institutional policy.
- Assess the insertion site for hematoma formation or bleeding.
- Assess the patient for delayed allergic reaction to the contrast medium, including rash and urticaria.
- Ask the patient to take increased fluids by mouth (unless contraindicated).
- Assess the patient for development of new symptoms of deep vein thrombosis.

(continued)

**TESTS USED TO DIAGNOSE DEEP
VEIN THROMBOSIS** (continued)

Doppler ultrasound

Purpose	• Identifies thrombi in the venous circulation • Particularly effective in diagnosing thrombi in proximal veins of lower extremities
Procedure	• Noninvasive procedure with minimal risks • May be done at the patient's bedside • Uses sound waves to detect abnormal venous flow patterns produced by an obstruction caused by a thrombus
Preparation	• This procedure involves little preparation. • The room should be comfortably warm to prevent venous constriction. • Patient should be in relaxed, supine position. • Explain to the patient in advance that he may be asked to deep-breathe or perform Valsalva's maneuver during the test.
Postprocedure	• None

Radioiodinated fibrinogen uptake test (RFUT)

Purpose	• Evaluates effectiveness of therapy designed to prevent the occurrence of deep vein thrombosis • Screening method for patients at high risk of developing deep vein thrombosis • Detects thrombi in calf veins accurately; may be used with other diagnostic methods to detect proximal vein thrombi
Procedure	• This procedure involves minimal risks. • After the radioisotope is injected I.V., it is taken up into the thrombus; definitive uptake may require 24 to 48 hours. • Patient is scanned 4 hours after injection, then every 24 hours for several days. • RFUT is contraindicated for pregnant or lactating women.
Preparation	• Make sure the patient has a patent I.V. access. • Explain the procedure to the patient.
Postprocedure	• None

Impedance plethysmography

Purpose	• Detects presence of thrombi in proximal veins in the legs
Procedure	• This procedure involves minimal risks. • With the patient supine, the involved leg is elevated 20 to 30 degrees with the knee flexed and calf supported on a pillow. • Electrodes are attached to the leg, and a thigh cuff is placed as far above the knee as is comfortable for the patient. • The thigh cuff is inflated for 15 seconds to 3 minutes and then released.

**TESTS USED TO DIAGNOSE DEEP
VEIN THROMBOSIS** (continued)

Impedance plethysmography (continued)

Procedure (continued)	• The rate of venous emptying in the calf after the release of the tourniquet is indirectly measured by recording changes in the electrical resistance of the leg. Results may be inaccurate if the patient is anxious, hypotensive, cold, or in pain. • Results may be interpreted as normal (no thrombosis) or abnormal (thrombosis present). Currently, researchers are using microcomputers to provide more specific information when abnormal results are obtained.
Preparation	• Explain the procedure to the patient. • If the procedure will be performed at the patient's bedside, make sure the room temperature is comfortably warm. Medicate the patient for pain, if indicated.
Postprocedure	• None

—Assess and report results of the patient's activated partial thromboplastin time (APTT), as ordered. (The APTT is used to regulate the dosage of heparin administered to each patient; it should be kept at approximately 1½ times that of normal.)

—Assess and report any signs of bleeding (see Anticoagulants, page 154).

• administration of warfarin, as ordered

—Assess and report results of prothrombin time (PT). (The PT is used to regulate the dose of warfarin for each patient; it should be kept at 1½ to 2 times the patient's control value.)

—Assess and report any signs of bleeding (see Anticoagulants, page 154).

• beginning the patient on an adjusted dosage of heparin subcutaneously, as ordered

—Change the patient from I.V. to subcutaneous dosages when ordered.

—Assess and report results of APTT, as ordered.

—Teach the patient and his family appropriate injection technique.

—Refer the patient and family to an appropriate home health agency, as needed, for help with injections. (Some patients are unable to administer their own heparin injections; referrals to the appropriate agency should be made before discharge.)

Rationale and comments: Heparin, the initial drug of choice to treat acute deep vein thrombosis, prevents thrombus growth and emboli formation by interfering with the normal clotting mechanism of the blood. Spontaneous bleeding or hemorrhage is a risk associated with heparin therapy.

Patients with deep vein thrombosis are usually discharged on anticoagulant therapy. Warfarin, often the drug of choice, takes at least 36 hours to affect the clotting cycle; therefore, it is started before the heparin is discontinued. The two medications are overlapped for several days. Pro-

COMMONLY PRESCRIBED MEDICATIONS	
ANTICOAGULANTS	
Examples	• Dicumarol (Dicoumarin): oral only • Heparin (Lipo Hepin, Panheprin): subcutaneous or I.V. only • Warfarin sodium (Coumadin): oral only
Actions	• Retards or slows clotting by interfering with the normal clotting cycle • Does not dissolve preexisting blood clots
Uses	• Prevents formation of blood clots in patients at risk • Prevents extension or growth of an existing blood clot
Side effects	• Spontaneous bleeding
Cautions	• Several drugs can increase the risk of bleeding when administered concurrently with anticoagulant therapy, including the following examples: —for heparin: aspirin —for warfarin: aspirin, ibuprofen (Motrin), sulfonamides, and cimetidine (Tagamet). —Consult a pharmacology text for a complete list.
Nursing responsibilities	• Assess the patient for signs of bleeding, including frank or occult bleeding in urine, feces, or aspirate from nasogastric tubes; bruising; petechiae; ecchymosis on skin; and changes in vital signs indicative of bleeding. • Monitor the patient's related laboratory tests. • See Intervention 5 in this care plan for additional nursing responsibilities.

longed anticoagulation is used to decrease the patient's risk of developing a recurrent thrombosis. Spontaneous bleeding and hemorrhage are also risks with warfarin therapy.

Some patients may be discharged on subcutaneous heparin instead of oral anticoagulants.

☑ **Intervention 6**

Implement measures to decrease the risk of thrombus development in another extremity (see "Deep Vein Thrombosis, Prevention of" in this section for details).

Rationale and comments: Bed rest is an important therapeutic measure in deep vein thrombosis to prevent emboli from breaking off; however, bed rest decreases the patient's mobility and increases the risk of further thrombus formation.

☑ **Intervention 7**

Assist with thrombolytic therapy, as prescribed, taking the following measures (see "Thrombolytic Therapy" in this section for more information):
• Start an I.V. line.
• Maintain the I.V. infusion for the time prescribed. (Infusion is usually maintained for 24 to 72 hours when treating deep vein thrombosis or pulmonary embolus.)

Rationale and comments: Some doctors recommend the use of thrombolytic therapy in deep vein thrombosis or pulmonary embolus because it can eliminate the source of emboli by dissolving the clot; prevent damage to the valves of the vein and decrease the risk of recurrent episodes of thrombosis; and, by decreasing the risk of pulmonary emboli, decrease the risk of damage to the pulmonary vascular bed.

☑ Intervention 8
Watch for development of pulmonary embolus.
• Assess for signs and symptoms, including:
—dyspnea
—cough
—chest pain that is affected by respiration
—hemoptysis
—tachypnea and tachycardia
—cyanosis
—fever.
• If signs and symptoms develop, notify the doctor and take the following measures:
—Assess the patient's vital signs and level of consciousness.
—Institute emergency measures, including cardiopulmonary resuscitation, as indicated.
• If no emergency measures are needed, implement the following interventions immediately:
—Return the patient to bed.
—Apply oxygen at a low flow rate.
—Notify the doctor.
—Stay with the patient to assess his condition for any rapid change, using appropriate measures to decrease his anxiety.
• Implement the prescribed medical orders, including the following:
—preparing the patient for prescribed diagnostic tests, such as pulmonary angiography, digital subtraction angiography, pulmonary perfusion scan, and ventilation lung scan (see *Tests used to diagnose pulmonary embolism*, pages 156 to 158)
—following the measures included in Interventions 4 and 5 above. (The care required for a patient with stable vital signs and a pulmonary embolus is similar to that needed for a patient with deep vein thrombosis.)

Rationale and comments: Pulmonary embolus is a common and potentially fatal complication of deep vein thrombosis. Some patients will develop signs and symptoms of a pulmonary embolus without having demonstrated any clinical signs and symptoms of deep vein thrombosis. Signs and symptoms associated with pulmonary embolus may be variable; two of the most common, dyspnea and coughing, are not always seen.

The patient's response to a pulmonary embolus depends on the size of the embolus, the size of the vessel occluded, and the amount of lung surface involved. A large pulmonary embolus can result in respiratory and cardiac arrest; patients who die from a pulmonary embolus frequently do so within 30 to 60 minutes of its occurrence.

(Text continues on page 158.)

TESTS USED TO DIAGNOSE PULMONARY EMBOLISM

Pulmonary angiography

Purpose	• Detects presence of pulmonary embolism • Evaluates pulmonary circulation
Procedure	• This procedure is invasive. • A catheter is inserted into the brachial or femoral artery and threaded to the pulmonary artery. Contrast medium is injected, and its movement through the pulmonary circulation is observed by fluoroscopy. • Continuous EKG monitoring is performed. • Risks include allergic reaction to contrast medium, cardiac dysrhythmias, rupture of the pulmonary artery, hemorrhage, and arterial occlusion at the insertion site.
Preparation	• Explain the procedure to the patient. • Assess the patient for allergies to shellfish, iodine, or other contrast media; notify the doctor if allergy is suspected. • Obtain an informed consent according to institutional policy. • Prepare the site, as ordered. • Make sure the patient receives nothing by mouth before the procedure. • Premedicate the patient, as ordered. • Complete other preprocedural care according to institutional policy. • Start an I.V. line.
Postprocedure	• Monitor the patient's vital signs every 15 minutes until he is stable; then monitor according to institutional policy. • Keep the patient flat in bed with the head of the bed elevated less than 30 degrees for 8 hours. Maintain a pressure dressing on the insertion site. • Observe the insertion site for bleeding or hematoma formation; if bleeding occurs, place direct pressure on the site, sufficient to control bleeding but not to occlude the distal pulse. • Monitor the pulse distal to the insertion site for changes; monitor the involved extremity for color or temperature changes. If the pulse decreases in strength or disappears or if the extremity becomes pale and cold, notify the doctor immediately. • Ask the patient to take increased fluids by mouth (unless contraindicated). • Observe the patient for delayed reaction to the contrast medium, including hives or rash.

TESTS USED TO DIAGNOSE
PULMONARY EMBOLISM *(continued)*

Digital subtraction angiography

Purpose	• Relatively new method for detecting clinically significant pulmonary emboli
Procedure	• This angiography method uses electronic enhancement of images. Images are obtained before and after injection of contrast dye; with the aid of a computer, these images are enhanced and manipulated to obtain the desired information. • Contrast medium is injected I.V. through a central line. • Contraindications to the procedure include renal failure, congestive heart failure, or decreased cardiac output because of the increased volume and concentration of contrast medium used in I.V. studies. • Excessive movement by the patient can interfere with results; the patient must be able to hold his breath when instructed to do so during imaging. • Risks include allergic reaction to contrast medium, transient renal failure, and development of phlebitis or thrombosis at the injection site.
Preparation	• Explain the procedure to the patient. • Obtain an informed consent according to institutional policy. • Assess the patient for allergies to shellfish, iodine, or other contrast media; notify the doctor if allergy is suspected. • Obtain any ordered diagnostic studies before the test, including such renal function studies as blood urea nitrogen or creatinine values. • Give the patient nothing by mouth for at least 6 hours before the test. • Premedicate the patient, as ordered. • Complete other preprocedural care according to institutional policy.
Postprocedure	• Maintain a pressure dressing on the injection site. • Activity is usually not restricted after the test. • Have the patient drink increased amounts of fluids (unless contraindicated). • Assess and record the patient's intake and output; notify the doctor if the patient has decreased urine output.

Pulmonary perfusion scan

Purpose	• Used with pulmonary ventilation scanning to detect pulmonary emboli • Assesses pulmonary arterial perfusion changes

(continued)

**TESTS USED TO DIAGNOSE
PULMONARY EMBOLISM** *(continued)*

Pulmonary perfusion scan *(continued)*

Procedure	• This procedure involves minimal risks. • After radionuclide is injected I.V., scanning is begun approximately 5 minutes later. • Chest X-ray is obtained for comparison with the scan.
Preparation	• Note that no restrictions on food or drink apply. • Explain the procedure to the patient. • Explain to the patient that he will need to lie still for approximately 30 minutes during the test.
Postprocedure	• None

Ventilation lung scanning

Purpose	• Used with perfusion scanning to detect pulmonary emboli
Procedure	• This procedure involves minimal risks. • Patient inhales radioactive gas, as directed. • Scans are taken.
Preparation	• Explain the procedure to the patient.
Postprocedure	• None

☑ Intervention 9

Evaluate the patient for indications of improvement in the following areas:
• deep vein thrombosis. Look for signs of the following:
—decreased edema in the affected extremity
—decreased pain in the affected extremity
—clotting studies that are within the desired parameters
—no indications of pulmonary embolus or new deep vein thrombi.
• pulmonary embolus. Look for signs of the following:
—decreased chest pain
—arterial blood gas levels that are within the desired parameters
—clotting studies within the desired parameters
—no indications of new emboli or deep vein thrombi.

Deep Vein Thrombosis, Prevention of*

ASSOCIATED STANDARD CARE PLANS
Deep Vein Thrombosis

ASSOCIATED TEACHING PLANS
Cardiac Anatomy and Physiology: Heart and Blood Vessels
Deep Vein Thrombosis: Disease Process and Prevention

Interventions and rationales
☑ **Intervention 1**
Assess the patient's risk of developing deep vein thrombosis (DVT). Factors to consider include the following:
• increasing age (Patients older than age 40 are considered more at risk than those under age 40.)
• history of deep vein thrombosis or pulmonary emboli
• complicated or lengthy surgical procedures
• chronic congestive heart failure, which is associated with decreased mobility and increased venous stasis
• history of varicose veins (Varicosities increase venous stasis.)
• obesity, which can increase venous stasis
• previous use of estrogens or previous pregnancy or cancer, which are associated with hypercoagulability of blood
• prolonged immobility, which increases venous stasis.

Rationale and comments: Prevention is crucial, because deep vein thrombosis is associated with a high risk of permanent vein damage and death from pulmonary embolism. Venous thrombi are thought to develop in the presence of venous stasis, damage to the vein's endothelial layer, or hypercoagulability of the blood. Any factor that results in one or more of those conditions increases the patient's risk of developing DVT.
• Deep vein thrombi damage the involved vessel and predispose the patient to recurrent episodes.
• A history of pulmonary emboli suggests a past history of DVT because most pulmonary emboli are thought to arise from thrombi in the deep veins above the knee.
• Prolonged surgical procedures, such as pelvic or abdominal surgery, major orthopedic surgery, and neurosurgery, can result in venous stasis during or after surgery or in damage to the veins distal to the surgical site.

---

*This care plan is for prevention of deep vein thrombosis in hospitalized patients.

☑ **Intervention 2**
Implement prescribed medical care to prevent deep vein thrombosis, which may include the following measures:
• Administer low-dose heparin, as ordered (see *Anticoagulants*, page 154, for additional information).
• Administer heparin and dihydroergotamine, as ordered.
• Institute external pneumatic compression of calves or legs, as ordered. Note the following information:
—Pneumatic pressure may be used until the patient is ambulatory.
—The nurse should follow institutional and manufacturer's guidelines for application.
—Prolonged use may cause patient discomfort.
• Administer oral anticoagulants, as prescribed. Keep in mind the following:
—Administer these drugs at the prescribed dose (see *Anticoagulants*, page 154, for additional information).
—Assess and report results of the patient's prothrombin time (PT), as ordered. (Warfarin's effectiveness is assessed by using the PT; the medication dosage is adjusted to keep the PT at 1½ to 2 times the control value.)
• Administer low molecular weight dextran, as ordered. Note the following:
—The usual dosage is 500 ml given I.V. over 4 to 6 hours.
—The dosage is repeated every 24 hours for 2 to 5 days.
—Signs of volume or circulatory overload should be assessed and reported.
• Assist the patient to ambulate, when ordered.
• Apply graded-pressure elastic hose (antiembolism stockings), as ordered. (Such stockings are used to apply a decreasing amount of pressure from the ankle to the thigh or knee; they prevent the formation of deep vein thrombosis by compressing superficial veins and increasing blood flow through the deep veins.) Take the following steps:
—Measure the patient for stockings as recommended by the manufacturer. (To effectively reduce venous stasis, stockings must fit correctly; incorrect fitting can impair arterial circulation or skin integrity.)
—Instruct the patient to apply stockings while lying supine in bed (since venous pooling occurs when the patient stands, the stockings should be applied before he gets up).
—Apply the stockings evenly and smoothly.
—Instruct the patient to avoid wearing the stockings partly rolled down or wrinkled.
—Remove the stockings only twice per day for 15 to 30 minutes to wash the feet and inspect the skin.
• Implement a combination of these orders as prescribed.

Rationale and comments: Low dose heparin is highly effective in preventing DVT in certain groups of patients; some surgeons prefer to avoid using heparin postoperatively because it increases the risk of postoperative bleeding. Heparin is strictly contraindicated for patients who have undergone neurosurgery.

Dihydroergotamine has undergone multicenter trials in the United States to evaluate its effectiveness and safety in preventing deep vein thrombi; it accelerates venous return through deep veins and prevents venous stasis by causing vasoconstriction of veins and venules.

External pneumatic compression of calves or legs is effective in patients for whom anticoagulant therapy is contraindicated. The major drawback is patient acceptance of the procedure (secondary to some discomfort experienced by patients).

Oral anticoagulants are effective in patients with hip fractures and in those undergoing hip or knee replacements or surgical repair of a fractured hip. The most commonly used oral agent is warfarin.

Low molecular weight dextran prevents the development of DVT by impairing platelet adhesion and preventing sludging of blood in microcirculation. More commonly used with surgical patients, dextran may be contraindicated for patients who are at risk for developing circulatory or volume overload.

Early ambulation helps to decrease the risk of DVT by increasing venous return to the heart and decreasing venous stasis.

Graded-pressure elastic hose is used to apply a decreasing amount of pressure from the ankle to the thigh or knee; it prevents the formation of DVT by compressing superficial veins and increasing blood flow through the deep veins.

✓ Intervention 3

Implement the following nursing measures to decrease the risk of deep vein thrombosis:

• Ask the patient to dorsiflex and plantar-flex his feet 5 to 10 times per hour while in bed.
• Ask the patient to avoid crossing his feet, ankles, or legs at all times.
• Position the patient to avoid putting pressure on the popliteal space.
• Position the patient with the foot of the bed elevated up to 30 degrees, unless contraindicated.

Rationale and comments: Active range of motion of the feet causes the gastrocnemius muscle in the leg to create a pumping action on the veins, which promotes venous return and decreases venous stasis.

Crossing feet, ankles, or legs impairs venous return from the lower extremities and causes venous stasis.

Pressure on the popliteal space can cause venous stasis by impairing venous return.

Elevating the foot of the bed increases venous return and decreases stasis; for some patients, such as those with severe occlusive arterial disease of the leg, elevation of the leg may be contraindicated.

✓ Intervention 4

Observe the patient for development of any clinical signs and symptoms of deep vein thrombosis or pulmonary emboli (see "Deep Vein Thrombosis" in this section).

Endocarditis, Infectious

ASSOCIATED NURSING DIAGNOSES
Anxiety
Depression, Reactive: Situational
Diversional Activity Deficit
Sleep-Pattern Disturbance

ASSOCIATED TEACHING PLANS
Cardiac Anatomy and Physiology: Heart and Blood Vessels
Endocarditis, Infectious: Disease Process and Prevention
Medication Guidelines

☑ Interventions and rationales
Intervention 1
Assess the patient for signs and symptoms of infectious endocarditis, an infection that typically takes one of two forms: subacute or acute. Signs and symptoms include:
• For subacute bacterial endocarditis (SBE)
—fever that is intermittent or continuous, low- or high-grade
—chills
—night sweats
—malaise and fatigue
—anorexia and weight loss
—cough
—complaints of aches and pains
—development of a new heart murmur or worsening of an existing one
—cutaneous symptoms, such as petechiae around the neck, shoulders, wrists, ankles, mucous membranes, and conjunctivae; and splinter hemorrhages on the distal third of the nail bed.
• For acute bacterial endocarditis (ABE)
—signs and symptoms are similar to those of SBE
—the course of disease is accelerated and signs are more overt.

Rationale and comments: Subacute bacterial endocarditis, which usually develops insidiously over a period of time, is caused by an organism of lesser virulence than ABE. The organism primarily harms the body by forming vegetation on the valve leaflets, which can permanently damage the valves. Also, pieces of the vegetation can break off, travel through the systemic circulation, and lodge in vessels in the brain, kidney, GI tract, heart, or lungs, resulting in infarct of the affected tissue or development of a mycotic or infectious aneurysm.

Acute bacterial endocarditis is caused by more virulent organisms than those that cause SBE. Besides damaging the valves and increasing the risk of systemic emboli, these organisms can directly invade other body tissues, causing increased infection.

☑ Intervention 2

Implement the prescribed medical care. Follow these measures:
• Make sure blood cultures are obtained, as ordered.
• Administer I.V. antibiotics, as ordered.
• Obtain repeat blood cultures, as ordered.

Rationale and comments: The causative microorganisms in infectious endocarditis live in the vegetation formed on the valves. Antibiotic therapy is the mainstay of treatment; specific agents are prescribed on the basis of the causative organisms.

Blood culture and sensitivity tests are used to identify the causative organisms and to determine the appropriate antibiotic therapy. The route of choice is intravenous. Because the organisms are well protected in the vegetation, prolonged antibiotic therapy is necessary to eradicate them effectively.

☑ Intervention 3

Take appropriate measures to promote physical and emotional rest, including the following:
• Make sure the patient has adequate rest periods throughout the day.
• Use measures to decrease patient discomfort from fever, chills, and aches and pains.
• Take measures to decrease the patient's anxiety.
• Promote a good night's sleep.
• Provide diversional activities.
• Make appropriate referrals, including a social worker for assistance with socioeconomic concerns and a home health agency for home administration of antibiotic therapy. (Although some patients may be discharged on home I.V. antibiotic therapy, others may be hospitalized, which could prove to be prolonged and costly.)

☑ Intervention 4

Observe the patient for complications, and notify the doctor if any occur. Complications include the following:
• congestive heart failure (CHF) (see "Congestive Heart Failure" in this section)
• systemic embolization such as in the following examples:
—In coronary arteries, such embolization results in myocardial infarction.
—In the pulmonary circulation, embolization results in a pulmonary embolus.
—In the cerebral circulation, embolization results in cerebrovascular accident.
—Emboli may also lodge in the spleen and mesenteric arteries or in the kidneys.

Rationale and comments: CHF can be a common complication in either form of bacterial endocarditis; it results from damage to a valve or its supporting structures.

Systemic embolization can result when pieces of the vegetation break off, travel, and lodge somewhere in systemic circulation. Specific signs depend on the tissue affected. For additional information, consult a medical-surgical nursing textbook.

Endocarditis, Infectious, Prevention of

ASSOCIATED CARE PLANS
Endocarditis, Infectious
Valve Replacement Surgery (Post ICU)

ASSOCIATED TEACHING PLANS
Endocarditis, Infectious: Disease Process and Prevention

Interventions and rationales
☑ **Intervention 1**
Assess the patient's risk of developing infectious endocarditis by assessing for the following:
• factors that predispose the patient to developing infectious endocarditis if exposed to the causative organism, including:
—history of congenital heart disease
—history of rheumatic or valvular heart disease
—previous history of endocarditis
—presence of prosthetic heart valves
• factors that increase the patient's risk of exposure to causative organisms, including:
—presence of invasive vascular lines, such as central catheters and transvenous pacemakers
—presence of a hemodialysis shunt or fistula
—I.V. drug use
—severe illness
—invasive procedures that can introduce bacterial microorganisms into the bloodstream, including dental procedures that result in gum bleeding, tonsillectomy, and diagnostic procedures or surgery of the genitourinary system or GI tract.

Rationale and comments: Bacterial endocarditis is an infection that develops on the heart valves or near defects on the endocardial layer of the heart. The structural defects that occur in valvular and congenital heart disease increase the patient's susceptibility to infectious endocarditis.

Residual damage to heart valves from an initial infection increases the patient's risk of developing a recurrent infection. Prosthetic valves are more susceptible to bacterial invasion.

Invasive lines, shunts, fistulas, and I.V. drug use provide direct access to the bloodstream for causative organisms. Severely debilitated patients are more at risk for developing infectious endocarditis.

COMMON ANTIBIOTICS TO PREVENT INFECTIOUS ENDOCARDITIS IN HIGH-RISK PATIENTS

Antibiotics prescribed for the prevention of infectious endocarditis vary, depending on the patient's condition and the proposed invasive procedure. This chart outlines some commonly used agents.

Aminoglycosides

Examples	• Gentamicin • Streptomycin
Actions	• Effective against gram-negative organisms
Side effects, toxic effects	• Hypersensitivity reactions • Neurotoxicity • Ototoxicity • Nephrotoxicity
Comments	• Poorly absorbed from the GI tract • Administered parenterally for most effective systemic effects • Administered orally for local effect in the GI tract

Cefazolin

Actions	• Effective against most gram-positive cocci and some gram-negative bacilli
Side effects, toxic effects	• Allergic reaction • Nausea, vomiting, and diarrhea • Phlebitis at the I.V. injection site
Comments	• Contraindicated for patients with history of moderate to severe penicillin allergy

Erythromycin

Actions	• Effective against gram-positive cocci • Spectrum of action similar to that of penicillin G
Side effects, toxic effects	• Nausea, vomiting, and diarrhea • Hepatotoxicity
Comments	• May be prescribed for patients with penicillin allergy • Not to be administered with food

Penicillin

Examples	• Amoxicillin • Ampicillin • Penicillin G • Penicillin V
Actions	• Broad-spectrum antibiotic • Active against gram-positive cocci and bacilli and some gram-negative cocci

COMMON ANTIBIOTICS TO PREVENT INFECTIOUS ENDOCARDITIS IN HIGH-RISK PATIENTS *(continued)*

Penicillin *(continued)*

Side effects, toxic effects	• Allergic reactions ranging from mild rash to anaphylaxis • Diarrhea, nausea, and vomiting
Comments	• Contraindicated for patients allergic to penicillin or cephalosporin

Vancomycin

Actions	• Effective against many strains of gram-positive bacteria, including staphylococci resistant to selected penicillins • Derived from *Streptomyces orientalis*
Side effects, toxic effects	• Nephrotoxicity • Tinnitus • Ototoxicity
Comments	• May be prescribed for patients with penicillin allergy • Poorly absorbed from the GI tract • Administered orally only when a local effect within the GI tract is desired • Usual route is I.V. • Elderly patients more susceptible to ototoxicity

☑ Intervention 2

Take measures to reduce the risk of introducing causative microorganisms into the patient, including the following:

• Use strict sterile technique when implementing the following procedures:
—starting an I.V. line
—inserting a urinary catheter
—changing a central line dressing
—changing a pacemaker dressing
—hanging or changing central line I.V. fluids
—caring for a dialysis shunt or fistula
—assisting with invasive diagnostic or surgical procedures.
• Use good hand-washing techniques at all times.
• Administer prophylactic antibiotics, as ordered. (These may be prescribed for individuals who are at high risk of developing infectious bacterial endocarditis. See *Common antibiotics to prevent infectious endocarditis in high-risk patients.*)

Rationale and comments: Stopping the entrance of causative microorganisms into the body is the most effective means of preventing infectious endocarditis.

☑ Intervention 3

Monitor the patient for any signs or symptoms of infection at sites of invasive lines.

• Signs and symptoms include:

—redness and warmth around the insertion site

—purulent drainage around the insertion site

—systemic signs of infection.

• If signs are present, obtain cultures (may require a doctor's order in some institutions).

☑ Intervention 4

Observe and report any signs or symptoms of infectious endocarditis (see "Endocarditis, Infectious" in this section for details.)

Rationale and comments: Infectious endocarditis is usually fatal if unrecognized and untreated.

☑ Intervention 5

Implement teaching on preventing infectious endocarditis at home (see "Endocarditis, Infectious: Disease Process and Prevention" in Section III).

Hypertension, Essential*

ASSOCIATED NURSING DIAGNOSES
Activity Intolerance, Potential for
Anxiety
Depression, Reactive: Situational
Noncompliance
Sexual Dysfunction

ASSOCIATED TEACHING PLANS
Atherosclerosis: Disease Process and Risk Factors
Blood Pressure Measurement
Cardiac Anatomy and Physiology: Heart and Blood Vessels
Cardiovascular Disease Risk Factors: Cigarette Smoking
Cardiovascular Disease Risk Factors: Diabetes Mellitus and Atherosclerosis
Cardiovascular Disease Risk Factors: Dietary Measures to Control
    Hyperlipidemia
Hypertension, Essential: Disease Process and Risk Factors
Medication Guidelines
Radial Pulse Measurement
Sodium-Restricted Diet
Stress Management

Interventions and rationales
☑ Intervention 1
Collect a baseline patient history, including the following data:
• signs and symptoms reported by the patient (the following signs and
symptoms occur with an elevation in blood pressure and are relieved with
a reduction in blood pressure):
　—occipital headaches on awakening and rising in the morning
　—migraine headaches
　—epistaxis without a local lesion or bleeding disorder.
• signs indicating damage to the heart, including:
　—chest pain caused by angina pectoris
　—dyspnea on exertion
　—paroxysmal nocturnal dyspnea
　—ankle edema
• signs indicative of brain damage, including:
　—vertigo
　—blurred vision
　—transient paresis
　—headache

*Some patients with hypertension may be admitted to the hospital to increase adherence to the prescribed
regimen when uncontrolled hypertension persists or to treat complications related to hypertension and/or
atherosclerosis; other hypertensive patients are usually cared for in outpatient settings.

- signs indicative of damage to kidneys, including:
—nocturia
—dysuria
—hematuria
- past history of hypertension, including:
—past treatment and its effectiveness
—the reason for cessation of treatment (Patients may choose to stop treatment for hypertension because of undesirable drug side effects or difficulties in maintaining prescribed life-style changes.)
- presence of nonmodifiable cardiovascular risk factors, such as:
—family history of hypertension or atherosclerotic diseases
—age (hypertension usually develops between ages 30 and 50)
—sex (hypertension develops early in males; risk increases after menopause with females)
—race (hypertension develops more frequently and severely in Black Americans)
- presence of modifiable cardiovascular risk factors, including:
—obesity
—sedentary life-style
—alcohol intake
—diet high in saturated fats and cholesterol
—diet high in sodium
—cigarette smoking
—hyperuricemia (history of gout or urinary tract stones)
—diabetes mellitus
- concurrent medical problems, including:
—angina pectoris
—post myocardial infarction
—congestive heart failure
—intermittent claudication
—post-cerebrovascular accident
—transient ischemic attacks
—nephrosclerosis
- accurate current drug history (use of some drugs may increase blood pressure or interfere with the action of antihypertensive drugs); assess for use of the following:
—antihypertensive drugs
—anti-inflammatory drugs
—nasal decongestants
—oral contraceptives
—appetite suppressants
—any other prescribed medications
—any other over-the-counter medications
- psychosocial factors, including:
—general coping patterns, such as how the patient handles anger
—stress tolerance, such as how easily the patient becomes upset
—self-perception, such as whether the patient is a hard-driving, impatient, or nervous person
—perception of the patient's roles in family settings and in interactions with others
—the patient's satisfaction with interactions with others.

Rationale and comments: Essential hypertension has been defined as a blood pressure greater than or equal to 140/90 mm Hg for persons under age 50, and a blood pressure equal to or greater than 160/95 mm Hg for persons age 50 and older. Patients are usually asymptomatic with mild to moderately severe hypertension. However, with prolonged duration of hypertension, signs of target organ damage can occur. The major target organs include the heart, brain, kidney, and retina of the eye.

☑ Intervention 2

Collect baseline physical assessment data, including the following:
- height and weight (see *Standard height-weight tables,* page 172).
- accurate blood pressure readings; be sure to:
  —check in both arms
  —check with the patient in the supine, sitting, and standing positions
  —record Korotkoff's sounds (phase I and phase V)
  —assess whether the patient has experienced a physically or emotionally stressful situation immediately before taking the blood pressure measurement. (Stress can cause a transient elevation in blood pressure.)
- funduscopic examination (This helps to detect the presence of retinal complications caused by hypertension.) Record this according to Keith-Wagener (K-W) grades I through IV:
  —Grade I: arterial narrowing or spasms
  —Grade II: arterioles compress venuoles where they cross (arteriovenous [A-V] nicking)
  —Grade III: flame-shaped hemorrhages or "cottonwool" (fluffy) exudates
  —Grade IV: papilledema (swelling of optic disk)
- signs of heart damage, including the following:
  —distended neck veins
  —displaced point of maximal impulse or precordial heave
  —ankle edema
  —tachycardia
  —murmurs
  —dysrhythmias
  —S_3 and S_4 heart sounds
  —rales and rhonchi
- signs of brain damage, including the following:
  —muscular asymmetry
  —muscular weakness
  —uncoordinated movements (unsteady gait, slurred speech)
  —unequal or abnormal deep-tendon reflex responses
- signs of kidney damage, including epigastric bruit.

☑ Intervention 3

Assist with prescribed diagnostic tests (see *Routine baseline diagnostic studies and indications,* page 173).

Rationale and comments: Diagnostic tests are used to rule out causes of secondary hypertension, confirm diagnosis of essential hypertension, and evaluate the extent of damage to the target organs.

(Text continues on page 174.)

STANDARD HEIGHT-WEIGHT TABLES

Desirable weights for men ages 25 to 59*

Height		Frame		
Feet	Inches	Small	Medium	Large
5	2	128-134	131-141	138-150
5	3	130-136	133-143	140-153
5	4	132-138	135-145	142-156
5	5	134-140	137-148	144-160
5	6	136-142	139-151	146-164
5	7	138-145	142-154	149-168
5	8	140-148	145-157	152-172
5	9	142-151	148-160	155-176
5	10	144-154	151-163	158-180
5	11	146-157	154-166	161-184
6	0	149-160	157-170	164-188
6	1	152-164	160-174	168-192
6	2	155-168	164-178	172-197
6	3	158-172	167-182	176-202
6	4	162-176	171-187	181-207

Desirable weights for women ages 25 to 59*

Height		Frame		
Feet	Inches	Small	Medium	Large
4	10	102-111	109-121	118-131
4	11	103-113	111-123	120-134
5	0	104-115	113-126	122-137
5	1	106-118	115-129	125-140
5	2	108-121	118-132	128-143
5	3	111-124	121-135	131-147
5	4	114-127	124-138	134-151
5	5	117-130	127-141	137-155
5	6	120-133	130-144	140-159
5	7	123-136	133-147	143-163
5	8	126-139	136-150	146-167
5	9	129-142	139-153	149-170
5	10	132-145	142-156	152-173
5	11	135-148	145-159	155-176
6	0	138-151	148-162	158-179

*Weight is in pounds, according to frame (in indoor clothing); height is measured in shoes with 1-inch heels.

©1983 Metropolitan Life Insurance Company. Source of basic data: 1979 Build Study. Society of Actuaries and Association of Life Insurance Medical Directories of America, 1980.

ROUTINE BASELINE DIAGNOSTIC STUDIES AND INDICATIONS

Diagnostic studies	Indications
Electrolytes	• Elevated sodium and potassium levels are noted in essential hypertension. • Potassium levels are a screening measure for secondary hypertension caused by primary aldosteronism.
Blood urea nitrogen and creatinine	• Elevation indicates renal insufficiency.
Uric acid	• Elevated levels are seen with diuretic therapy; may result in development of clinical gout.
Cholesterol and triglycerides	• Elevations may indicate the presence of cardiovascular risk factors, such as hypercholesterolemia. • Serum lipid levels may increase slightly after prolonged diuretic therapy.
Hemoglobin	• Decreased levels indicate possible anemia. • Decreased levels may cause symptoms common to hypertension and anemia, including headache, dyspnea, and dizziness.
Hematocrit	• Elevation indicates high blood viscosity that increases peripheral resistance and elevates blood pressure.
Urinalysis	• Proteinuria usually indicates renal disease possibly related to essential or secondary hypertension. • Granular casts indicate renal disease. • Glycosuria may indicate diabetes, a cardiovascular risk factor.
EKG	• Left ventricular hypertrophy or myocardial ischemia indicates hypertensive cardiovascular disease.
Chest X-ray	• Enlarged heart size and presence of congestive heart failure indicate hypertensive cardiovascular disease.
24-hour vanillyl-mandelic acid	• Elevated catecholamine excretion in urine has been found in some patients with essential hypertension.

☑ Intervention 4
Implement the prescribed medical care.
• Check the patient's vital signs with serial blood pressure readings.
—Record blood pressure in the arm that had the higher blood pressure during the initial assessment.
—Chart which arm is used for each reading.
—Check the blood pressure every 8 hours; this may advance to every 12 hours (unless ordered more frequently by the doctor). (Blood pressure may show a diurnal variation with a circadian pattern reflecting highest readings in midmorning, a progressive fall to lower readings during sleep, and a high reading on awakening.)
—If the patient has experienced emotional or physical stress, allow him to rest and relax before taking his blood pressure.
—Measure the patient's blood pressure while he is lying, sitting, and standing during each measurement.
—Keep the patient's forearm at heart level and in a relaxed state during measurement.
—Avoid upper-arm constriction, such as occurs with a rolled-up sleeve.
—Tell the patient his blood pressure measurements.
• Monitor the patient's activity.
—Orders vary depending on the patient's condition (see "Activity Intolerance, Potential for" in Section I and "Hypertension, Essential: Disease Process and Risk Factors" in Section III).
—Teach the patient to use relaxation therapy in activities of daily living (see "Stress Management" in Section III).
• Monitor the patient's diet. The diet may be:
—sodium-restricted (Decreasing sodium intake is a general measure used to control hypertension.)
—low in fat and cholesterol. (This helps to decrease the patient's risk of developing atherosclerosis.)

☑ Intervention 5
Administer antihypertensive medications as prescribed.
• Commonly prescribed medications include:
—diuretics (see *Diuretics,* page 132)
—adrenergic antagonists (see *Adrenergic antagonists* and *Beta-adrenergic blocking agents,* page 191)
—arterial vasodilators (see *Vasodilators,* page 133)
—angiotensin-converting enzyme inhibitors (see *Angiotensin-converting enzyme inhibitors,* page 134)
—calcium channel blockers (see *Calcium channel blockers,* page 120).
• Obtain orders for specific parameters for withholding antihypertensive drugs or notifying the doctor (acceptable guidelines for withholding medication until the doctor sets specific parameters are <120 mm Hg systolic and/or <80 mm Hg diastolic).
• Measure and record the patient's blood pressure before administering antihypertensive medications.

ADRENERGIC ANTAGONISTS

The adrenergic antagonists are categorized below according to their antihypertensive properties. For a discussion of beta-adrenergic blockers, another category within this classification, see *Beta-adrenergic blocking agents,* page 191.

Centrally acting agents

Examples	• Clonidine hydrochloride (Catapres) • Methyldopa (Aldomet)
Actions	• Reduces blood pressure by inhibiting selected sympathetic nervous system activity
Side effects	• Drowsiness • Dry mouth • Fatigue • Sexual dysfunction
Nursing responsibilities	• Monitor the patient's blood pressure response, and observe for signs of orthostatic hypotension. • Teach the patient how to take medication correctly at home. • With clonidine, if blood pressure drops below parameters preset by the doctor, notify the doctor immediately. Marked rebound hypertensive reaction may occur if medication is abruptly stopped.

Peripherally acting agents

Examples	• Guanethidine (Ismelin) • Reserpine (Serpasil, Sandril) • Rauwolfia alkaloids
Actions	• Lowers blood pressure by depleting stores of catecholamines in the sympathetic nerve endings
Side effects	• Sexual dysfunction • Reserpine or rauwolfia alkaloids: drowsiness, weight gain, and GI distress • Guanethidine: orthostatic hypotension and fluid retention
Nursing responsibilities	• Follow the measures outlined in care plan.

Alpha-adrenergic blocking agents

Examples	• Prazosin (Minipress)
Actions	• Lowers blood pressure by reducing total peripheral vascular resistance
Side effects	• Syncope with initial doses • Orthostatic hypotension
Nursing responsibilities	• Follow the measures outlined in care plan.

ANTIHYPERTENSIVE DRUG THERAPY: STEPPED-CARE APPROACH TO CONTROLLING HYPERTENSION

Step	Therapy
1	• Begin treatment with a low dosage of either a thiazide diuretic or a beta blocker. Dosage of drug is increased if patient's blood pressure does not successfully respond. • Proceed to next step if blood pressure remains uncontrolled.
2	• Add another antihypertensive drug: —Add propranolol (or methyldopa, clonidine, reserpine, or prazosin) if a diuretic was initiated in Step 1. —Add or substitute a diuretic if a beta blocker was initiated in Step 1. • Dosages are gradually increased, as needed, to control high blood pressure. • Proceed to next step if blood pressure remains uncontrolled.
3	• Add other antihypertensive drugs (hydralazine or minoxidil). • Proceed to next step if blood pressure remains uncontrolled.
4	• Add or substitute guanethidine.

• If the blood pressure is lower than the preset parameters, assess the patient for signs that he is not tolerating the blood pressure, including such signs of decreased cerebral and cardiovascular blood flow as:
—restlessness
—confusion
—irritability
—light-headedness
—slurred speech
—unsteady gait
—rapid heart and respiratory rates
—pale, cool skin.
• If any of the above signs and symptoms are present, check vital signs every 5 minutes, adjusting the frequency as blood pressure stabilizes, and notify the doctor.

Rationale and comments: The goals of the pharmacologic management of hypertension include controlling the patient's blood pressure as close to normal as possible and as tolerated, minimizing side effects, and keeping the medication regimen prescribed for home use as simple as possible to promote compliance. For additional information about a common pharmacologic approach to controlling hypertension, see *Antihypertensive drug therapy: Stepped-care approach to controlling hypertension.*

☑ Intervention 6
Administer other medications, as prescribed, which may include:
• mild tranquilizing medications
• other cardiovascular medications as indicated by the patient's condition.

Rationale and comments: Mild tranquilizers are prescribed to reduce anxiety. Patients with hypertension may also have other concurrent cardiovascular diseases, including angina pectoris and congestive heart failure.

☑ Intervention 7

Assess the patient's response to prescribed antihypertensive therapy.
• Assess his blood pressure response; notify the doctor if the patient experiences continued hypertension.
• Assess for side effects of prescribed medications (see Interventions 8 to 11 below for specific side effects and related interventions).

Rationale and comments: Individual response to prescribed antihypertensive medications can vary. Continued hypertension suggests that the patient's medication regimen may need to be altered to achieve optimal blood pressure control. Negative side effects of drug therapy may diminish over a period of a few days to months; if they do not diminish, attempts should be made to alter the prescribed therapy.

☑ Intervention 8

Assess the patient for orthostatic hypotension (a common complication with many antihypertensive medications); implement appropriate measures if it is present.
• Assess for the following signs when the patient changes positions from supine to sitting to standing:
  —fainting
  —dizziness or light-headedness
  —changes in blood pressure
  —nausea and vomiting.
• If any of the above signs are present, implement the following measures:
  —Have the patient lie down until the symptoms disappear.
  —Apply support stockings or elastic stockings, as ordered, to decrease venous pooling in the legs.
  —Instruct the patient to change positions slowly.
  —Take appropriate measures to decrease the patient's risk of falling.

☑ Intervention 9

If the patient experiences fatigue, drowsiness, lack of energy, or lethargy, implement the following measures:
• Tell the patient that these feelings will decrease as his body adjusts to a lowered blood pressure and drug effects.
• Assess ordered laboratory tests or abnormal results indicating hyperglycemia, hypokalemia, or signs of liver damage; notify the doctor if these signs are present (alternate drug therapy may be prescribed).

☑ Intervention 10

If the patient has a dry mouth, take the following measures:
• Promote good oral hygiene.
• Suggest that the patient chew sugarless gum or candy.
• Tell the patient that these symptoms will diminish.

☑ Intervention 11

If the patient reports sexual dysfunction, implement the following measures:
• Tell the patient that sexual functioning may be decreased with initial lowering of blood pressure and may return to normal as his body adjusts to a lowered blood pressure.

**DISTINCTION BETWEEN HYPERTENSIVE CRISES:
EMERGENCIES AND URGENCIES**

	Emergencies	Urgencies
Description	• Life-threatening blood pressure elevations • Requires immediate reduction in blood pressure	• Life-threatening blood pressure elevations • Requires reduction in blood pressure that can be obtained safely within 24 hours
Treatment	• Parenteral antihypertensive drug therapy	• Parenteral or oral antihypertensive drug therapy

---

• Notify the doctor (sometimes a change in drug therapy may decrease this side effect).

☑ **Intervention 12**
Monitor the patient for development of the complication of hypertensive crisis.
• Assess the patient for signs and symptoms, including:
—life-threatening blood pressure elevations
—headache that is occipital or increasing in frequency
—restlessness, increased anxiety, irritability, extreme apprehension, and confusion
—blurred vision
—pain in the chest or abdomen that may increase in severity and radiate to the back
—dyspnea
—nausea and vomiting
—hematuria
—seizure activity or unconsciousness
—epistaxis.

Rationale and comments: Hypertensive crises are caused by life-threatening elevations in blood pressure, which compromise cerebral, renal, or cardiovascular functioning. These may be caused by accelerated or malignant hypertension or other conditions, such as toxemia of pregnancy, endocrine problems, postoperative reaction to surgical procedures, or drug-induced hypertension (see *Distinctions between hypertensive crises: Emergencies and urgencies*).

☑ **Intervention 13**
If the patient demonstrates signs of hypertensive crisis, implement the following measures:
• Institute bed rest with the patient placed in a comfortable position.
• Notify the doctor immediately.

MEDICATIONS USED TO MANAGE HYPERTENSIVE EMERGENCIES AND URGENCIES

Diazoxide (Hyperstat)

Action	• Direct vasodilator
Administration	• I.V. administration only for management of hypertension • Begins to act within 3 to 5 minutes of I.V. administration
Side effects	• Nausea and vomiting • Hypotension • Hyperglycemia • Sodium or water retention
Nursing responsibilities	• Assess the patient closely for hyperglycemia. • Monitor the patient's blood pressure response. • Notify the doctor if the patient has continued hypertension or significant hypotension.

Sodium nitroprusside (Nipride)

Action	• Mixed arterial and venous vasodilator
Administration	• Continuous I.V. infusion (mixed in dextrose 5% in water); dosage titrated by patient response • Begins to act immediately
Side effects	• Nausea and vomiting • Muscle twitching • Thiocyanate intoxication
Nursing responsibilities	• Prepare a fresh solution every 24 hours. • Mix the medication with dextrose 5% in water only. • Protect the medication from light, as directed. • Monitor the patient's blood pressure response. • Notify the doctor if continued hypertension or significant hypotension occurs. • Monitor serum thiocyanate levels, as ordered; notify the doctor about abnormal values.

Hydralazine hydrochloride (Apresoline)

Action	• Direct vasodilator
Administration	• Administer either I.M. or I.V. • I.M. administration begins to work within 20 to 30 minutes. • I.V. administration begins to work within 10 to 12 minutes. • I.V. dose should be administered in total volume of at least 20 ml and given no faster than 0.5 ml/minute.
Side effects	• Sodium or water retention • Headache • Tachycardia • Vomiting and diarrhea

(continued)

MEDICATIONS USED TO MANAGE HYPERTENSIVE EMERGENCIES AND URGENCIES (continued)

Hydralazine hydrochloride (Apresoline) (continued)

Nursing responsibilities	• Assess the patient's blood pressure response. • Monitor the patient's blood pressure continuously during I.V. administration. • Notify the doctor if the patient experiences continued hypertension or significant hypotension.

Trimethaphan camsylate (Arfonad)

Action	• Lowers blood pressure by blocking transmission of nerve impulses through the ganglia
Administration	• Continuous I.V. infusion (diluted in dextrose 5% in water); begins to act within 5 to 10 minutes
Side effects	• Orthostatic hypotension • Blurred vision • Dry mouth • Respiratory depression • Tachycardia
Nursing responsibilities	• Carefully monitor the patient's blood pressure for desired drop in pressure during administration. • Notify the doctor if the patient experiences continued hypertension or significant hypotension.

Methyldopa (Aldomet)

Action	• Lowers blood pressure by inhibiting sympathetic nervous system activity
Administration	• I.V., every 4 to 6 hours • Takes 2 to 3 hours to begin to work
Side effects	• Drowsiness • Headache • Impotence • Bradycardia • Changes in bowel habits
Nursing responsibilities	• Carefully monitor the patient's blood pressure for desired drop in pressure during administration. • Notify the doctor if the patient experiences continued hypertension or significant hypotension.

Labetalol hydrochloride

Action	• Lowers blood pressure through beta- and selective alpha-adrenergic blockade
Administration	• I.V. bolus • Continuous I.V. infusion

**MEDICATIONS USED TO MANAGE HYPERTENSIVE
EMERGENCIES AND URGENCIES** *(continued)*

Labetalol hydrochloride *(continued)*

Side effects	• Nausea and vomiting • Postural hypotension • Dizziness • Fatigue
Nursing responsibilities	• Keep the patient supine during I.V. administration. • Monitor the patient's blood pressure closely before, during, and after administration. • Notify the doctor if the patient experiences continued hypertension or significant hypotension.

Reserpine

Action	• Lowers blood pressure by blocking peripheral sympathetic nervous system activity
Administration	• I.M. • Takes 2 to 3 hours to begin to work
Side effects	• Drowsiness • Mental depression • Gastric distress
Nursing responsibilities	• Monitor the patient's blood pressure. • Notify the doctor if the patient experiences continued hypertension or significant hypotension.

• Prepare to initiate the prescribed medical care, which may include the following:
—starting an I.V. access to administer parenteral drugs
—administering prescribed parenteral medications (see *Medications used to manage hypertensive emergencies and urgencies,* page 179)
—monitoring the patient's blood pressure every 5 minutes until it stabilizes at a desired level
—monitoring the patient's intake and output
—transferring the patient to the intensive care unit for continuous monitoring of blood pressure and infusion of potent antihypertensive medications.

☑ Intervention 14
Teach the patient and family how to manage the patient's hypertension at home (see "Hypertension, Essential: Disease Process and Risk Factors" and "Blood Pressure Measurement" in Section III).

Myocardial Infarction, Acute

ASSOCIATED NURSING DIAGNOSES
Activity Intolerance
Activity Intolerance, Potential for
Anxiety
Bowel Elimination, Alteration in: Constipation
Depression, Reactive: Situational
Family Processes, Alteration in
Grieving, Family
Grieving, Individual Patient
Noncompliance
Self-Concept, Alteration in
Sexual Dysfunction
Sleep-Pattern Disturbance

ASSOCIATED TEACHING PLANS
Atherosclerosis: Disease Process and Risk Factors
Cardiac Anatomy and Physiology: Heart and Blood Vessels
Cardiovascular Disease Risk Factors: Cigarette Smoking
Cardiovascular Disease Risk Factors: Diabetes Mellitus and Atherosclerosis
Cardiovascular Disease Risk Factors: Dietary Measures to Control
    Hyperlipidemia
Exercising after Myocardial Infarction or Heart Surgery
Hypertension, Essential: Disease Process and Risk Factors
Medication Guidelines
Myocardial Infarction: Disease Process and Home Care
Radial Pulse Measurement
Sexual Activity and Heart Disease
Stress Management

Interventions and rationales
☑ Intervention 1
Assess the patient for the following indications of acute myocardial infarction
(AMI):
• chest pain
   —often described as crushing, constricting, squeezing, viselike, or heavy;
    may also be described as stabbing, knifelike, boring, or burning dis-
    comfort
   —usually described as severe in quality; if patient has experienced angina
    in the past, he may describe pain as more severe than anginal pain.
   —frequently located in the retrosternal region; may spread to both sides
    of the anterior chest (left side more than the right)

—may also radiate to the shoulder, arms, neck, jaw, and interscapular area (left side more than the right)

—also may radiate down the ulnar side of the left arm (Patient may report tingling sensation in the left wrist, hand, and fingers.)

—may be experienced less frequently as severe substernal or precordial discomfort accompanied by a dull ache or dullness in the wrist

—usually lasts more than 30 minutes

—is unrelieved by rest or sublingual nitroglycerin

• other signs and symptoms

—nausea and vomiting

—feeling of profound weakness or dizziness

—palpitations

—cold perspiration

—sense of impending doom

—restlessness (Patient appears in acute distress.)

—clenching of fist over chest

—changes in vital signs, such as dysrhythmias, transient hypertension, hypotension, or tachypnea

• less common signs and symptoms

—complaint of a strange sensation (not pain) in the chest area

—cold and clammy skin

—cyanosis

—dyspnea (Patient complains of feeling short of breath.)

—confusion

—elevated temperature

—hypertension or hypotension

—irregular pulse rate

—bradycardia or tachycardia

—rales on auscultation of the lung fields

—distended external jugular veins when head of bed is elevated more than 15 degrees

—pedal or sacral edema

—nausea

—acute fatigue

• additional supporting data

—cardiac enzyme levels, if ordered

—12-lead EKG, if ordered.

Rationale and comments: AMI results from a prolonged, substantial, acute reduction in blood flow to the myocardium.

• Chest pain, the classic symptom of AMI, requires careful assessment to help differentiate pain associated with AMI from anginal pain or pain of noncardiac origin. (See "Angina Pectoris" in this section for a complete discussion of chest pain associated with angina; also see *Characteristics of noncardiac chest pain,* pages 184 and 185.)

• The chest pain in AMI often is accompanied by other signs and symptoms that are related to either the body's response to deep visceral pain or the drop in cardiac output that can occur in AMI.

CHARACTERISTICS OF NONCARDIAC CHEST PAIN

Pulmonary embolus	• May mimic the chest pain of acute myocardial infarction • Has severe, abrupt onset; may persist for hours • Described as stabbing or knifelike pain that is aggravated by breathing • With massive embolus, pain located in retrosternal area; with smaller embolus, pain more laterally located • Accompanied by acute dyspnea, tachypnea, cyanosis, and tachycardia • May be accompanied by cough with hemoptysis
Acute dissection of the aorta	• Severe, excruciating; begins abruptly; may persist for many hours • Described as tearing, lacerating, throbbing, or ripping pain • Pain experienced more often in back, but location may vary • Is not aggravated when patient turns or breathes deeply • Accompanied by sudden absence of peripheral pulse in one extremity • Blood pressure may be significantly lower in one arm than in the other. • Patient may appear to be in shock.
Spontaneous pneumothorax	• Described as tearing sensation; does not radiate • Aggravated by breathing • Abrupt onset • Accompanied by dyspnea and diminished or absent breath sounds over the involved lung field • Trachea deviated away from the affected side • Diagnosis confirmed by X-ray
Reflux esophagitis and hiatal hernia	• Described as heartburn or indigestion • Experienced as a burning sensation in the retrosternal area between the xiphoid and suprasternal notch • May also be experienced as a sensation of localized pressure or squeezing pain across the middle of the chest, radiating to the back • Aggravated by eating • Relieved by belching or antacids • Sometimes accompanied by regurgitation of sour, bitter fluid or food
Diffuse esophageal spasm	• Described as burning, dull, sharp, or squeezing pain • Located in retrosternal area with radiation to back, arms, or jaw • May last minutes to hours • May be relieved by sublingual nitroglycerin • Accompanied by dysphagia • Occurs during or after a meal, especially after ingesting cold liquids • May also be precipitated by position changes, such as lying down or bending over

CHARACTERISTICS OF NONCARDIAC CHEST PAIN (continued)

Cholecystitis and cholelithiasis	• Located in epigastric area or right upper quadrant of abdomen • Abrupt onset • May be steady or intermittent • May be referred to back or right scapular area • Tenderness present in right upper quadrant on palpation • Accompanied by nausea and vomiting, fever and chills, dyspepsia, flatulence, indigestion, and intolerance to fatty, spicy foods • Diagnosis confirmed by X-ray or ultrasound studies
Pericarditis	• Sharp, knifelike pain that is aggravated by coughing, deep-breathing, lying flat, or swallowing • May be referred to neck, shoulder, or upper abdomen • Often relieved when patient sits up and leans forward • Accompanied by pericardial friction rub and characteristic ST segment elevation • If effusion present, may be diagnosed by echocardiography
Chest wall pain and tenderness	• May be reproduced by palpating area of pain or by movement of the thoracic cage, such as by bending, stooping, twisting, or turning • May last seconds to hours • Is unrelieved by sublingual nitroglycerin • Other symptoms variable (depends on specific etiology) • Causes numerous; common example is incisional pain after surgery

• Some patients with AMI don't experience severe chest pain. Instead, they have symptoms resembling those of congestive heart failure (CHF). AMI should be suspected in any patient who has no history of CHF but who presents with its signs and symptoms.

• The patient's temperature may become elevated within 24 to 48 hours after infarction as part of the inflammatory response and may remain elevated for up to 1 week.

• Certain enzymes rise and fall in a predictable pattern after myocardial injury; these enzymes may be used to definitively diagnose the presence of AMI. Also, the degree of elevation of some of these enzymes may provide a relative indication of the extent of the infarct. (See *Cardiac enzymes*, pages 186 and 187, for more information.)

• Characteristic changes in a patient's EKG may assist with the diagnosis of AMI as well as provide information about the type and location of the damage. These changes may occur within hours after the onset of symptoms or may take several days to develop.

CARDIAC ENZYMES

Creatine kinase, total (CK)

Onset of elevation	• 4 to 6 hours after onset of symptoms
Peak	• 12 to 24 hours after onset
Return to normal	• 72 to 96 hours after onset
Normal value	• Men: 50 to 180 IU/liter • Women: 50 to 160 IU/liter
Comments	• Will be elevated in typical pattern if the patient has acute myocardial infarction (AMI) • Is nonspecific for cardiac damage; may also be elevated in response to injury to skeletal muscle or brain tissue

Creatine kinase MB isoenzyme (CK-MB)

Onset of elevation	• 3 to 4 hours after onset of symptoms
Peak	• 12 to 24 hours after onset
Return to normal	• 36 hours after onset
Normal value	• <3 IU/liter or 0%
Comments	• Will be elevated in typical pattern in AMI • Highly specific for myocardial damage • Positive CK-MB (sometimes called MB bands) diagnostic for AMI even in presence of normal total CK

Aspartate aminotransferase (formerly serum glutamic-oxaloacetic transaminase [SGOT])

Onset of elevation	• 8 to 12 hours after onset of symptoms
Peak	• 18 to 36 hours after onset
Return to normal	• 72 to 96 hours after onset
Normal value	• 0 to 36 IU/liter
Comments	• Will rise in a predictable pattern in AMI • Elevation not specific for myocardial damage

Lactate dehydrogenase, total (LDH)

Onset of elevation	• 24 to 48 hours after onset of symptoms
Peak	• 48 to 72 hours after onset
Return to normal	• 7 to 10 days after onset

CARDIAC ENZYMES *(continued)*

Lactate dehydrogenase, total (LDH)*(continued)*	
Normal value	• Men: 63 to 155 units • Women: 62 to 131 units
Comments	• Will usually be elevated in AMI • Is nonspecific for cardiac damage

Lactate dehydrogenase-1 isoenzyme (LDH-1)	
Onset of elevation	• 12 to 24 hours after symptom onset
Peak	• 48 to 60 hours after symptom onset
Return to normal	• 7 to 10 days
Normal value	• 25% to 40%
Comments	• More specific than total LDH for cardiac damage • Most useful in patients who present with significant delay after the onset of symptoms

---

☑ **Intervention 2**

Implement the following measures to relieve pain and limit myocardial damage:

• Administer sublingual nitroglycerin, as ordered (*see* "Angina Pectoris" in this section for details).

• If chest pain is unrelieved by sublingual nitroglycerin, administer morphine sulfate I.V. (or other prescribed medication), as ordered.

—Monitor vital signs for hypotension and respiratory depression.

—Assess the patient for relief of chest pain.

—Common dosage of morphine sulfate is 2 to 4 mg I.V. every 5 minutes until chest pain is relieved, the maximum prescribed total dose has been administered, or respiratory depression or significant hypotension occurs.

• Be prepared to administer an I.V. nitroglycerin drip, as ordered.

—Monitor the patient for relief of chest pain.

—Take vital signs every 5 to 15 minutes until vital signs stabilize at the desired level; monitor the patient for hypotension.

• Administer oxygen by nasal cannula according to institutional policy or as ordered.

• Use measures to decrease the patient's anxiety.

Rationale and comments: Immediate treatment of AMI focuses on limiting myocardial damage by decreasing oxygen consumption and increasing myocardial oxygen supply to the ischemic area. Research has shown that the area of infarction is surrounded by a zone of ischemic tissue. If the

balance between oxygen supply and demand is restored rapidly enough to this border zone, the size of the infarct may be limited. Limiting the size of the infarct reduces subsequent complications and mortality.
• Pain relief should be the nurse's top priority. Severe pain triggers the release of catecholamines, which increase myocardial oxygen demand and the risk of dysrhythmias, thus increasing myocardial ischemia.
• Nitroglycerin decreases the myocardium's oxygen demands and increases blood flow and oxygen supply through collateral vessels, particularly in the ischemic area of the myocardium. Administration of I.V. nitroglycerin has been found to limit infarct size and relieve pain. Because it can cause significant hypotension, it is started at a low dose and increased gradually to achieve pain relief as long as the patient's blood pressure remains within the limits set by the doctor.
• Morphine decreases oxygen demand by decreasing pain and anxiety as well as by decreasing myocardial work load.
• Use of supplemental oxygen helps to prevent hypoxia, which increases myocardial ischemia and subsequent myocardial damage.

☑ **Intervention 3**
Assess the patient for presence of complications frequently seen during the initial period, including:
• CHF (see "Congestive Heart Failure" in this section); notify the doctor if signs and symptoms develop.
• dysrhythmias (see "Coronary Artery Bypass Surgery [Post ICU]" in this section for details); notify the doctor if signs and symptoms develop.
• cardiogenic shock; notify doctor if symptoms occur.
Signs and symptoms include:
—extreme hypotension (<80 mm Hg systolic)
—rapid, thready pulse
—oliguria (<20 ml/hr)
—tachypnea
—cold, moist skin
—cyanosis and pallor
—dulled sensorium
—failure to improve with oxygen administration or relief of chest pain.

Rationale and comments: CHF, a common complication during the acute period, results from damage to the ventricular wall. Dysrhythmias frequently cause death during the initial period. However, their rapid detection and treatment improves the patient's prognosis. Cardiogenic shock, another leading cause of death in AMI, results from massive death of left ventricular tissue. Prognosis for a patient with cardiogenic shock is poor.

☑ **Intervention 4**
Assist with implementing aggressive medical therapy, as directed, including:
• thrombolytic therapy (see "Thrombolytic Therapy" in this section for details)
• percutaneous transluminal coronary angioplasty (see "Percutaneous Transluminal Coronary Angioplasty" in this section for details).

Rationale and comments: Research has shown that restoring blood flow and oxygen supply to the ischemic area of the myocardium within hours after the onset of symptoms can be effective in limiting infarct size and subsequent complications.

☑ Intervention 5
Assist with implementing conventional medical therapy, as ordered.
• Transfer the patient to the coronary care unit (CCU) or telemetry unit, as ordered, until he is stable.
• Common medical orders for patients during CCU stay include:
—monitoring the patient's EKG continuously
—maintaining a patent I.V. or heparin lock
—monitoring the patient's vital signs as indicated by his condition
—limiting the patient's activity to bed rest with use of a bedside commode
—providing a liquid or soft diet for first 24 hours
—prohibiting the patient from smoking
—limiting visitors and telephone calls according to unit policy
—providing oxygen, as ordered
—administering medications, as ordered (see Intervention 6).

Rationale and comments: Goals during the initial period include recognizing and treating complications rapidly, decreasing stress (physical and emotional) and myocardial oxygen demand, and preventing complications. The usual length of stay in the CCU for uncomplicated AMI is 1 to 3 days. Once stable, the patient may be transferred to a step-down or telemetry unit or to a regular unit.

Initially, the patient's diet is restricted to easy-to-digest foods, served in small, frequent meals, to decrease the stress on the heart and the risk of vomiting.

☑ Intervention 6
After the patient's transfer from the CCU, implement the following orders:
• Maintain continuous EKG monitoring, as ordered.
• Maintain a patent I.V. or heparin lock, as ordered.
• Monitor the patient's vital signs every 4 hours or as needed.
• Provide an appropriate diet, as ordered.
—Diet may be regular with no restrictions.
—Diet may be restricted to one low in saturated fats and cholesterol.
—Caffeine intake may be restricted.
• Continue the patient with low-level activity, increasing activity according to the exercise plan (see "Activity Intolerance, Potential For" in Section I for details).
• Discourage the patient from smoking.
• Limit visitors and telephone calls as indicated by the patient's condition.
• Provide oxygen, as ordered.

Rationale and comments: Limiting the patient's activity reduces myocardial work load and oxygen demands.

Once the patient stabilizes, he may be placed on a regular diet without restriction. Patients who have had an AMI need adequate nutrition to heal well. An abrupt change in diet coupled with stress may result in anorexia and may interfere with the healing of the heart. A diet low in saturated fat and cholesterol usually is started before the patient's discharge and is prescribed for home use. Caffeine is a stimulant that can increase myocardial oxygen demand.

Inhaled smoke serves as a stimulant that increases heart rate and blood pressure, thereby increasing oxygen consumption. It causes constriction of coronary arteries, which can increase the risk of additional myocardial ischemia. It also increases platelet aggregation, which increases the risk of thrombus formation.

Visits by close friends or family can serve as an important source of support; however, prolonged visits or too many visits can tire the patient and increase stress on the heart.

☑ Intervention 7
Administer prescribed medications, including:
• cardiovascular medications (as indicated by the patient's condition), including:
—beta-adrenergic blocking agents (see *Beta-adrenergic blocking agents*)
—antiarrhythmic medications (see *Antiarrhythmic medications,* pages 144 and 145)
—diuretics (see *Diuretics,* page 132)
—long-acting nitrates (see *Nitrates,* page 119, and *Vasodilators,* page 133)
—calcium channel blockers (see *Calcium channel blockers,* page 120)
• antiplatelet medications (see *Antiplatelet medications,* page 143)
• antianxiety medications
• stool softeners and laxatives.

Rationale and comments: Use of specific cardiovascular medications varies, depending on the patient's condition, presence of concurrent cardiovascular diseases, and presence of complications. Because the body's response to anxiety increases myocardial oxygen demand, antianxiety medications are used. Stool softeners and laxatives are used to ease straining with defecation, which also increases myocardial oxygen demand as well as the risk that the patient will use Valsalva's maneuver (Valsalva's maneuver can result in bradycardia and a reduction of blood flow to the myocardium).

☑ Intervention 8
Assess for complications that may occur during the rehabilitation period, including:
• dysrhythmias (see "Coronary Artery Bypass Surgery (Post ICU)" in this section for assessment and interventions)
• CHF (see "Congestive Heart Failure" in this section for assessment and interventions)
• extension of the original infarct or reinfarction; assess for the following signs:
—recurrent signs and symptoms of AMI
—second elevation of cardiac enzyme (creatine kinase MB) levels
—new EKG changes indicating that an infarct has occurred

BETA-ADRENERGIC BLOCKING AGENTS

Examples	• For angina pectoris: —Atenolol (Tenormin) —Nadolol (Corgard) —Propranolol (Inderal) • After myocardial infarction: —Metoprolol (Lopressor) —Propranolol (Inderal) —Timolol (Blocadren) • Antiarrhythmic: —Propranolol (Inderal) • Antihypertensives: —Atenolol (Tenormin) —Labetalol (Normodyne, Trandate) —Nadolol (Corgard) —Pindolol (Visken) —Timolol (Blocadren)
Actions	• Decrease heart rate and myocardial contractility • Decrease myocardial oxygen demand and improve balance between oxygen supply and demand • Increase refractory period of atrioventricular node
Use	• Limit infarct size and decrease mortality • Prevent or reduce acute ischemic attacks in patients with angina pectoris • Control dysrhythmias, including supraventricular tachydysrhythmias (such as atrial fibrillation) and ventricular tachycardias • Control hypertension
Side effects	• Bronchospasm (especially in patients with underlying lung disease) • Bradycardia and heart block • Nausea, vomiting, and diarrhea
Cautions	• Should be used cautiously in patients with congestive heart failure, bronchial asthma, or chronic obstructive pulmonary disease • Can mask symptoms of hypoglycemia in patients with diabetes mellitus • Do not discontinue medication abruptly, gradually reduce; abruptly stopping medication may exacerbate angina or cause a myocardial infarction or dysrhythmias.
Nursing responsibilities	• Monitor the patient's pulse rate and rhythm carefully. • Monitor diabetic patients carefully for indications of hypoglycemia; monitor blood glucose levels.

• postinfarct angina
—Assess for symptoms of angina.
—Implement measures as outlined in "Angina Pectoris" in this section.
• pericarditis
—Assess for symptoms (see Characteristics of noncardiac chest pain, pages 184 and 185).
—Notify the doctor if signs are present.
—Administer medications, as ordered, including mild analgesics, nonsteroidal anti-inflammatory agents, and steroids (for pericarditis unresponsive to other medication).
—Explain the cause and treatment to the patient and his family.
• deep vein thrombosis (see "Deep Vein Thrombosis" and "Deep Vein Thrombosis, Prevention of" in this section for details)
• systemic arterial embolus (signs and symptoms and treatment depend on the tissue affected).

Rationale and comments: Several complications can develop during the rehabilitation period.
• Dysrhythmias may develop for many reasons, including electrolyte imbalances, hypoxia, or damage to the electrical conducting system.
• CHF may develop later in the rehabilitation period secondary to damage to the ventricular wall.
• If extension of the original infarct or reinfarction develops, it frequently occurs about 5 days after the original infarct.
• Postinfarct angina usually indicates the presence of multivessel coronary artery disease. It may occur at rest or with activity. Further medical intervention (such as coronary artery bypass grafting or percutaneous transluminal coronary angioplasty) may be necessary to prevent a second infarct.
• Pericarditis, a common cause of noncardiac chest pain after AMI, is caused by extension of the infarction to the pericardial surface, resulting in local, sometimes extensive inflammation. Pericarditis produces chest pain that can mimic the pain of AMI and can be frightening to the patient and his family; explaining its cause and treatment can help alleviate some of their fears.
• In some patients, mural thrombi form in the left ventricle after AMI. Emboli break off, travel through arterial circulation, and may lodge in any artery, including those which supply the brain, kidneys, and intestines. Consult a medical-surgical textbook for details.

☑ **Intervention 9**
Assist with evaluating the patient's progress.
• Monitor the patient's response to increasing activity (see "Activity Intolerance, Potential for" in Section I for specific parameters).
• Monitor the development or progression of complications.

☑ **Intervention 10**
Assist with prescribed diagnostic tests used to evaluate the extent of myocardial damage and probable patient prognosis. Commonly used diagnostic tests include:
• exercise stress test
• exercise stress test with radionuclide imaging

• Holter monitor
• multiple-gated acquisition study (MUGA) (resting or exercise)
• technetium pyrophosphate scan
• thallium scan (resting or exercise)
• cardiac catheterization.

See *Diagnostic tests: coronary artery disease, angina, myocardial infarction, congestive heart failure*, pages 122 to 127, for details about these tests.

Rationale and comments: A patient's home activity prescription is based on assessment of the amount of damage to the myocardium. Diagnostic measures can provide valuable information about the safe level of activity for each patient, the patient's degree of risk for experiencing a second cardiac event, and left ventricular function. Specific information can help decrease the patient's and his family's anxiety before discharge.

Occlusive Arterial Disease

ASSOCIATED NURSING DIAGNOSES
Activity Intolerance
Anxiety
Bowel Elimination, Alteration in: Constipation
Comfort, Alteration in: Acute Pain
Depression, Reactive: Situational
Family Processes, Alteration in
Grieving, Individual Patient
Self-Concept, Alteration in
Skin Integrity, Impaired
Skin Integrity, Potential for Impairment
Sleep-Pattern Disturbance

ASSOCIATED TEACHING PLANS
Atherosclerosis: Disease Process and Risk Factors
Cardiac Anatomy and Physiology: Heart and Blood Vessels
Cardiovascular Disease Risk Factors: Cigarette Smoking
Cardiovascular Disease Risk Factors: Diabetes Mellitus and Atherosclerosis
Cardiovascular Disease Risk Factors: Dietary Measures to Control
    Hyperlipidemia
Hypertension, Essential: Disease Process and Risk Factors
Medication Guidelines
Occlusive Arterial Disease: Disease Process and Home Care

Interventions and rationales
☑ **Intervention 1**
Assess the patient for the following signs and symptoms of occlusive arterial disease:
• intermittent claudication
  —pain that occurs with walking and disappears when the patient stops walking and stands quietly
  —often described as an ache, a cramp, severe fatigue, or numbness usually occurring in the calf or leg
  —may radiate to the thigh, buttock, or foot
• rest pain
  —pain that occurs in the foot or toes while the patient is at rest
  —may be relieved or lessened when the foot is placed in a dependent position
  —described as severe or unrelenting
  —often disturbs the patient at night

• complaint of cold feet or legs
• diminished or absent peripheral pulses in the affected leg
• postural color changes (With moderate to severe disease, feet turn pale when legs are elevated; when returned to a dependent position, feet develop rubor in response to hypoxia that develops when legs are elevated.)
• trophic changes including:
—feet cold to the touch
—hair loss noted on the leg
—brittle toenails
—dry, scaly skin
—development of ischemic ulcers on the toes and heels
• edema in the lower leg when the leg is placed in a dependent position for a prolonged period.

Rationale and comments: Occlusive arterial disease is caused by atherosclerosis in one or more peripheral arteries. Intermittent claudication may be one of the first symptoms the patient notices. It occurs when the exercising muscles demand more oxygen than the diseased arteries can supply. Pain at rest indicates increasing severity of disease; the blood supply is no longer adequate to prevent ischemia, even at rest. Trophic changes occur as the disease progresses secondary to impaired cellular nutrition caused by the reduced blood flow.

Impaired circulation to the legs and feet can also result from other causes (see *Selected causes of impaired arterial circulation,* page 196).

☑ Intervention 2
Implement the prescribed medical orders regarding:
• smoking
—Discourage the patient from smoking (smoking causes vasoconstriction, which can further impair circulation to the legs).
• activity; orders commonly include:
—allowing patients with mild to moderate disease and no open lesions to ambulate as condition permits
—restricting patients with significant open lesions or ulcers to bed rest with bathroom privileges (bed rest helps to promote healing by decreasing oxygen demand of the legs)
• diet; often restricted to one low in saturated fats and low cholesterol.

☑ Intervention 3
Administer the prescribed medications, which may include:
• analgesics to relieve the severe pain of occlusive arterial disease; those prescribed may range from salicylates or propoxyphene hydrochloride (Darvon) to morphine sulfate.
• pentoxifylline (Trental); some doctors believe this drug will reduce intermittent claudication.
• vasodilators; this is controversial. Some doctors believe that selected vasodilators improve peripheral circulation; others, that they show no positive effect and may increase ischemia by decreasing blood pressure.

SELECTED CAUSES OF IMPAIRED ARTERIAL CIRCULATION

Acute arterial occlusion

Signs and symptoms	• Pain • Pallor below the level of occlusion • Paresthesias • Paralysis • Decreased pulse or loss of pulse distal to the point of occlusion • Skin temperature cold below the level of occlusion
Causes	• Emboli generated as complication of mural thrombus formation after acute myocardial infarction, atrial fibrillation, valve replacement surgery, or cardiac bypass surgery • Thrombosis in artery at the site of atherosclerotic lesion, resulting in total occlusion of artery • Thrombus formed at arterial puncture site after arteriogram
Treatment	• Embolectomy • Thromboendarterectomy • Arterial bypass graft • Conservative measures, including I.V. heparin, bed rest, elevation of head of bed, relief of spasm and pain

Thromboangiitis obliterans (Buerger's disease)

Signs and symptoms	• Intermittent claudication, initially in the feet; may later spread to the calf • Pain at rest (often worse at night) • Pain in the fingers or toes • Sensitivity to cold in the hands • Ulcers at the tips of toes or fingers
Causes	• Occurs only in smokers; thought to be some type of sensitivity reaction to tobacco • May result in chronic occlusive arterial disease
Treatment	• No smoking • Conservative measures similar to those used for occlusive arterial disease • Amputation if conservative measures fail or severe gangrene or infection occurs

Raynaud's disease

Signs and symptoms	• Intermittent color changes of the fingers or toes; initially, digits become pale or white, then turn cyanotic • Bilateral involvement • May occur spontaneously or in response to cold or stress • No evidence of occlusive arterial disease • In later stages, possibility of bilateral gangrene
Causes	• Symptoms caused by vasospasm of unknown etiology • May or may not be accompanied by a connective tissue disorder, such as systemic lupus erythematosus or scleroderma
Treatment	• Avoidance of exposure to thermal, mechanical, or chemical trauma • Medication to control spasm

☑ Intervention 4

Take appropriate measures to control diabetes mellitus, when applicable. (Consult a medical-surgical textbook for a complete discussion on care of patients with diabetes mellitus.)
• Monitor the patient's blood glucose levels and report abnormal results.
• Administer prescribed hypoglycemic agents.
• Provide a calorie-restricted diet, as ordered.

☑ Intervention 5

Prepare the patient for prescribed diagnostic tests, including:
• segmental plethysmography
• Doppler ultrasound
• angiography.
(See *Tests used to diagnose occlusive arterial disease in the legs,* pages 198 to 200.)

☑ Intervention 6

Implement measures to increase blood flow to the legs and to prevent injury (see "Skin Integrity, Potential for Impairment" in Section I for specific interventions).

Rationale and comments: Taking measures to increase blood flow and prevent injury decreases the risk of serious complications for the patient with occlusive arterial disease.

☑ Intervention 7

If an ischemic ulcer or other wounds are present, implement the following measures:
• Follow the interventions outlined in "Skin Integrity, Impaired" in Section I.
• Observe ulcers or wounds for indications of deterioration, including:
—signs of infection, such as redness, warmth, and purulent drainage
—failure of ulcers or wounds to heal
—development of blackened areas (infarcted tissue) on heels or toes (dry gangrene).

Rationale and comments: Ischemic ulcers may occur spontaneously or after some type of trauma. Common sites include the heels, ankles, and toes. Ulcers may become infected or progress to gangrene. Patients with severe disease may develop dry gangrene, which may be caused by trauma, acute arterial occlusion, or overwhelming infection.

☑ Intervention 8

Implement prescribed measures used in the long-term medical management of occlusive arterial disease, including:
• a walking program (see "Activity Intolerance" in Section I)
• alteration of the patient's risk factors for atherosclerosis
• measures to promote blood flow and prevent injury to legs.

(Text continues on page 200.)

TESTS USED TO DIAGNOSE OCCLUSIVE ARTERIAL DISEASE IN THE LEGS

Plethysmography

Purpose	• Evaluates blood flow through the arteries of the leg and identifies abnormalities • May confirm diagnosis of occlusive arterial disease • Provides little information about arterial anatomy
Procedure	• This noninvasive procedure involves minimal patient risk. • Blood pressure cuffs are applied to arms, ankles, calves, and thighs. The cuffs are inflated and pressures are taken according to a set protocol.
Preparation	• Explain the procedure to the patient. • If the test is to be done at the patient's bedside, make sure the room is comfortably warm to prevent vasoconstriction. • Medicate the patient for pain before the test, if indicated.
Postprocedure	• None

Doppler flow studies or ultrasound

Purpose	• Helps to determine the presence of arterial occlusion
Procedure	• This noninvasive procedure involves minimal patient risk. • Procedure uses sound waves to evaluate blood flow. • Procedure may be done at the patient's bedside.
Preparation	• Explain the procedure to the patient. • Tell the patient that he will need to lie still during the test. • If procedure is to be done at the patient's bedside, make sure the room is comfortably warm.
Postprocedure	• None

Angiography

Purpose	• Identifies specific areas of occlusion in peripheral arterial circulation • Provides information about the anatomy of the involved arteries, which assists in evaluating the patient for possible bypass surgery
Procedure	• A catheter is placed in the patient's arterial circulation and advanced to a designated spot (depends on artery to be evaluated). • When the catheter is in place, contrast medium is injected and serial pictures of the movement of the medium are taken. • The patient may feel a sensation of warmth or flushing when the contrast medium is injected. • Procedure can last 30 to 60 minutes. • Risks of the procedure include allergic reaction to the contrast medium, hemorrhage, arterial occlusion at the insertion site, and cerebrovascular accident.

TESTS USED TO DIAGNOSE OCCLUSIVE
ARTERIAL DISEASE IN THE LEGS *(continued)*

Angiography *(continued)*

Preparation
- Obtain the patient's informed consent according to institutional policy.
- Assess the patient for allergies to shellfish, iodine, or other contrast media. Notify the radiologist if allergy is suspected.
- Scrub and shave the insertion site according to institutional policy.
- Depending on the institution's policy, the patient may have full liquids or may be given nothing by mouth.
- Premedicate the patient with a mild sedative, as ordered.
- Start an I.V. line or heparin lock, as ordered.
- Complete other preprocedure routines according to institutional policy.

Postprocedure
- Maintain a pressure dressing at the insertion site.
- Check the patient's vital signs every 15 minutes until he is stable.
- Keep the patient on bed rest for 4 to 8 hours, as ordered, with the head of the bed elevated less than 30 degrees.
- Check the patient's pulse distal to the insertion site; evaluate for changes from preprocedure to postprocedure.
- Check the leg for changes in warmth and color, comparing preprocedure with postprocedure findings.
- Check the insertion site for bleeding or hematoma formation. If significant bleeding occurs, notify the doctor and apply direct pressure that is sufficient to control bleeding but not occlude the distal pulse.
- Unless contraindicated, instruct the patient to drink increased amounts of fluids.
- Medicate the patient for pain, as indicated and as ordered.

Digital subtraction angiography

Purpose
- Screening measure for occlusive arterial disease
- Evaluates the effectiveness of percutaneous transluminal angioplasty (PTA) or arterial bypass surgery
- Aids in defining anatomy and lesions before PTA or arterial bypass surgery

Procedure
- This angiography procedure uses electronic enhancement of images.
- Images are obtained before and after injection of contrast medium. With the aid of a computer, these images are enhanced and manipulated to obtain the desired information.
- Contrast medium may be injected I.V. through a peripheral or central line or intra-arterially.
- Patient may experience a feeling of warmth or flushing when contrast medium is injected.

(continued)

TESTS USED TO DIAGNOSE OCCLUSIVE ARTERIAL DISEASE IN THE LEGS *(continued)*

Digital subtraction angiography *(continued)*

Procedure *(continued)*	• I.V. administration is contraindicated for patients with renal failure, congestive heart failure, or decreased cardiac output because of the increased volume and concentration of contrast medium used in I.V. studies. • Excessive movements by the patient can interfere with test results. The patient must be able to cooperate for a successful study. • Risks of the procedure may include allergic reaction to contrast medium, transient renal failure, and development of phlebitis or thrombosis at the insertion site.
Preparation	• Explain the procedure to the patient. • Obtain the patient's informed consent per institutional policy. • Assess the patient for allergies to shellfish, iodine, or other contrast media; notify the doctor if allergy is suspected. • Obtain any ordered diagnostic studies before the test, including such renal function studies as blood urea nitrogen or creatinine levels. • Give the patient nothing by mouth for at least 6 hours before the test. • Shave and prepare the site, as ordered. • Administer premedication, as ordered. • Complete other preprocedure care per institutional policy.
Postprocedure	• For arterial administration, see the postprocedure care for *Angiography,* above. • For I.V. administration: —maintain a pressure dressing at the injection site. —instruct the patient to drink increased amounts of fluids, unless contraindicated. —assess and record the patient's intake and output; notify the doctor of decreased urine output. —resume activity according to preprocedure orders.

Rationale and comments: Long-term management will depend on the severity of the disease and the patient's overall health. Medical management may be prescribed for patients with mild to moderate disease and for those who are not considered good surgical risks.

☑ **Intervention 9**

Assist with prescribed care of the patient undergoing surgical treatment for occlusive arterial disease; common surgical management includes:
• peripheral vascular bypass surgery (see "Peripheral Vascular Bypass Surgery" in this section)
• amputation (see "Amputation, Leg [for Vascular Disease]" in this section)
• percutaneous transluminal angioplasty (PTA).

Rationale and comments: Peripheral vascular bypass surgery has become the treatment of choice to restore blood flow past the point of an athero-sclerotic lesion. Percutaneous transluminal angioplasty is used for selected patients, including those for whom bypass surgery poses too great a risk. Amputation is used as a last resort.

☑ **Intervention 10**
Implement appropriate care for patients undergoing PTA.
• Assess the patient and his family regarding their knowledge about the procedure.
• Assess the patient's and family's anxiety level.
• Implement teaching as follows:
—Explain that a balloon-tipped catheter will be inserted into the arterial circulation. Under fluoroscopy, the catheter will be advanced to the point of the atherosclerotic lesion. Then, when the catheter is correctly positioned, the balloon will be inflated to compress the lesion to open the arterial lumen, then deflated.
—Also explain that several cycles of inflation and deflation may be nec-essary to open the artery to the fullest extent possible.
—Tell them the risks associated with the procedure, including rupture of the vessel and emboli formation caused by a piece of the lesion breaking off and entering arterial circulation.
• Implement preprocedure measures (see Intervention 3 in "Percutaneous Transluminal Coronary Angioplasty" in this section for specific information).

☑ **Intervention 11**
Implement appropriate, immediate postprocedure care after PTA, including:
• checking the patient's vital signs every 15 minutes until he is stable
• implementing measures to decrease the risk of bleeding from the puncture site, including:
—keeping the patient in bed with the head of the bed elevated less than 30 degrees for 8 hours or as ordered (Patients who were taking anti-coagulants before undergoing PTA may be on bed rest for up to 18 hours.)
—instructing the patient to minimally flex his hip for 24 hours
—maintaining a pressure dressing over the puncture site
—assessing the puncture site closely for signs of bleeding or hematoma formation
—if significant bleeding occurs from the puncture site, applying direct pressure to the site sufficient to control bleeding but not to totally occlude the distal pulse
• monitoring the patient closely for development of an arterial occlusion at the puncture site, which includes:
—checking the pulse distal to the puncture site frequently
—assessing the extremity for color and temperature changes
—notifying the doctor if any of the above signs occur.
Rationale and comments: Hemorrhage from the puncture site is one complication that can occur following PTA. Abrupt occlusion of the artery at the puncture site is another complication. Signs of an abrupt occlusion

include loss of the pulse distal to the puncture site, a change in skin color from normal to pale or mottled, and a change in skin temperature from warm to cold.

☑ Intervention 12

After the patient has undergone PTA, implement the following measures:
• Assess the quality of arterial circulation in the patient's affected extremity every 4 hours or as needed; assess for:
—presence and quality of peripheral pulses; if peripheral pulse is not palpable, check for the pulse with a Doppler transducer, if available
—color and temperature of the extremity.
• Notify the doctor if the patient has:
—a decreased pulse rate or loss of pulse
—changes in skin color and temperature to pale and cold
—increased or recurrent pain in the extremity.
• Administer medications, as prescribed, including anticoagulants to decrease the risk of reocclusion (see *Anticoagulants,* page 154).

Rationale and comments: Reocclusion may occur after PTA. Loss of the peripheral pulse, change in skin temperature from warm to cold, and change in skin color from normal to pale or mottled are classic signs of arterial reocclusion.

Pacemaker Insertion, Permanent

ASSOCIATED NURSING DIAGNOSES
Anxiety
Depression, Reactive: Situational
Self-Concept, Alteration in

ASSOCIATED TEACHING PLANS
Cardiac Anatomy and Physiology: Heart and Blood Vessels
Medication Guidelines
Pacemaker, Permanent: Home Care
Radial Pulse Measurement

Interventions and rationales
☑ **Intervention 1**
Assist in collecting preoperative data, including:
• vital signs
• reason for pacemaker insertion (including underlying rhythm disturbance)
• recent history of such clinical signs and symptoms as:
—decreased activity tolerance and fatigue
—dizziness and syncope
—convulsive seizure activity
—slowed heart rate
• patient and family knowledge about pacemaker insertion and pacemakers in general
• patient and family emotional response to the need for a permanent pacemaker and to the impending surgical procedure.

Rationale and comments: A pacemaker is inserted because the heart's intrinsic electrical conducting system is not functioning effectively.
• Knowing the specific underlying problem can assist in evaluating pacemaker function postoperatively. Many clinical signs are related to a drop in cardiac output secondary to the rhythm disturbance.
• Patients may know little about pacemakers and their function, or they may be misinformed because of what family and friends have told them. Lack of information or misinformation about the care and functioning of pacemakers in current use may increase anxiety.
• Patients may respond to changes in body image caused by the insertion of a permanent pacemaker. Knowing how the patient feels, the nurse can help the patient and family adjust.

☑ Intervention 2

Assist with preoperative preparation.

• Obtain the patient's informed consent according to institutional policy.

• Give the patient nothing by mouth before the procedure.

Based on the following information about endocardial insertion, explain the procedure to the patient.

—After administration of a local anesthetic, a 3″ to 4″ (7.6 to 10.2 cm) incision will be made in the subcutaneous tissue of the upper chest for pacemaker insertion. Then, the pacemaker leads will be inserted through a major vein and positioned in the correct part of the heart under fluoroscopy.

—The patient may be asked to cough or to deep-breathe to verify lead placement, as correct positioning is essential for proper functioning.

—Warn the patient that he will be covered in sterile drapes but that he will be able to communicate. (Patients sometimes complain of feeling smothered or isolated during this procedure.)

—EKG monitor leads and an I.V. line will be attached during the procedure.

—Pacemaker functioning and programming will be tested before the patient is moved out of the operating room (OR). (Pacer functioning will be tested several times during the healing process; the initial check occurs in the OR.)

—If the patient is admitted only for pacemaker insertion, the usual length of stay is 3 to 4 days.

• Implement other preoperative teaching and care, as indicated.

• Take appropriate measures to decrease the patient's anxiety (see "Anxiety" in Section I).

☑ Intervention 3

Obtain baseline data on the patient after his return from the OR or recovery room, including such information as:

• the type of pacemaker and leads inserted, including:

—manufacturer's name and the model number

—type of leads (endocardial or epicardial)

—unipolar or bipolar

• pacemaker programming, including:

—lower rate limit

—upper rate limit (when applicable)

—mode of function (inhibited or triggered)

—programmed intervals

—other pertinent programming information

• end-of-life characteristics for the specific pacemaker inserted.

Rationale and comments: Several types of pacemakers are currently in use (see *Selected pacemaker types* and *Pacemaker coding*, page 208, for information). Manufacturers make pacemakers that are similar in function but that vary in some characteristics. To evaluate and correct any pacemaker malfunction, the specific model and setting must be known. This information should be readily available on the the patient's chart and should be given to the patient on discharge.

SELECTED PACEMAKER TYPES

VVI or ventricular demand pacemaker

Description
- Single-chamber pacing mode
- Paces the ventricle only
- Senses electrical activity in the ventricle only
- Inhibited by electrical activity sensed in ventricle only

Indications
- Patients with atrial fibrillation, atrial flutter, atrial standstill, or greatly hypertrophied atria
- Patients who would not benefit hemodynamically from atrial contraction
- Patients with many types of bradydysrhythmias

Mechanisms
- Pacemaker contains an internal clock that times each cardiac cycle. The clock is started when:
  —the pacemaker senses the heart's intrinsic electrical activity in the ventricle; if the next beat does not occur by the end of the prescribed interval (which is controlled by setting the pacemaker's rate), the pacemaker fires to stimulate the ventricles to contract. The clock then resets. If an appropriate beat occurs within the prescribed interval, the pacemaker does not fire and the clock is again reset.
  —the pacemaker senses a paced ventricular beat; if the next beat does not occur by the end of the prescribed interval, the pacemaker fires to stimulate the ventricles to contract. The clock then resets. If an appropriate intrinsic beat occurs within the prescribed interval, the pacemaker does not fire and the clock resets.

Rate settings
- Lower rate limit only

Advantages
- Pacemaker is easily inserted with minimal associated risks.
- Maintenance and follow-up are easy.
- Unit is economical to insert and maintain.
- Pacemaker unit is small and cosmetically acceptable to most patients.
- Pacemaker generator has long life.

Disadvantages
- Onset of VVI pacing may induce pacemaker syndrome in some patients.
- Pacemaker rate cannot change in response to increased or decreased metabolic demands.

DVI or AV sequential pacemaker

Description
- Single-chamber sensing; dual-chamber pacing mode
- Paces atrium or atrium and ventricle in correct sequence
- Senses electrical activity in ventricle only; does not sense any intrinsic electrical activity in atrium
- Inhibited when unit senses intrinsic ventricular activity

(continued)

SELECTED PACEMAKER TYPES *(continued)*

DVI or AV sequential pacemaker *(continued)*

Indications	• Patients who require atrial and ventricular contraction in the correct sequence to maintain sufficient cardiac output • Patients who do not have atrial fibrillation or flutter
Mechanisms	• Pacemaker stimulates the atrium and ventricle to contract in the correct sequence when the intrinsic ventricular rate drops below the programmed rate. • Pacemaker is inhibited when the intrinsic ventricular rate exceeds the programmed rate.
Rate settings	• Lower rate limit only
Advantages	• Pacemaker increases cardiac output in some patients by preserving atrial contraction. • Unit can prevent pacemaker syndrome by preserving atrial contraction.
Disadvantages	• Because the pacemaker does not sense intrinsic atrial electrical activity, it may produce atrial dysrhythmias by stimulating the atria at a vulnerable time in the cardiac cycle. • Unit has a shorter pacemaker generator life. • Pacemaker cannot be reprogrammed to other modes as the DDD pacemaker can (see below). • Pacemaker rate cannot increase in response to increased metabolic demands.

DDD or universal pacemaker

Description	• Can pace the atrium, ventricle, or both as needed • Senses electrical activity in both the atrium and ventricle • Uses triggered and inhibited modes of response as needed • Dual-chamber pacing and sensing
Indications	• Patients who will benefit from a paced rate that increases or decreases in response to the body's metabolic demands, such as those with an active life-style • Patients who have stable atrial electrical activity (that is, no atrial fibrillation or atrial flutter) • Patients who have documented deterioration with another type of pacing • Patients with pacemaker syndrome
Mechanisms	• DDD pacemakers can function in several different ways: —When the patient's intrinsic atrial rate drops below the programmed rate, the pacemaker stimulates the atrium to contract at a preset rate. —If a ventricular response does not occur by the end of a programmed interval after the pacemaker's stimulation of the atrium, the pacemaker then stimulates ventricular contraction.

SELECTED PACEMAKER TYPES *(continued)*

DDD or universal pacemaker *(continued)*

Mechanisms *(continued)*	—If the patient's intrinsic atrial rate exceeds the minimum programmed rate, the pacemaker senses in the ventricle for appropriate ventricular electrical activity after each atrial impulse. —If appropriate ventricular activity does not occur by the end of the programmed interval, the pacemaker stimulates ventricular contraction. An upper rate limit is programmed into the pacemaker; the pacemaker will stimulate ventricular contraction at the rate determined by the atrial rate unless the atrial rate exceeds the programmed upper limit. —If the atrial rate exceeds the upper limit, the pacemaker gradually slows the ventricular response (using complex mechanisms) to prevent the patient's rate from exceeding that limit. —If the patient's intrinsic atrial rate exceeds the programmed rate and appropriate ventricular response occurs by the end of the programmed interval, the pacemaker is inhibited and does not fire.
Rate settings	• Upper and lower rate limits set
Advantages	• Pacemaker can fire at increased or decreased rates as indicated by the patient's metabolic demands. • Pacemaker preserves the normal sequence of atrial-ventricular contraction. • Unit may prevent pacemaker syndrome. • Pacemaker may increase cardiac output by preserving the atrial contraction in the normal sequence. • Pacemaker may be reprogrammed into another mode using noninvasive techniques, if needed.
Disadvantages	• Pacemaker is more difficult to insert and monitor correctly. • Pacemaker is also more expensive to insert and maintain. • Pacemaker may cause dysrhythmias. • Unit may pace the heart at a rate faster than the patient can tolerate (may be corrected by lowering the upper rate limit). • Unit has a shorter pacemaker generator life.

• All pacemakers give warning signs that the pulse generator (usually lithium-powered) needs to be replaced. These characteristics vary from pacemaker to pacemaker. To permit prompt battery replacement, the individual characteristics should be known.

• See *Glossary of pacemaker-related terms,* pages 209 and 210, for an explanation of commonly used terminology.

☑ **Intervention 4**

Implement the prescribed medical orders.

• Take the patient's vital signs as follows:

—every 15 minutes until the patient is stable

—when stable, every 4 hours or as indicated by the patient's condition.

PACEMAKER CODING

The following coding is based on Intersociety Commission for Heart Disease guidelines. The first three letters are most commonly used in coding.

First letter	Identifies which chamber(s) are paced V = ventricle A = atrium D = both
Second letter	Identifies the chamber(s) in which intrinsic electrical activity can be sensed by the pacemaker V = ventricle A = atrium D = both 0 = none
Third letter	Identifies the mode of response or interaction between the pacemaker activity and the intrinsic electrical activity of the heart I = inhibited T = triggered D = dual R = reverse 0 = no response to sensed beats
Fourth letter	Identifies programmability P = simple programming changes may be made noninvasively M = multiple programming changes may be made noninvasively 0 = no changes may be made noninvasively
Fifth letter	Describes special features that may treat or prevent dysrhythmias

• Keep the patient on continuous EKG monitoring.
• Maintain a patent I.V. or heparin lock, as ordered.
• Have the patient ambulate on the 1st postoperative day unless contraindicated by other medical problems.
• Administer any prescribed medications, which often include:
—mild analgesics for incisional pain
—prophylactic antibiotics (usually I.V.)
—other medications as indicated by concurrent medical problems.

☑ **Intervention 5**
Implement the following measures to prevent infection:
• Check the patient's vital signs every 4 hours.
• Assess the patient's wound incision over the pacemaker pocket daily for signs of infection.
• Use strict sterile technique with any dressing changes or invasive procedures.

GLOSSARY OF PACEMAKER-RELATED TERMS

Capture	Designated chamber of the heart depolarizes appropriately when stimulated to do so by pacemaker stimulus. Failure to capture can be a serious type of pacemaker malfunction.
Demand pacemaker	Type of pacemaker currently in use that senses patient's own intrinsic electrical activity; it does not compete with the patient's underlying rhythm.
Dual mode of response	Seen in newer, more complex pacemakers. These pacemakers use a combination of inhibited and triggered modes of response; they respond to some sensed stimuli in the heart by inhibiting pacemaker-initiated depolarization of the designated chamber; to other stimuli, they respond by triggering the chamber to depolarize.
Endocardial leads	Type of pacemaker leads that are inserted through a major vein into the inside layer of the heart.
Epicardial leads	Type of pacemaker leads that are inserted through a thoracic incision and attached to the outside of the heart.
Fixed rate or asynchronous pacemaker	Type of pacemaker rarely used currently for permanent insertion. Paces ventricle at a set rate; does not sense intrinsic activity. Serious dysrhythmias can develop as a result of competition between paced rhythm and patient's intrinsic rhythm.
Inhibited	Describes one form of interaction between pacemaker activity and intrinsic electrical activity in designated chamber(s) of the heart. With this type of response, the pacemaker does not fire when it senses appropriate electrical activity. Pacemaker then resets itself and continues to sense for appropriate electrical activity.
Intervals	One of the parameters that can be programmed or set in the pacemaker. It is related to rate-limit settings.
Leads and electrode system	Delivers a generated impulse to the cardiac muscle. It connects a pulse generator to the heart.
Pacer artifact	Marking or deflection on EKG tracing that indicates electrical energy has been delivered by the pacemaker.
Pacemaker pocket	Incision in subcutaneous tissue (usually of the upper chest) where the pulse generator is implanted.
Pacemaker syndrome	Group of symptoms that may occur in patients after undergoing insertion of a venticular demand pacemaker. Symptoms include fatigue, dizziness, dyspnea, and postural hypotension. The syndrome is thought to result from the loss of atrial-ventricular synchrony that occurs in ventricular demand pacing.

(continued)

GLOSSARY OF PACEMAKER-RELATED TERMS (continued)

Programmability	Characteristic of some more recently developed pacemakers that allows the settings, functions, and parameters of the pacemaker to be changed noninvasively.
Pulse generator	Consists of the power source (usually lithium) for the pacemaker and electronic circuitry necessary for the pacemaker to perform its specified functions.
Refractory period	Interval of time during which the pacemaker is nonresponsive to any incoming stimuli.
Sensing	Pacemaker's ability to detect intrinsic electrical activity in the designated heart chambers.
Sensitivity setting	Setting on the pacemaker that determines the ability of the pulse generator to recognize intrinsic electrical activity of the heart.
Stimulation threshold	Amount of electrical current or energy needed to stimulate the desired depolarization of the paced chamber.
Telemetry	Ability of the pacemaker to transmit information back from the pacemaker to the doctor or programmer. Several different types of information can be obtained, including the date and reason for implantation, a "read back" of newly programmed changes so the programmer can verify accuracy, and information regarding the functional state of the pacemaker system.
Triggered	Another type of interaction between pacemaker activity and intrinsic cardiac electrical activity in the designated heart chambers. When the pacemaker senses the appropriate stimulus in the designated heart chamber, it responds by stimulating the chamber to depolarize.

• Administer prophylactic antibiotics, as ordered.
• If signs and symptoms of infection develop, notify the surgeon immediately.

Rationale and comments: Infection, a serious complication that may occur after pacemaker insertion, can result in reoperation for the removal of the infected pacemaker and reinsertion of a replacement. It can also result in septicemia or endocarditis.

☑ Intervention 6
Assess the patient for proper pacemaker function.
• Maintain continuous EKG monitoring, as ordered. (Correct EKG interpretation of the pacemaker requires specialized knowledge, which exceeds the scope of this text.)
• Obtain a 12-lead EKG, as ordered.
• Check the patient's pulse rate and rhythm every 4 hours, and assess for the following:
  —the rate dropping below the lower rate limit of the pacemaker (With proper pacemaker functioning, the pulse rate should never drop below

the minimum rate set. Rates that are consistently or significantly below minimum indicate malfunction.)
—the rate exceeding the upper rate limit, when applicable (With DDD pacing, the fastest rate at which the heart can be paced is set. If the patient's intrinsic rate exceeds the upper rate limit, the EKG pattern should be checked; the patient may have developed a tachydysrhythmia.)
—development of an irregular pulse rate (Dysrhythmias may indicate pacemaker malfunction.)
—complaint of palpitations.
• Assess for signs of decreased cardiac output, including:
—fatigue
—dizziness
—malaise or weakness
—postural hypotension
—sporadic sensation of fullness in the chest or neck
—continued or worsening symptoms experienced before pacemaker insertion.
• Assess for exacerbation of congestive heart failure (CHF); see "Congestive Heart Failure" in this section for details. (In patients with CHF or myocardial damage, a paced heart rate that is too high can precipitate signs of acute pump failure.)

Rationale and comments: Assessing the patient's clinical status is important in evaluating pacemaker functioning. Decreased cardiac output may result from pacemaker failure, inappropriate pacemaker settings, loss of normal atrial and ventricular sequential contraction (seen with some types of pacemakers), and inability of some types of pacemakers to meet increased metabolic demands of the body.

☑ **Intervention 7**
Assist the patient and family to adapt emotionally to the permanent pacemaker.

Rationale and comments: Some patients may use denial or anger or feel a loss of control with pacemaker insertion.

☑ **Intervention 8**
Assess for socioeconomic or financial concerns, and make appropriate referrals, as needed. Areas of concern may include:
• change in employment or employability secondary to insertion of permanent pacemaker
• obtaining new or additional life insurance.

Rationale and comments: Some research has indicated that employability and insurance present problems for patients with permanent pacemakers.

Percutaneous Transluminal Coronary Angioplasty

ASSOCIATED NURSING DIAGNOSES
Activity Intolerance
Activity Intolerance, Potential for
Anxiety
Noncompliance
Self-Concept, Alteration in
Sleep-Pattern Disturbance

ASSOCIATED TEACHING PLANS
Atherosclerosis: Disease Process and Risk Factors
Cardiac Anatomy and Physiology: Heart and Blood Vessels
Cardiovascular Disease Risk Factors: Cigarette Smoking
Cardiovascular Disease Risk Factors: Diabetes Mellitus and Atherosclerosis
Cardiovascular Disease Risk Factors: Dietary Measures to Control
    Hyperlipidemia
Hypertension, Essential: Disease Process and Risk Factors
Medication Guidelines
Stress Management

Interventions and rationales
☑ **Intervention 1**
Assist in the preoperative assessment of:
• the patient's and family's knowledge about percutaneous transluminal coronary angioplasty (PTCA)
• the patient's and family's level of anxiety
• pertinent baseline data including:
—vital signs
—presence and quality of peripheral pulses
—EKG, if ordered
—cardiac enzyme studies, if ordered
—type and cross match for ordered blood transfusions.

Rationale and comments: PTCA may be an elective, scheduled procedure to prevent myocardial infarction. It may also be an emergency procedure to limit the size of an evolving infarction.

☑ **Intervention 2**
Implement preprocedure teaching using the following information:
• The goal of PTCA is to restore blood flow to areas of the myocardium by mechanically dilating one or more occluded coronary arteries.

• With the patient under local anesthesia, a catheter will be inserted through the skin into the femoral artery. Through the use of fluoroscopy, the catheter will be threaded through the vascular system until it is correctly positioned at the site of a blockage in the coronary artery.

• Once the catheter is positioned correctly, a balloon on the tip of the catheter will be inflated for 5 to 7 seconds; this inflation compresses the blockage, thereby opening the lumen of the artery and improving blood flow through it.

• Several cycles of inflation and deflation may be necessary to open the lumen optimally; the procedure may be repeated for more than one blockage.

• The patient may experience angina during the time that the balloon is inflated.

• The patient may be mildly sedated during the procedure, which may last 2 to 3 hours.

• Major risks associated with PTCA include:

—possible emergency coronary artery bypass grafting (CABG) surgery because of acute coronary occlusion or acute dissection of a coronary artery

—possible death (although this rarely occurs).

• Because of the risk that CABG surgery may be needed, patient teaching should include a brief description of intensive care unit procedures. This teaching should be carefully individualized; for some, discussion of CABG surgery may be too anxiety provoking.

Rationale and comments: Knowledge of the procedure and what to expect may help to decrease the patient's and family's anxiety and increase their ability to cope with a highly stressful situation.

☑ Intervention 3
Implement preparation for the procedure.

• Obtain the patient's informed consent according to institutional policy. (The operative permit often includes permission not only for PTCA but also for CABG surgery in the event that an emergency occurs.)

• Give the patient nothing by mouth before the procedure (6 to 8 hours, if possible).

• Prepare the insertion site (usually femoral); scrub and shave the site, as ordered.

• Start an I.V. line or heparin lock.

• Administer a mild sedative before the procedure, as ordered.

• Initiate other preoperative care according to institutional policy.

☑ Intervention 4
Implement appropriate, immediate postprocedural care.

• Check the patient's vital signs every 15 minutes until he is stable, assessing for changes indicative of complications, such as hemorrhage, acute myocardial infarction, or congestive heart failure.

• Maintain continuous EKG monitoring.

• Implement the following measures to decrease the risk of bleeding from the puncture site. (Note that heparin is administered during the procedure; it is not reversed. It may also be administered after the procedure for a period of time.)
—Keep the patient flat in bed until the catheter sheath is removed (usually, 2 to 8 hours after completion of the procedure, although this may vary).
—Keep the patient flat in bed (or with the head of the bed elevated less than 30 degrees) for 6 to 12 hours after sheath removal.
—Maintain a pressure dressing over the puncture site when the sheath is removed.
—Instruct the patient to flex his hip minimally during the first 24 hours.
—Observe the puncture site closely for bleeding and for hematoma formation.
—If significant bleeding occurs, place direct pressure on the site (sufficient to control bleeding but not enough to occlude the peripheral pulse), and notify the doctor immediately.

Rationale and comments: At the beginning of the PTCA procedure, a catheter sheath is introduced into the femoral artery to facilitate catheter insertion. At the end of the procedure, the sheath is often left in place for a period of time to permit rapid reinsertion of the catheter, if needed. Acute reocclusion and coronary artery spasm are two complications that may require reinsertion of the catheter to prevent myocardial damage. To prevent injury, the patient should be kept flat until the sheath is removed.

☑ Intervention 5
Monitor the patient for development of an arterial occlusion at the puncture site.
• Check the pulse distal to the puncture site every 15 minutes until the patient is stable, then every 1 to 4 hours as needed.
• Assess the extremity for changes in color and temperature.
• Notify the doctor if any changes occur.

Rationale and comments: After PTCA, a clot may form on the inside of the artery at the site used for catheter insertion. This clot can occlude the lumen of the artery and prevent blood flow to the distal part of the extremity. Signs and symptoms of occlusion include loss of the pulse distal to the occlusion, a change in the temperature in the extremity from warm to cold, and a change in skin color from normal to pale or mottled.

☑ Intervention 6
Monitor the patient for any signs of angina.
• Assess the patient for any complaints of chest pain and any signs or symptoms commonly associated with angina (see "Angina Pectoris" in this section for details).
• If an episode of chest pain occurs:
—Implement care as outlined in "Angina Pectoris" in this section.
—Check the patient's vital signs.
—Obtain a 12-lead EKG (may require a doctor's order in some institutions).
—Notify the doctor immediately.

—Be prepared to implement additional orders, including administering an I.V. nitroglycerin drip, administering sublingual nifedipine, and preparing the patient for repeat angiography or angioplasty.

—Take appropriate measures to reduce the patient's and family's anxiety.

Rationale and comments: Chest pain that occurs after PTCA may represent acute myocardial ischemia. The most common causes in the immediate postoperative period include acute coronary occlusion by spasm or embolus or dissection of the coronary artery resulting from damage to the intimal layer during the procedure. Immediate treatment is necessary to prevent myocardial damage.

✅ Intervention 7

Implement prescribed medical care regarding the patient's:

• activity

—Initially, the patient will be on bed rest, which may be advanced after 24 hours if his condition is stable.

—For patients who have had an acute myocardial infarction (AMI), see "Activity Intolerance, Potential for" in Section I for guidelines.

—Patients who have not had an MI may ambulate out of bed as tolerated.

• diet; the patient may be put on a low cholesterol, low saturated fat diet (commonly ordered).

• prescribed medications, including:

—antiplatelets (Antiplatelet medications may decrease the risk of acute coronary thrombosis after PTCA as well as the occurrence of reocclusion; see *Antiplatelet medications,* page 143.)

—calcium channel blockers (These may be used to decrease coronary artery spasm in selected patients; see *Calcium channel blockers,* page 120.)

—other medications as indicated by the patient's cardiovascular status.

✅ Intervention 8

Assist with measures to assess the patient's progress and the effectiveness of PTCA, including:

• monitoring the patient's response to activity

• preparing the patient for a stress test.

Rationale and comments: A stress test may be performed before or after discharge to evaluate the status of the coronary arteries (see *Diagnostic tests: coronary artery disease, angina, myocardial infarction, congestive heart failure* pages 122 to 127, for details).

Peripheral Vascular Bypass Surgery

ASSOCIATED NURSING DIAGNOSES
Anxiety
Comfort, Alteration in: Acute Pain
Nutrition, Alteration in: Less Than Body Requirements
Respiratory Function, Alteration in
Respiratory Function, Potential Alteration in
Skin Integrity, Impaired
Skin Integrity, Potential for Impairment
Sleep-Pattern Disturbance

ASSOCIATED TEACHING PLANS
Atherosclerosis: Disease Process and Risk Factors
Cardiac Anatomy and Physiology: Heart and Blood Vessels
Cardiovascular Disease Risk Factors: Cigarette Smoking
Cardiovascular Disease Risk Factors: Diabetes Mellitus and Atherosclerosis
Cardiovascular Disease Risk Factors: Dietary Measures to Control
    Hyperlipidemia
Hypertension, Essential: Disease Process and Risk Factors
Medication Guidelines
Occlusive Arterial Disease: Disease Process and Home Care
Stress Management
Vascular Bypass Surgery: Home Care

Interventions and rationales
☑ **Intervention 1**
Upon transfer of the patient to the unit, obtain the following information about the postoperative course in the recovery room or intensive care unit, including:
• type of surgical procedure performed (see *Common arterial occlusion sites and surgical bypass procedures*)
• date of surgery
• patient's response to surgery
• presence and status of any postoperative complications
• concurrent medical problems
• mental status
• pattern of vital signs
• activity level and response to activity

COMMON ARTERIAL OCCLUSION SITES AND SURGICAL BYPASS* PROCEDURES

In a bypass procedure, the diseased arterial segment (lesion) is bypassed with the graft material of choice; the graft is anastomosed (connected) above and below the lesion.

Arterial disease	Bypass procedure	Graft preferred†
Aortoiliac	Aortofemoral	Synthetic (Dacron)
	Aortobifemoral	Synthetic (Dacron)
	Axillofemoral‡	Synthetic (Dacron or PTFE**)
Iliac	Same as above	Synthetic (Dacron or PTFE)
	Femorofemoral††	Synthetic (Dacron or PTFE)
Superficial femoral	Femoropopliteal	Autogenous (saphenous vein)
Femoropopliteal	Femorotibial	Autogenous
Femorotibial	Femorotibial	Autogenous

* Decisions to use bypass procedures rather than other procedures (e.g., thrombo-endarterectomy, transluminal angioplasty, profundoplasty) depend on the extent of the disease and doctor preference.

† This does not exclude the use of alternative graft materials.

‡ May be procedure of choice when transabdominal approach is contraindicated (e.g., patient has severe anesthetic risk or intraabdominal disease or disorder)

** PTFE (polytetrafluoroethylene, a Teflon fabric)

†† May be procedure of choice for unilateral iliac disease in elderly patients.

• fluid volume status, including:
—ability to take fluids or food by mouth
—presence of nasogastric tube and usual amount of drainage
—presence of I.V. lines (including rate and type of fluid)
—urine output
• information about the extent of circulation to the limbs involved in the surgery, including:
—peripheral pulses
—skin temperature and color
—movement of distal extremities (feet and toes)
—presence of edema in the involved limb(s)
—reports of pain and the effectiveness of pain relief measures
—status of incision(s), including dressings and presence of drainage tubes.

• Assemble any necessary equipment in the patient's room before his arrival, including:
—sheepskin for the lower half of the bed (This helps to prevent skin breakdown to pressure areas and areas with compromised circulation.)
—heel protectors or bunny boots
—lamb's wool or cotton balls (Placed between toes, this helps to prevent pressure areas from skin-to-skin contact and promotes air circulation to decrease moisture between toes.)
—bed or foot cradle (This prevents linens from applying pressure to the legs with compromised circulation.)
—suction apparatus as indicated for gastric decompression or wound drainage. (Nasogastric tubes are often inserted after abdominal surgical procedures.)

☑ **Intervention 2**
Immediately after the patient's transfer, assess:
• vital signs
• mental status
• ability to communicate
• comfort level
• status of involved extremities; compare bilaterally for symmetry and assess for:
—skin color and temperature
—size and shape
—sensation in distal part of extremity
—movement of distal extremity (such as feet and toes)
—capillary refill
—peripheral pulses for quality and amplitude; use a Doppler probe to auscultate pulses that cannot be palpated. Mark the location of each pulse clearly (distal pulses may be difficult to locate; marking the location will indicate where the strongest impulse can be assessed).
• condition of the incision, including dressings, drains, and amount of drainage
• presence of leg ulcers
• invasive lines, including:
—nasogastric tube
—Foley catheter
—I.V. lines
• laboratory findings, including:
—electrolyte levels
—blood urea nitrogen and creatinine levels
—complete blood count
—platelet count
—prothrombin time and partial thromboplastin time
—urinalysis
—chest X-ray reports
—EKG readings.

☑ Intervention 3

Implement the prescribed medical care.
• Check the patient's vital signs every 4 hours or as indicated by patient status.
• Monitor the patient's activity, positioning him as follows:
—After surgery involving the legs, make sure the patient keeps his legs straight, avoids crossing of legs, and avoids bending at the graft site; he may elevate the head of the bed less than 45 degrees (or as ordered by the doctor).
—After surgery involving the arms, make sure the patient does not lie on the operative side (because of the risk of increased external compression of the graft).
• Begin ambulation when ordered. (This is usually started as early as possible to decrease complications associated with immobility.)
—Assist the patient in standing and ambulating. (Such assistance helps to prevent prolonged bending at the graft site and reduces the risk of injury from falls.)
—Initially, have the patient avoid sitting. Advance his activity, as ordered, to bathroom privileges and later to include sitting during mealtimes. (Prolonged periods of sitting increase the risk of thrombus or embolus formation during the early postoperative period.)
• Administer any prescribed medications, including:
—antibiotics (to prevent infection at the graft site or incision lines and to treat infected ulcers, if present)
—analgesics (to promote comfort and compliance with prescribed treatments)
—other medications as prescribed by the doctor (the patient may have other medical problems including those resulting from atherosclerosis).
• Monitor the patient's diet.
—Initially, patients are usually given nothing by mouth until bowel sounds return.
—When bowel sounds are present, the patient may advance to ice chips, then clear liquids, then to a regular diet, as tolerated.
—When the diet has advanced past clear liquids, a diet low in saturated fat or cholesterol may be prescribed. (Vascular bypass surgery does not cure atherosclerosis; alteration of risk factors is necessary to decrease the patient's chance of developing recurrent atherosclerosis.)
• Administer I.V. fluids as prescribed, including:
—maintenance I.V. fluids for maintaining intravascular volume and adequate hydration while the patient is receiving nothing by mouth
—replacement fluids for nasogastric drainage. (Replacement fluids maintain electrolyte balance by replacing gastric fluid losses and are usually prescribed to replace milliliter for milliliter the amount drained.)
• Monitor fluid losses, including urine output, gastric drainage, wound drainage, and bowel movements. (Urine output indicates renal functioning that reflects adequate blood flow to the kidneys.)
• Discourage the patient from smoking. (Smoking causes vasoconstriction, which can impair circulation to the legs; it also increases platelet aggregation, thereby increasing the risk of thrombus formation.)

☑ Intervention 4
Implement measures to prevent or treat the following common postoperative problems:
• pain (see "Comfort, Alteration in: Acute Pain" in Section I)
• atelectasis (see "Respiratory Function, Potential Alteration in" in Section I)
• impaired skin integrity (see "Skin Integrity, Potential for Impairment" in Section I).

☑ Intervention 5
Implement measures to manage edema in the affected arm(s) or leg(s), including:
• assessing the affected extremity for:
—swelling or a change in the usual contour of the distal part of the extremity
—redness or discoloration of the extremity
—failure of the area over a bony prominence to refill rapidly after being manually depressed for a few seconds
• if edema is present, taking the following measures:
—elevating the affected extremity (unless contraindicated or otherwise ordered)
—keeping the skin clean and dry
—keeping the distal extremity warm
—assessing for increased swelling
—notifying the doctor.

Rationale and comments: Edema may result from increased capillary permeability caused by prolonged tissue ischemia to affected arms or legs or by lymphatic obstruction. Significant edema can impair circulation in the affected limb.

☑ Intervention 6
Monitor the patient's GI function.
• Assess for the return of peristalsis, checking for:
—presence of bowel sounds in all four quadrants
—passage of flatus and bowel movements.
• Assess the nasogastric (NG) tube for the amount and type of drainage.
• Assist the patient with ambulation as soon as orders permit (ambulation promotes peristalsis).
• After peristalsis has returned, continue to assess for the following:
—presence of bowel sounds in all four quadrants
—patient's oral intake (amount ingested and his tolerance of the diet)
—amount and consistency of bowel movements.
• Notify the doctor if the patient experiences:
—prolonged absence of bowel sounds
—continued large amounts of drainage from the NG tube
—decrease or loss of bowel sounds
—nausea and vomiting
—copious diarrhea
—constipation.

Rationale and comments: Depending on the procedure performed, peristalsis may be absent for several days after surgery. Return of peristalsis is indicated by the presence of normal bowel sounds in all four quadrants and by the passage of flatus and bowel movements. Patients may develop an ileus postoperatively. An ileus is characterized by continued absence of bowel sounds (past the expected period), loss of bowel sounds after the initial return of peristalsis, nausea and vomiting, and abdominal distention. Copious diarrhea can sometimes occur after abdominal aortic aneurysm repair.

☑ Intervention 7
Monitor the patient for development of abrupt arterial occlusion.
• Assess for the following signs at least every 4 hours and as needed (this may be done once per shift when the patient stabilizes):
—diminished or absent pulses
—pale, cyanotic, or mottled skin
—skin that is cool or cold to the touch
—decreased capillary refill
—complaints of tingling, numbness, or painful sensations in the affected extremities.
• If any of the above signs are present:
—Notify the doctor at once.
—Institute bed rest.
—Anticipate preparing the patient for surgery.

Rationale and comments: A serious complication after surgery, arterial occlusion can occur from a thrombus or an embolus. Surgical intervention may be required to remove the thrombus or embolus and to restore circulation.

☑ Intervention 8
Monitor the patient for signs of bleeding.
• Check for signs of bleeding (hematoma formation) in the incision sites, including:
—swelling
—bluish discoloration
—tenderness at the site.
• Check for changes in vital signs indicative of hemorrhage.
• For patients who have had abdominal surgery involving the aorta or iliac arteries, check for:
—abdominal distention (may indicate internal bleeding)
—increased abdominal girth (may indicate internal bleeding).
• If any of the above signs are present:
—Notify the doctor immediately.
—Institute bed rest.
—Continue to monitor the patient closely for signs of increased bleeding and deterioration in vital signs.
• For a hematoma in the incision, apply manual pressure to the site.
• Implement measures to treat shock, if indicated, as prescribed.

Rationale and comments: Hemorrhage can be a serious complication after peripheral bypass surgery. Additional surgery may be required to control the bleeding and evacuate the hematoma.

☑ Intervention 9

Monitor the patient and implement measures to control the complication of postoperative wound infection.
• Perform routine incision line care using strict sterile technique.
• Implement measures to control diabetes mellitus when applicable, including:
  —monitoring blood glucose levels and reporting abnormal results
  —administering antidiabetic agents as ordered
  —providing calorie-restricted meals as ordered.
• Assess the patient's incision(s) for:
  —swelling
  —tenderness or pain
  —reddened discoloration
  —foul odor
  —elevated skin temperature
  —drainage.
• Assess for systemic signs of infection, including:
  —fever
  —elevated white blood cell count.
• Notify the doctor if signs or symptoms are present.
• If infection is present, assist with implementing the following as ordered:
  —Obtain a wound culture.
  —Administer prescribed antibiotics.
  —Implement prescribed dressing changes.
  —Continue to implement measures to control diabetes as indicated.
  —Assess for signs of continued infection or of healing.

Rationale and comments: Wound infection can be a serious complication for a patient with an arterial graft. It can interfere with healing; surgical removal of the infected graft may be required to resolve the infection. Many patients who require peripheral bypass surgery because of occlusive arterial disease are also diabetic. Maintaining strict control of diabetes facilitates healing.

Thrombolytic Therapy

ASSOCIATED NURSING DIAGNOSIS
Anxiety

ASSOCIATED STANDARD CARE PLANS
Coronary Artery Bypass Surgery (Post ICU)
Myocardial Infarction, Acute
Percutaneous Transluminal Coronary Angioplasty

Interventions and rationales
☑ **Intervention 1**
Assist with determining the patient's eligibility for thrombolytic therapy.
• Criteria for eligibility include:
  —episode of chest pain lasting more than 30 minutes
  —onset of signs and symptoms occurring less than 6 hours before the start of thrombolytic therapy
  —EKG report showing specific changes indicative of ischemia
  —patient under age 76.
• Possible contraindications to thrombolytic therapy include:
  —any current problems with active bleeding
  —history of bleeding or a coagulation disorder
  —invasive neurologic diagnostic procedure within the previous 2 months
  —cerebrovascular accident within the last 2 months
  —recent surgery or trauma
  —current use of anticoagulants
  —recent history of cardiopulmonary resuscitation
  —allergy to streptokinase
  —recent streptococcal infection
  —administration of streptokinase within the previous 6 months.

Rationale and comments: The goal of thrombolytic therapy is to restore blood flow to the ischemic area of the myocardium and to limit the size of the infarct by dissolving any clots occluding the coronary arteries. Only patients who meet strict criteria are currently eligible for this therapy. Research has shown that thrombolysis is most effective if begun within 6 hours of the onset of chest pain.

Hemorrhage is a major risk associated with thrombolytic therapy. Any condition that further increases the risk of serious hemorrhage can be a contraindication for thrombolytic therapy.

Because streptokinase is derived from a foreign protein, an allergic reaction (ranging from mild to anaphylactic) can occur.

Recent administration of streptokinase or a recent streptococcal infection can result in a high titer of streptokinase antibody, which neutralizes streptokinase and inhibits its ability to lyse clots.

☑ **Intervention 2**

Collect baseline data before the procedure, including:
• vital signs
• head-to-toe assessment that includes:
—neurologic status
—peripheral pulses
—skin lesions or bruising
—any evidence in excretions of occult bleeding
• characteristics of the patient's angina pain
• patient's and family's knowledge of thrombolysis
• patient's and family's anxiety level.

Rationale and comments: The major complication associated with thrombolytic therapy is bleeding. Bleeding can occur as overt hemorrhage from the catheter insertion site. It can also occur in other parts of the body, including the GI tract and the brain. A baseline assessment provides data that can assist the nurse in evaluating the patient's condition after the procedure.

☑ **Intervention 3**

Implement preprocedure teaching.
• Take appropriate measures to reduce the patient's anxiety.
• Based on the following information, briefly explain the procedure to the patient and family.
—The amount of myocardial tissue damaged by acute occlusion of a coronary artery is not fixed at the exact time of the occlusion. The damage increases over a period of time (often 4 to 6 hours).
—Fresh clots superimposed on atherosclerotic lesions in coronary arteries are thought to be a major cause of occlusion and myocardial infarction.
—If these clots can be dissolved before damage to the myocardium is complete, the infarct size may be limited.
—Limiting infarct size decreases the risk of later complications or death.
—Thrombolytic therapy does not replace coronary artery bypass grafting (CABG) surgery or percutaneous transluminal coronary angioplasty (PTCA). Although thrombolytic agents dissolve the clots, they do not affect the underlying atherosclerotic disease process. If further measures are not taken, an acute occlusion may again develop at the point of the atherosclerotic lesion.
—The procedure may take up to 6 hours to complete.
—Patient preparation depends on the thrombolytic agent's route of administration.
—For the I.V. route, an I.V. line is started and continuous EKG monitoring begun.
—For the intracardiac route, a catheterization laboratory and catheterization laboratory team are required.
—For information on the thrombolytic agents used, see *Comparing thrombolytic drugs.*

Rationale and comments: Knowledge about the procedure and what to expect can help the patient and family cope better.

COMPARING THROMBOLYTIC DRUGS

	Streptokinase	Tissue plasminogen activator (t-PA)
Action	• Dissolves clots	• Dissolves clots
Systemic effects	• Produces a systemic lytic state; depletes clotting factors	• Does not produce a systemic lytic state or deplete clotting factors
Route of administration	• I.V. • Intracoronary	• I.V. • Intracoronary
Effectiveness	• Intracoronary more effective than I.V.	• Both routes are equally effective. • I.V. t-PA has been found to be as effective as intracoronary streptokinase.
Side effects and risks	• Hemorrhage secondary to systemic effects on coagulation • Allergic reaction varying from mild to anaphylactic	• Decreased risk of hemorrhage • No risk of allergic reaction
Source	• Streptococcal bacterial protein	• Naturally occurring substance in humans
Other information	• Lytic effects longer lasting than those of t-PA • Prolonged risk of hemorrhage secondary to long half-life	• Has shorter half-life than streptokinase; normal coagulation state restored more rapidly • Does not delay further procedures, such as percutaneous transluminal coronary angioplasty.

☑ **Intervention 4**

If the patient is undergoing I.V. thrombolytic therapy, follow these measures:

• Assess for indications that clots have been successfully dissolved; signs include:

—abrupt cessation of chest pain—a sign that ischemia has been relieved

—rapid fall of a previously elevated ST segment noted on the EKG (Elevation of ST segments indicates injury; their return to normal indicates relief of ischemia, the cause of injury.)

—Creatine kinase (CK) levels that peak early (After successful thrombolysis, CK levels will peak 3 to 4 hours after conclusion of the procedure.)

—reperfusion dysrhythmias, indicated by new or increased premature ventricular beats (Although the cause of such dysrhythmias is unclear,

they occur when blood flow is restored to the ischemic area of the myocardium and may require emergency treatment with such antiarrhythmic medications as lidocaine.)
—bradycardia and hypotension. (If these occur, immediate treatment is initiated to stabilize vital signs.)

Rationale and comments: With intracoronary administration, clots are visualized by means of fluoroscopy and the actual dissolution is observed. With I.V. administration, the doctor must rely on indirect signs (sometimes called markers of perfusion) to indicate successful clot lysis.

☑ **Intervention 5**
Implement the appropriate postprocedure care.
• Observe the patient carefully for signs of hemorrhage or occult bleeding; notify the doctor if any occur.
—Check the patient's vital signs every 15 minutes until he is stable.
—Check neurologic signs every 15 minutes until the patient is stable.
—Assess the patient's skin for new bruising, petechiae, or other indications of subcutaneous bleeding.
—Check all puncture sites for overt bleeding.
—Perform a guaiac test (Hemoccult) on all excretions for occult blood.
—Observe the patient for hemoptysis or epistaxis.
• Report and record results of any ordered hematology and coagulation tests, which may include:
—activated prothrombin time
—fibrinogen
—fibrin split products
—thrombin time
—platelet count
—complete blood count.
• Implement the following measures to decrease the risk of hemorrhage:
—Limit venous punctures and injections as much as possible.
—Administer antacids prophylactically, as ordered, to decrease the risk of GI bleeding.
• Maintain continuous EKG monitoring to assess for:
—dysrhythmias
—new ST wave changes indicating recurrent ischemia, which can indicate reocclusion of the involved artery.
• Take measures to decrease the patient's and family's anxiety.

☑ **Intervention 6**
Monitor the patient for any signs of recurrent angina.
• Assess for any complaints of chest pain and any signs or symptoms commonly associated with angina (see "Angina Pectoris" in this section for details).
• If an episode of chest pain occurs:
—notify the doctor immediately
—implement care as outlined in "Angina Pectoris" in this section

—check the patient's vital signs
—obtain a 12-lead EKG (may require a doctor's order in some institutions)
—be prepared to assist with repeat thrombolysis or other procedures.

☑ Intervention 7

After intracoronary administration, implement additional measures.
• Use appropriate measures to decrease the risk of hemorrhage, including:
—maintaining a pressure dressing on the site, as ordered
—assessing the puncture site closely for signs of bleeding or hematoma formation
—if significant bleeding occurs, applying direct pressure to site sufficient to control bleeding but not to occlude the pulse; notify the doctor immediately.
—positioning the patient with the head of the bed elevated no more than 30 degrees
—telling the patient to flex his hip minimally during the first 24 hours or as directed.
• Monitor the patient for the development of an arterial occlusion at the puncture site by:
—checking the pulse distal to the puncture site every 15 minutes until the patient is stable, then every 1 to 4 hours as needed.
—assessing the extremity for changes in color and temperature
—notifying the doctor immediately if any of the above signs occur.

Rationale and comments: For intracoronary administration, a catheter is introduced into an artery (usually the femoral) and threaded through the arterial circulation into the heart. One complication that can occur with intracoronary administration is hemorrhage from the arterial puncture site. A clot can also form on the inside of the artery at the puncture site. This clot can occlude the lumen of the artery and prevent blood flow to the distal part of the extremity. Signs and symptoms of occlusion include loss of the pulse distal to the occlusion, a change in temperature in the extremity from warm to cold, and a change in skin color from normal to pale or mottled.

☑ Intervention 8

Administer prescribed medications, as ordered, including:
• heparin
• sodium warfarin (Coumadin)
• antiplatelet medications, such as dipyridamole
• other medications as indicated by the patient's condition.

Rationale and comments: I.V. heparin is often administered immediately after thrombolysis to decrease the risk of another clot forming in the coronary artery. After the immediate period, the patient may be started on oral anticoagulants or antiplatelet medications. (See *Anticoagulants,* page 154, and *Antiplatelet medications,* page 143.)

✅ Intervention 9

Assist with the prescribed follow-up care.

• Implement the interventions outlined in "Myocardial Infarction, Acute" in this section, as indicated.

• Prepare the patient for diagnostic tests to help evaluate the need for further procedures, such as PTCA and CABG.

Rationale and comments: Although thrombolytic therapy can help limit the size of an infarct, it does not reverse tissue death that occurred before circulation was restored. Because patients usually sustain some degree of infarction, follow-up care is similar to that for acute myocardial infarction.

Also, thrombolytic therapy is insufficient to restore full blood flow through a diseased artery. Therefore, PTCA or CABG surgery is often necessary to prevent a second infarction from occurring at a later date.

Valve Replacement Surgery (Post ICU)

ASSOCIATED NURSING DIAGNOSES
Activity Intolerance
Activity Intolerance, Potential for
Anxiety
Bowel Elimination, Alteration in: Constipation
Comfort, Alteration in: Acute Pain
Depression, Reactive: Situational
Family Processes, Alteration in
Grieving, Family
Grieving, Individual Patient
Respiratory Function, Alteration in
Respiratory Function, Potential Alteration in
Sleep-Pattern Disturbance

ASSOCIATED TEACHING PLANS
Cardiac Anatomy and Physiology: Heart and Blood Vessels
Endocarditis, Infectious: Disease Process and Prevention
Exercising after Myocardial Infarction or Heart Surgery
Medication Guidelines
Radial Pulse Measurement
Stress Management
Valve Replacement Surgery: Home Care

Interventions and rationales
☑ **Intervention 1**
Obtain baseline data on the patient after his transfer from the intensive care unit (ICU), including information on:
• type of valve replacement
• complications during or after surgery, including:
—low cardiac output
—dysrhythmias, which may include chronic atrial dysrhythmias and various types of heart block (see *Common dysrhythmias seen in patients with cardiovascular disease*, pages 139 to 142)
—respiratory complications
—reoperation for excessive bleeding
—cerebrovascular accident
• vital sign pattern
• presence of invasive lines (Invasive lines are discontinued as rapidly as possible after valve surgery to decrease the risk of infectious endocarditis.);

such invasive lines may include:
—a heparin lock
—pacemaker wires
• chest tubes (rarely present after transfer from ICU)
• status of the midline incision
• fluid and electrolyte balance, including:
—most recent electrolyte values
—current weight
—urine output.

Rationale and comments: Complications that occur during or after surgery can influence the patient's later postoperative course. For example, low cardiac output occurring in the immediate postoperative period can cause such later complications as renal failure and myocardial ischemia. Reoperation (for bleeding) increases the patient's risk of developing a wound infection. A cerebrovascular accident (CVA), although considered a relatively rare complication after surgery, will significantly alter the medical and nursing management of the patient.

Temporary pacemaker wires may be inserted during surgery; they may or may not be connected to an external pacemaker. If they are not connected, they are protected in some type of dressing. Should the patient develop rhythm disturbances that require the use of a pacemaker, the wires may be rapidly and easily attached to an external pacemaker. These wires are often removed before the patient is transferred from the ICU.

☑ Intervention 2
Implement the prescribed medical care regarding the patient's:
• activity; the patient may:
—sit out of the bed and ambulate to the bathroom on the day of transfer.
—advance activity according to exercise prescription. (see "Activity Intolerance, Potential for" in Section I).
• diet; the diet may be sodium-restricted or fluid-restricted for patients with congestive heart failure (CHF)
• continuous EKG monitoring, as ordered.
• respiratory care measures, including use of oxygen.

☑ Intervention 3
Administer medications as ordered. Prescribed medications may include:
• cardiovascular medications, such as:
—cardiac glycosides (see *Cardiac glycosides,* page 131)
—diuretics (see *Diuretics,* page 132)
—antiarrhythmics (see *Antiarrhythmic medications,* pages 144 and 145)
• anticoagulants and antiplatelets (see *Anticoagulants,* page 154, and *Antiplatelet medications,* page 143)
• analgesics

• prophylactic antibiotics (may be limited to the first 48 hours postoperatively)
• stool softeners or laxatives.

Rationale and comments: Patients with a history of valvular heart disease may also have other cardiovascular problems that commonly include significant dysrhythmias and CHF. Anticoagulants and antiplatelets are prescribed to decrease the risk of thromboembolic complications associated with prosthetic valves. Stool softeners and laxatives are prescribed because straining with defecation increases the stress on the heart and can result in bradycardia and hypotension.

✓ Intervention 4
Implement measures to prevent or treat the following common postoperative problems:
• constipation (see "Bowel Elimination, Alteration in: Constipation" in Section I)
• pain (see "Comfort, Alteration in: Acute Pain" in Section I)
• depression (see "Depression, Reactive: Situational" in Section I)
• postoperative atelectasis (see "Respiratory Function, Potential Alteration in" in Section I)
• postoperative wound infection
  —Perform routine incision line care.
  —Instruct the patient to avoid using lotions, creams, or powders on the incision line.
  —Assess the incision once per shift for signs of inflammation.

✓ Intervention 5
Implement measures to decrease the patient's risk for developing prosthetic valve endocarditis, including:
• obtaining doctor's orders to discontinue all invasive lines as soon as possible
• implementing the measures outlined in "Endocarditis, Infectious, Prevention of" in this section and "Endocarditis, Infectious: Disease Process and Prevention" in Section III.

Rationale and comments: Prosthetic valves are more susceptible than normal valves to bacterial endocarditis. Infected prosthetic valves are difficult to treat; they usually must be replaced surgically.

✓ Intervention 6
Implement measures to decrease the risk of thromboembolic events.
• Administer warfarin as prescribed (see *Anticoagulants,* page 154).
• Assess the patient for signs and symptoms of systemic emboli. (Specific symptoms depend on the tissue affected.) Notify the doctor if any are present.

Rationale and comments: Prosthetic valves are associated with an increased risk of thromboembolic complications. Warfarin is usually the drug of choice to decrease the patient's risk.

☑ Intervention 7

Monitor the patient for development of congestive heart failure (see "Congestive Heart Failure" in this section).

☑ Intervention 8

Monitor the patient for additional complications, including:
- dysrhythmias
- pericarditis
- pulmonary vascular congestion
- postoperative wound infection.

See "Coronary Artery Bypass Surgery (Post ICU)" in this section for a discussion of these complications.

SECTION III: TEACHING PLANS

Note: The emphasis of Section III is on teaching patients and their families how to manage cardiovascular disease successfully at home. Although an extensive discussion of the teaching-learning process exceeds the scope of this text, a summary of major points is provided in the plan of care for the nursing diagnosis Knowledge Deficit. In this plan, the interventions outline the steps of the teaching process, and major teaching-learning principles are included as part of the interventions or rationale and comments sections. The reader is encouraged to review this material before implementing any of the teaching interventions outlined in the subsequent teaching plans.

Knowledge Deficit

Knowledge Deficit related to:
• new diagnosis
• new medications
• treatments
• newly prescribed home care measures
• expressed lack of understanding of current treatment regimen
• expressed lack of understanding of how to effectively incorporate prescribed treatment into usual life-style

SUPPORTING DATA
Patient or family:
• states lack of knowledge about information related to the disease process, prescribed treatment, or home care management.
• asks questions or expresses concern about how to implement the prescribed measures successfully at home.

PLAN OF CARE
Outcome criteria
Patient and family demonstrate acquisition of new knowledge and skills. (Specific outcome criteria are listed for each teaching plan.)

Interventions and rationales
☑ Intervention 1
Identify appropriate learners, including:
• the patient
• specific family members
• a designated caregiver.

Rationale and comments: Unless medically unable to participate in the teaching session, the patient should always be included. Family members should also be included because their life-styles may be affected by the patient's condition and prescribed treatment. Also, the family can play an instrumental role in promoting compliance to the prescribed regimen. Teaching will be most effective if the person who will actually be performing or managing the care is included.

☑ Intervention 2
Assess those involved in the teaching session for the following:
• educational level and ability to read and write (Knowing this may affect your teaching strategies.)
• vision and hearing (Special approaches may be needed with patients who have impaired sight or hearing.)

• any psychomotor deficits (Because patients with psychomotor deficits will have trouble learning psychomotor skills, you may need to modify your teaching.)
• cultural background (Cultural background can affect the patient's or family's response to illness and the prescribed treatment.)
• financial status (Be sure to modify home care measures to fit the patient's budget; for example, when helping to plan the patient's meals, be sure to recommend foods he can routinely afford.)
• previous knowledge of topic (Presenting information that the patient or family already knows is an inefficient use of teaching time.)
• current interest in topics to be discussed (Teaching is more effective when the patient and family are interested in topics or sense the need to know the information.)
• current areas of concern in relation to topics to be discussed (The patient's or family's areas of concern are often a good place to begin teaching.)
• emotional response to the patient's illness and prescribed treatment (Such emotional responses as anger, depression, and denial can interfere with learning.)
• fatigue or pain. (The patient's fatigue or pain will decrease his ability to learn.)

☑ Intervention 3
Determine what information to include in the teaching session.
• Collaborate with the doctor and health care team for discharge orders and planned follow-up.
• Identify what information is primarily the nurse's responsibility to teach.

Rationale and comments: An organized plan facilitates effective teaching. Because several clinicians, including dietitians, cardiac rehabilitation nurses, pharmacists, staff nurses, and doctors, may be involved in teaching the cardiovascular patient, careful collaboration and coordination are necessary to ensure consistent instruction.

☑ Intervention 4
Prioritize the information you will present in the teaching session.
• Consider the amount of time available for teaching.
• Begin with information the patient or family *must* know for safe home care. Such information may include administration of medications and the prevention, recognition, and treatment of major complications.
• Continue with information that will help the patient or family to better manage the patient's cardiovascular disease independently at home. This information may include understanding of the disease process, knowledge of cardiac anatomy and physiology, and knowledge of how to modify the patient's risk factors.

Rationale and comments: Because teaching time is frequently limited in the hospital, setting priorities helps to ensure that the most important information is taught first.

☑ Intervention 5
Identify the appropriate strategy to use in the teaching session, such as:
• a didactic presentation with question and answer time (Useful for explaining disease processes, treatments, and medications, this type of presentation is usually combined with another method and can be used for groups or individuals.)
• a presentation using illustrations, models, or diagrams (This may be combined with any method to facilitate understanding of content.)
• a demonstration and return demonstration (This is an effective method of teaching a skill, activity, or exercise.)
• a presentation using problem-solving with the patient and family (Home management of most cardiovascular diseases involves life-style changes. Simply presenting factual material is usually insufficient; patients and families often need help in determining realistic ways to incorporate the changes into their individual life-styles.)
• a presentation using written materials (Remember to provide written information regardless of which teaching strategy you use. You can use it to supplement other forms of teaching and to ensure that the patient receives essential information, especially if you haven't had time to cover a specific topic during your teaching session.)

Rationale and comments: The strategy chosen should be based on the nurse's assessment of the patient and family as well as the information she needs to teach.

☑ Intervention 6
Set measurable goals; goals may be stated in terms of:
• behavioral objectives
• outcome criteria.

Rationale and comments: Goals may be used to evaluate teaching effectiveness.

☑ Intervention 7
Implement the teaching plan, paying particular attention to the following details:
• Schedule the teaching for a time when you won't be interrupted.
• Ensure that everyone requiring instruction is present.
• Reschedule the teaching if the patient is fatigued or in pain.
• Conduct the teaching session in a private, quiet environment, away from all distracting sights and sounds.

Rationale and comments: Carefully selecting the time and location for teaching greatly enhances the effectiveness of instruction.

☑ Intervention 8
Evaluate your teaching's effectiveness by:
• asking the patient and family to repeat, in their own words, specific information or instructions (Use this method to evaluate their understanding of the factual content discussed.)

• asking the patient and family to give a return demonstration (Use this method to evaluate their ability to perform skills, activities, or exercises.)
• having the patient and family develop specific plans for implementing the teaching at home. (Use this method to evaluate their problem-solving ability for a given situation.)

Rationale and comments: The type of evaluation method should correspond to the goals and teaching strategy used.

☑ Intervention 9
Revise and reinforce the teaching, as necessary.

Rationale and comments: Home management of cardiovascular disease can be complex and confusing to the patient and family. Presenting the information more than once is often necessary for learning.

Amputation, Leg: Home Care

TEACHING PLAN
Assessment
• Assess the patient's and family's knowledge about home care after amputation, including residual limb care, care of the unaffected limb, exercises, and positioning.
• Collaborate with the doctor, physical therapist, prosthetist, and occupational therapist regarding the patient's discharge orders and planned rehabilitation to ensure the patient and family receive consistent instructions.

Materials needed
• Elastic wrap or shrinker sock, if ordered
• Sample stump sock
• Hand mirror

Strategies to use
• Demonstrate care of the residual limb to the patient and his family; have the patient or family member care for the residual limb in the hospital under a nurse's supervision.
• Demonstrate care of the unaffected limb; have the patient or a family member care for the unaffected limb in the hospital under a nurse's supervision.

Patient-teaching aids
See *Caring for yourself at home after amputation,* page 241; and *Caring for your prosthesis,* page 245.

Evaluation method
Have the patient or family member demonstrate the following:
• proper positioning of the patient on the bed and chair to prevent contractures
• washing, rinsing, and drying procedures for the residual limb
• care procedure for the stump sock and prosthesis
• prescribed exercises to use at home
• procedures for inspecting the incision and residual limb for any signs of infection or injury
• foot care procedures for the unaffected limb
• precautions to prevent injuring the unaffected limb.

Interventions and outcome criteria
☑ **Intervention 1**
Demonstrate daily care of the residual limb, including these procedures:
• bathing
   —Use tepid water and mild soap.

—Rinse the limb thoroughly.
—Dry the limb thoroughly but gently.
—Use lotion for extremely dry skin only.
—Instruct the patient to perform these procedures at night before retiring.
• daily inspection
—Use a hand mirror to view the entire residual limb.
—Inspect for signs of infection or injury; notify the doctor if any appear.
• daily massage.

☑ Intervention 2

Have the patient or a family member perform daily care of the residual limb under a nurse's supervision.

Outcome criteria: The patient and family demonstrate correct procedures for bathing, rinsing, and drying the limb as well as the correct procedures for applying lotion, inspecting for any signs of infection, and massaging the limb without assistance from the nurse.

☑ Intervention 3

Demonstrate how to position the patient properly to avoid contractures; include the following positions:
• lying supine in bed
• lying prone in bed
• sitting in chair.

☑ Intervention 4

Have the patient and family demonstrate the correct sitting, supine, and prone positions.

Outcome criteria: The patient and family position the patient correctly in the above positions without assistance from the nurse.

☑ Intervention 5

Instruct the patient to continue exercises at home, as directed by the physical therapist.
• Have the patient and family demonstrate the prescribed exercises.
• If the patient and family are unable to demonstrate exercises, notify the physical therapist and collaborate for further patient teaching.

Outcome criteria: The patient and family correctly demonstrate prescribed exercises.

☑ Intervention 6

Instruct the patient and family on the use of a prescribed shrinkage device, including:
• how to apply the device
• when to wear the device
• when to notify the doctor.

☑ Intervention 7

Have the patient and family apply the prescribed shrinkage device under the supervision of a nurse or physical therapist.

Outcome criteria: The patient and family demonstrate correct application of the shrinkage device without assistance.

☑ Intervention 8

Discuss phantom limb sensation with the patient and family.

Outcome criteria: The patient and family describe phantom limb sensation correctly.

☑ Intervention 9

Demonstrate proper care for the unaffected limb and foot.

Outcome criteria: The patient and family demonstrate proper care for the unaffected limb and foot.

☑ Intervention 10

Discuss general management of the prosthetic device, including:
• procedures for washing and drying the socket
• use and care of socks
• storage of the prosthesis.

☑ Intervention 11

Have the patient and family demonstrate care of the prosthesis.

Outcome criteria: The patient and family demonstrate correct care of the prosthesis.

Caring for Yourself at Home after Amputation

This patient-teaching aid answers some common questions patients have about caring for themselves at home after amputation. If you have other questions, be sure to ask your doctor, nurse, or physical therapist.

DAILY CARE
• Wash your residual limb daily using tepid (barely warm) water and mild soap. Do not use hot water. Test the water on your wrist before using it on your limb. If it feels too hot or warm, add more cool water before washing your limb.
• Rinse your limb well after washing with soap, making sure that all the soap is rinsed off. Residual soap can damage your skin.
• Gently dry your limb well. Excess moisture can also damage your skin.
• Wash and dry your limb at night before going to bed.
• Use lotion on your skin only if it is extremely dry. Apply it at night.
• Carefully massage your limb each day. Your nurse will show you how to do this correctly.
• Keep your residual limb dry. If you perspire heavily, you may need to change your sock or elastic bandage during the day to help keep your limb dry.

DAILY INSPECTION
• Look at your limb carefully each day, using a hand-held mirror to see the bottom and back of the limb.
• Inspect the limb for reddened areas, blisters, scrapes, or other injuries.
• Also check for increased redness or tenderness around the incision, drainage from the incision, or any separation of the wound edges.
• Contact your doctor immediately if you notice any of the above signs.

PROPER POSITIONS
How you sit in a chair and lie in bed can affect your recovery. Use of incorrect positions can damage your joints and make it much more difficult or impossible for you to wear a prosthesis.

Sitting position
• When sitting, always keep your residual limb straight.
• If you have a below-the-knee amputation, always keep your knee straight. You may need to support the knee on another chair.
• If you have an above-the-knee amputation, do not use a pillow to prop up your residual limb.
• Do not sit for long periods of time.
• Do not allow the foot of your unaffected leg to droop. Place your foot firmly on the floor or against the footrest of your wheelchair.

(continued)

Lying position

- When lying in bed, keep your residual limb straight. Do not let your foot turn inward or outward. Use a small blanket rolled up and placed next to your ankle to keep your leg in the correct position. The nurse can show you how to do this.
- Do not prop up your residual limb on a pillow.
- Do not let your foot droop while you are in bed. You may use a footboard or place a rolled up blanket against the sole of your foot to keep your foot in a normal position. The nurse can show you how.
- Spend some time lying on your stomach each day. With your doctor's permission, you should spend up to 4 hours each day on your abdomen. The nurse can show you and your family how to help you turn.

EXERCISES

Continue to do your exercises at home as your physical therapist has told you. These exercises strengthen the muscles that you will need to move yourself in bed and to get out of bed.

DRESSINGS

Your doctor may want you to use some type of special dressing or elastic wrap on your residual limb. These dressings or wraps are used to decrease the swelling and pain in your residual limb. Be sure to use them exactly as your doctor has ordered. The nurse or physical therapist will show you how to apply the dressing.

The type of dressing that your doctor wants you to use is:

☐ elastic wraps

☐ shrinker sock

☐ other

☐ none

You should wear this dressing:

☐ all of the time except when bathing the residual limb

☐ other: _____

- If you use an elastic wrap (Ace bandage), apply it evenly and without wrinkles. Rewrap your residual limb whenever the wrap slips or becomes too loose. You will probably need to rewrap your limb several times throughout the day.
- If you use a shrinker sock, apply it evenly and without wrinkles. Suspend it from your waist or shoulder harness as directed; do not roll it down from the top to hold it in place. Keep in mind that you will need to buy a new shrinker sock when the one you are using becomes too big. You may need to buy several socks before you are finally fitted for your prosthesis.

(continued)

In the spaces below, list where you can buy the correct shrinker sock when needed.

Pharmacy or medical supply: ———————————————————

Phone: ————————————————————————————

Address: ————————————————————————————

Hours: —————————————————————————————

PHANTOM LIMB SENSATION
• After surgery, you may feel that your lost limb is still there. Such phantom limb sensations are normal and may gradually disappear over time. Usually, these sensations are painless; sometimes they are described as a tingling feeling or a feeling of pressure or numbness.
• If you experience a severe, constant burning pain or a stabbing, crushing pain in your residual limb, notify your doctor immediately. This is not phantom limb sensation; it should be checked immediately.

YOUR PROSTHESIS
When you are ready to be fitted with a permanent prosthesis, your doctor will refer you to a prosthetist, a specialist who makes artificial limbs. You will have to go to the prosthetist's office or center to be fitted for your new limb. Because your first visit may be fairly long, plan ahead how you will manage your usual medications, meals or snacks, or other parts of your daily routine while you are away from home.
• When you get your permanent prosthesis, learn to care for it properly. Some general guidelines are attached to this patient-teaching aid. Review these when you get your prosthesis. You or your prosthetist may also write down additional instructions for your specific prosthesis.
• When you receive your prosthesis, a physical therapist will teach you how to walk and move around.
• Contact your prosthetist or physical therapist if you have any questions.

In the spaces provided below, write down pertinent names and other information.

Prosthetist: ————————————————————————

Phone: ————————————————————————————

Address: ————————————————————————————

Hours available: ——————————————————————

(continued)

Physical therapist: _____

Phone: _____

Address: _____

Hours available: _____

FOLLOW-UP

Finally, keeping your follow-up appointments is important. Your first appointment is:

Doctor: _____

Phone: _____

Address: _____

Date and time: _____

PATIENT-TEACHING AID

Caring for Your Prosthesis

GENERAL CARE

• Wash the socket of your prosthesis every day with a damp cloth, allowing it to dry thoroughly. It usually is best to wash and dry the socket at night so that it has time to dry completely.
• Keep any leather parts of your prosthesis clean and dry.
• When you are not wearing your prosthesis, store it flat to avoid any damaging falls.
• If you notice any problems with your prosthesis, such as the fit or working condition, contact your prosthetist as soon as possible.
• Keep all scheduled appointments with your prosthetist for routine maintenance of your prosthesis.

Other instructions: _____

_____

_____

_____

_____

_____

_____

_____

_____

_____

CARING FOR SOCKS

• Change your socks at least once a day—more often if you perspire heavily.
• Wash all socks after wearing them, using cool water and mild soap. Thoroughly rinse them. Dry the socks flat and block them to maintain their correct shape.
• Use enough socks to keep your prosthesis correctly fitted to your residual limb.
• Replace your socks when they start to wear out or become too thin.

Angina Pectoris: Disease Process and Home Care

TEACHING PLAN
Assessment
• Identify the extent of the patient's angina, including:
—the amount of activity the patient can usually perform before experiencing an angina attack
—the frequency with which angina attacks occur during a day
—any consistent precipitating factors
—what usually relieves the patient's acute attacks.
• Review any pertinent diagnostic tests for information about the degree of occlusion in the coronary arteries.
• Identify the signs and symptoms associated with the patient's acute attacks.
• Assess the patient's and family's knowledge of angina, its signs and symptoms, and home management.
• Assess the patient's and family's past experience with managing angina at home; identify areas of concern.
• Collaborate with the doctor regarding the patient's discharge orders, including the number of sublingual nitroglycerin tablets he should take before seeking medical care.

Materials needed
• Diagram and model of a heart, normal artery, and diseased artery
• Bottle of sublingual nitroglycerin tablets

Strategies to use
• Stimulate interest in the topic by beginning with the patient's and family's areas of concern.
• Assist the patient and his family to problem-solve the following:
—specific situations that may precipitate an angina attack
—measures that help to limit angina attacks at home
—how to recognize when the patient is having an acute angina attack
—where the patient will keep nitroglycerin
—who will know the location of the nitroglycerin tablets
—when and how to obtain additional medical help.

Patient-teaching aid
See *Managing angina pectoris at home*, page 250.

Evaluation method
Have the patient and family:
• explain in their own words what occurs in angina pectoris, including its major signs and symptoms

• identify when additional medical help is needed and how they will obtain that care
• state how to manage an acute angina attack
• state plans for limiting the patient's angina attacks at home.

Interventions and outcome criteria

☑ Intervention 1

Explain that angina pectoris is an imbalance in cardiac oxygen supply and demand.

Outcome criteria: The patient and family state that angina occurs when the heart does not get enough oxygen to meet its needs.

☑ Intervention 2

Review the highlights of cardiac anatomy and physiology and coronary circulation.

☑ Intervention 3

Explain the role of atherosclerosis in the development of angina.

Outcome criteria: The patient and family state that atherosclerosis narrows coronary arteries and decreases the amount of blood and oxygen traveling to the myocardium.

☑ Intervention 4

Describe the signs and symptoms associated with angina, including:
• general symptoms, such as chest pain and its associated signs and symptoms
• the patient's individual symptoms.

Outcome criteria: The patient and family state major signs indicative of an acute angina attack.

☑ Intervention 5

Describe how to manage acute angina attacks, including:
• the need for the patient to stop all activity and sit down
• ways of taking or giving sublingual nitroglycerin.

Outcome criteria: The patient and family state that, if an acute attack occurs, the patient should stop all activity, sit down, and take sublingual nitroglycerin. They also state the correct way to take or give sublingual nitroglycerin.

☑ Intervention 6

Instruct the patient and family to obtain additional medical help if the acute angina attack is not relieved by the prescribed amount of nitroglycerin.

Outcome criteria: The patient and family state that additional medical help is needed if an acute attack is unrelieved by nitroglycerin.

☑ Intervention 7

Have the patient and family determine how they will obtain additional medical help, including:
• who they will call (including weekends and nights)
• how they will get there.

Outcome criteria: The patient and family state how they will obtain additional medical help.

☑ Intervention 8
Discuss how to care for and store nitroglycerin tablets, including:
• proper storage
• the need for a family member and co-worker to also know where tablets are kept.

Outcome criteria: The patient and family state that nitroglycerin should be stored in a light- and moisture-resistant container and kept in several locations at home and work.

☑ Intervention 9
Have the patient identify where he will keep the nitroglycerin and who will know its location.

Outcome criteria: The patient and family state where nitroglycerin will be kept and who will know its location.

☑ Intervention 10
Discuss how to limit acute angina attacks at home, including:
• factors that can precipitate acute attacks
• the importance of taking all medications as prescribed
• other measures to limit acute attacks, such as:
—pacing activities
—getting sufficient rest and sleep
—avoiding overeating
—stopping smoking
—using prophylactic sublingual nitroglycerin
—taking measures to decrease myocardial oxygen demand during sexual intercourse
—participating in a cardiac rehabilitation program (with doctor's permission).
Have the patient problem-solve ways to limit his acute attacks using the above guidelines.

Outcome criteria: The patient and family state which measures to use to decrease acute angina attacks at home.

☑ Intervention 11
Describe the signs of worsening angina, including:
• increased attacks during the day or week
• attacks precipitated by lessened stress or activity
• attacks that occur at night or at rest
• attacks that require more nitroglycerin tablets to obtain relief.

Outcome criteria: The patient and family state major signs that indicate worsening angina.

✅ Intervention 12

Describe signs and symptoms associated with acute myocardial infarction, including:

- characteristics of chest pain
- accompanying symptoms
- atypical presentation, such as:
  —absence of chest pain
  —signs and symptoms of congestive heart failure.

Outcome criteria: The patient and family state signs indicative of myocardial infarction.

✅ Intervention 13

Have the patient and family identify where and how they will obtain emergency medical care if needed.

Outcome criteria: The patient and family plan how to get medical help in the event of a myocardial infarction.

Managing Angina Pectoris at Home

DESCRIPTION

Angina pectoris occurs when the heart muscle does not get enough oxygen to meet its needs. You remember that the heart is a muscle. It needs oxygen to work correctly. Normally, the oxygen is supplied through blood that travels to the heart through the coronary arteries. When your heart does not receive enough oxygen, angina occurs. The most common cause of angina is coronary artery disease (CAD).

CAD is caused by a disease known as atherosclerosis. Atherosclerosis causes the buildup of fatty deposits in your coronary arteries. As these deposits grow bigger, the artery becomes smaller, and less blood gets through to your heart. This results in less oxygen getting through to your heart. When the amount of oxygen supplied to the heart is less than the amount that the heart needs, you have angina.

SIGNS AND SYMPTOMS

Chest pain is the most common symptom of angina. How the pain feels may differ from person to person. You might describe this chest pain as a feeling of tightness or pressure in your chest. Or you might think that it feels like indigestion. The pain is often felt on the left side of the chest; it may travel down your left arm or up the left side of your neck. It may also travel to the right side (although this is not as common). Chest pain caused by angina usually goes away by taking nitroglycerin and resting. Besides chest pain, you may also feel dizzy, perspire heavily, or feel short of breath or weak.

MANAGING ACUTE ATTACKS

Chances are, you will have an angina attack at home. It can be very frightening. However, with careful planning, you will be able to handle the situation.

When you first notice any symptoms of chest pain, immediately take the following actions:
• Stop what you are doing and sit down.
• Take your sublingual nitroglycerin. Take one tablet and place it under your tongue; let it dissolve. If your chest pain is unrelieved within 5 minutes, take a second tablet. Place it under your tongue and let it dissolve. If your chest pain is still unrelieved, you may continue to take one nitroglycerin tablet every 5 minutes up to _____ tablets.
• If the nitroglycerin relieves your chest pain, continue to rest for a while. Taking nitroglycerin may make you dizzy; if you feel dizzy, change positions carefully until the dizziness passes. Nitroglycerin may also cause a headache. If this occurs, take acetaminophen (Tylenol) to relieve the headache.

(continued)

• If your chest pain is unrelieved after you have taken _____ nitroglycerin tablets, you must seek medical attention. You may be having a heart attack. Immediate treatment is extremely important to limit permanent heart damage.

TAKING NITROGLYCERIN

Always have nitroglycerin tablets with you. Be sure to:
• carry a bottle of nitroglycerin in your purse or in your shirt or jacket pocket
• keep bottles of nitroglycerin tablets in several places in your home and office.

Nitroglycerin tablets will become damaged if exposed to light, moisture, or air. Always carry the tablets in a closed, airtight, dark container. The bottle in which you originally received the tablets is small and easily carried; it protects the tablets well. If you carry the tablets loose, they will not work well and may not relieve your attack of chest pain.

Always check the expiration date on your bottle of nitroglycerin. Do not use the tablets after the expiration date has passed.

Another person should always know where you keep your nitroglycerin tablets. This person can be your spouse, a family member, co-worker, or supervisor. You may need that person's help to get your nitroglycerin when you are having an attack.

In the spaces below, list where you will keep your nitroglycerin tablets.

At home: _____

At work: _____

When away from home: _____

In the spaces below, list other people who will know where you keep your nitroglycerin and how to help you take it.

_____

_____

_____

LIMITING ATTACKS

Although you may not be able to completely avoid having attacks of chest pain at home, you can take certain measures to limit the attacks that you have.
• Take your prescribed medications as ordered. These medications help increase the oxygen supply to your heart. They also help to decrease the amount of oxygen that your heart needs. These medications will help to limit your attacks of chest pain. The nurse will give you more information about each medication you will be taking at home.

(continued)

• Pace your activities. Spread them out through the course of the day; avoid doing a number of activities rapidly without resting in between. Remember to plan your activities ahead of time to save steps and energy.
• Include adequate rest in your daily schedule. Get enough sleep at night. Plan several scheduled rest periods during the day. Recommended times for resting include immediately after a meal, after returning from work, and after engaging in some strenuous activity. Do not let yourself become too tired; stop your activity when you first begin to become tired.
• Avoid overeating. When you overeat, your heart has to work harder and needs more oxygen. You might want to eat smaller meals, about three or four times a day, rather than eating fewer, larger meals.
• Avoid smoking. Smoking can bring on an acute angina attack. Chemicals in the smoke can increase the amount of oxygen your heart needs. They can also cause the blood vessels supplying your heart to become smaller; this reduces the amount of blood and oxygen to your heart.
• If you frequently have chest pain with any activity, try taking one nitroglycerin tablet before beginning the activity.
• Talk with your doctor about the possibility of participating in an outpatient cardiac rehabilitation exercise program. Supervised, planned exercise may help you increase the amount of activity you can do before experiencing chest pain and may help reduce the major risk factors for atherosclerosis. Exercise can also help with weight control, stress reduction, decreasing the amount of fatty substances circulating in your bloodstream, and promoting feelings of relaxation and well-being.

What sort of activities do you think might bring on an acute attack when you get home? Think about what you might do to change each situation. List each situation and your plans in the space provided below.

_____

_____

_____

_____

_____

_____

_____

_____

_____

(continued)

ENGAGING IN SEXUAL ACTIVITY

Some patients with angina are concerned that they will have chest pain during sexual intercourse. To decrease the risk of chest pain during intercourse, follow these guidelines:
• Have intercourse in a familiar place that is comfortable for you. The room temperature should be neither too hot nor too cold.
• Have intercourse at a time when you are well rested. Wait at least 3 hours after eating a large meal or drinking alcoholic beverages before having intercourse.
• Use positions that are familiar and comfortable for you and your partner.
• Take a nitroglycerin tablet before engaging in sexual activity.

DEVELOPING WORSENING ANGINA

Some patients will develop increased or worsening angina. You will know if your angina is getting worse if you develop any of the following signs or symptoms:
• you suddenly start having acute attacks of chest pain at night when you are asleep or resting quietly
• you have to take more nitroglycerin to relieve each angina attack
• you have more and more attacks each day or each week
• you can't do as much as you used to without bringing on an acute attack of chest pain.

Sometimes, increasing chest pain is a warning that you may soon have a heart attack. If you have any of these symptoms, you need to obtain medical care.

HOW TO RECOGNIZE A HEART ATTACK

Some patients with angina may have a heart attack. You will know you are having a heart attack if:
• you have chest pain that feels crushing, viselike, sharp, or stabbing. Often more severe than your usual angina pain, this pain is frequently in the same place as your angina pain; it may travel down your right or left arm or up the right or left side of your neck. With this chest pain you may also feel short of breath, sweat heavily, feel dizzy, or have palpitations. You may also feel very nervous or restless.
• you have chest pain that is not relieved after you have stopped your activity and taken _____ nitroglycerin tablets.

Some patients do not experience any chest pain with a heart attack; if you have any of the following signs or symptoms—with or without chest pain—you may also be having a heart attack:
• you become extremely short of breath
• your skin becomes cold to the touch and you break out in a cold sweat
• you become nauseated or feel extremely tired
• your family notices that you have become very confused.

If you develop any of these signs and symptoms, you must get to the hospital immediately. Getting treatment quickly is very important. It can help limit the damage to your heart and prevent later problems.

(continued)

Plan now how you will get additional medical care. Use the space provided below.

Person to call (include name and telephone number):

during the day: _____

on the weekend: _____

at night: _____

How I will get to the doctor's office/clinic/hospital (include telephone numbers if needed):

during the day:_____

on the weekend: _____

at night: _____

I will keep my emergency numbers (specify location):

_____

_____

_____

_____

Atherosclerosis: Disease Process and Risk Factors

TEACHING PLAN
Assessment
• Determine the patient's and family's knowledge about atherosclerosis and its associated risk factors.
• Assess the patient and family for presence of risk factors; identify any specific risk factors present.

Materials needed
• Diagram or model showing normal and diseased arteries
• Diagram of major arteries in body

Strategies to use
• To stimulate interest in the topic, explain to the patient and family that, if measures are not taken, atherosclerosis can worsen or recur. Explain that understanding a few facts about atherosclerosis can help them identify appropriate measures to limit or halt further growth of atherosclerotic plaques.
• Present the information using didactic teaching with the opportunity for questions and answers; use a model or diagram to illustrate major points.
• Individualize teaching by identifying the patient's and family's specific risk factors.

Patient-teaching aid
See *Understanding atherosclerosis,* page 257.

Evaluation method
Have the patient or a family member:
• describe, in his own words, what occurs in atherosclerosis
• list risk factors for atherosclerosis (both general factors and those specific to the individual patient and his family).

Interventions and outcome criteria
☑ Intervention 1
Describe the growth of an atherosclerotic plaque in an artery using the diagram or model for an illustration.

Outcome criteria: The patient and family state that atherosclerosis narrows the arteries by causing fatty deposits to build up on the inside of the artery.

☑ Intervention 2

Explain how atherosclerosis damages the artery, including loss of elasticity and narrowing of the lumen.

Outcome criteria: The patient and family state that narrowed arteries may be unable to supply all the oxygen that a tissue needs in order to function properly.

☑ Intervention 3

Explain the effects of arterial damage on tissue functioning, including:
• decreased oxygen supply available to meet tissue's needs
• development of tissue ischemia
• development of tissue infarct.

Outcome criteria: The patient and family state that permanent damage to a tissue can result from inadequate oxygen supply.

☑ Intervention 4

Describe modifiable risk factors for atherosclerosis, including:
• cigarette smoking
• diet high in saturated fats and cholesterol
• hypertension
• diabetes mellitus
• obesity
• sedentary life-style
• stress.

Outcome criteria: The patient and family state risk factors associated with atherosclerosis.

☑ Intervention 5

Explain that risk factors are cumulative.

☑ Intervention 6

Have the patient and family identify any individual risk factors present.

Outcome criteria: The patient and family state their individual risk factors.

Understanding Atherosclerosis

Atherosclerosis is a disease of the arterial blood vessels in which fatty deposits attach to the inside of the arteries. These deposits grow larger and larger and thereby narrow the artery. This results in less blood and oxygen passing to the tissue normally supplied by that artery.

When your arteries become quite narrowed (usually more than 70%), the amount of blood with its oxygen supply that can pass through the artery is not enough to meet the demands of the tissue. When the tissue's demands for oxygen are not met, the tissue may become damaged. Sometimes, the damage is temporary; however, if the oxygen supply drops too low for too long a time, the damage will be permanent.

When the tissue does not get sufficient oxygen to meet its needs, you may experience signs and symptoms. The specific signs and symptoms depend on which artery is narrowed and on the tissue it supplies.

Most arteries in your body can be damaged by atherosclerosis. Some of the most common include the coronary arteries on the outside of your heart, the carotid arteries that supply your brain, and some arteries that supply your legs and feet.

RISK FACTORS

The reason fat deposits begin to stick to an artery is still uncertain. However, researchers do know that certain factors known as risk factors increase the chances of developing atherosclerosis. Major risk factors for atherosclerosis include:

• cigarette smoking. Your risk increases with each cigarette you smoke.

• high levels of fatty substances in the bloodstream. This results in an increased chance that some of those fats will stick to the wall of an artery.

• hypertension, or high blood pressure. High blood pressure damages the inside of the arteries; fatty deposits are attracted to these areas of damage and cause narrowing of the arteries.

• diabetes mellitus. People with diabetes have an increased risk of developing atherosclerosis, especially in the arteries taking blood and oxygen to the legs and feet.

• obesity. No direct link between being overweight and atherosclerosis has been found. However, obesity can lead to hypertension or diabetes mellitus, both major risk factors associated with atherosclerosis.

• tension and stress. No direct link between tension and stress and atherosclerosis has been found. However, these factors can lead to hypertension and increased levels of fatty substances circulating in the bloodstream, both major risk factors associated with atherosclerosis.

(continued)

In the spaces below, list your personal risk factors.

_____

_____

_____

_____

_____

_____

_____

_____

• The more risk factors you have, the greater your chances are of developing atherosclerosis.
• You can lessen your risk of getting atherosclerosis by taking measures to control your personal risk factors. The nurse will give you more information on how to change each one.

Blood Pressure Measurement

TEACHING PLAN
Assessment
• Assess the patient's and family's understanding of the importance of monitoring blood pressure after discharge.
• Assess the patient's and family's previous experience with monitoring blood pressure.
• Assess the patient's and family's ability to read and write numbers.
• Assess the patient's and family's ability to see numbers on the sphygmomanometer (mercury, aneroid, electronic, or digital models).
• Assess the patient's and family's ability to hear Korotkoff sounds with a stethoscope (unless an electronic or digital model is used).
• Assess the patient's and family's ability to manually manipulate the sphygmomanometer and stethoscope (a stethoscope is not needed with an electronic or digital model).
• Collaborate with the doctor regarding setting desired parameters for the patient's blood pressure.

Materials needed
• Sphygmomanometer (the model that will be used at home)
• Stethoscope (if needed)
• Step-by-step diagram of person checking another person's blood pressure
• Example of blood pressure record for home use

Strategies to use
• Stimulate interest in the topic by explaining why monitoring blood pressure at home is essential for controlling hypertension.
• Present the information using a demonstration and return demonstration format.

Patient-teaching aid
See *How to take your blood pressure*, page 261.

Evaluation method
Have the patient and a family member:
• state the importance of monitoring the blood pressure at home
• take and record blood pressure measurements under a nurse's supervision
• state which blood pressure readings indicate a need for notifying the doctor.

Interventions and outcome criteria
☑ **Intervention 1**
Explain the basic meaning of systolic and diastolic blood pressure measurements.

Outcome criteria: The patient and family state the basic meaning of systolic and diastolic blood pressure measurements.

☑ **Intervention 2**
Explain general guidelines for measuring blood pressure, including:
• frequency of measurement
• when to measure
• parameters for notifying the doctor
• how to record blood pressure values.

Outcome criteria: The patient and family state when and how often blood pressure should be taken and which readings indicate the need for notifying the doctor.

☑ **Intervention 3**
Demonstrate the correct technique for measuring blood pressure, including:
• using the equipment needed
• explaining how to work the parts of the equipment, for example:
—how to inflate the cuff
—how to read the gauge
—how to deflate the cuff
—how to position the stethoscope
• explaining what sounds should be noted
• measuring blood pressure
• recording blood pressure correctly.

☑ **Intervention 4**
Have the patient and family take and record the patient's blood pressure under a nurse's supervision.

Outcome criteria: The patient and family correctly take and record blood pressure without assistance from the nurse.

How to Take Your Blood Pressure

Knowing how to take your blood pressure at home is important. It tells you whether the medications and risk factor control measures are, in fact, controlling your hypertension and lowering your blood pressure. It also tells you when your blood pressure is too high or too low so that you can notify the doctor to prevent damaging your body.

You have already discussed with the nurse the type of equipment that will be best for you to use in checking your blood pressure. In the spaces below, you or the nurse may write down exactly what you will need.

Type of sphygmomanometer
(blood pressure checking device): _____

Size of cuff (standard, small, oversized): _____

Stethoscope (yes/no): _____

You may obtain this equipment at: _____

_____

_____

_____

_____

_____

Remember these general guidelines when taking a blood pressure measurement:
• Take the blood pressure in the same arm each time.
• Make sure the arm is resting comfortably on a surface that raises the arm to the level of the heart.
• Make sure you are in a comfortable sitting position.
• Take the blood pressure reading at approximately the same time each day.

(continued)

Your nurse has already explained how to take a blood pressure measurement. The steps are outlined here as a guide for you to use at home.

1. Wrap the cuff snugly, about 1″ above the bend in the elbow. Do not wrap it too tightly.

2. Place the stethoscope earpieces in your ears.

3. Tighten the screw on the bulb, making sure you can easily loosen it with the fingers of one hand.

4. Pump up (inflate) the cuff while feeling the pulse at the wrist. When you can no longer feel the pulse, inflate the cuff 30 points higher on the gauge. Or inflate the cuff until _____ mm Hg is reached on the gauge.

5. Position the diaphragm of the stethoscope flatly and firmly on the inner part of the arm at the bend in the elbow. Do not press down hard on the diaphragm.

6. Loosen the screw slightly, allowing the air to slowly reduce the pressure of the cuff on the arm.

7. Listen and note the number on the gauge when you hear the first beating sound.

8. Continue to listen and note the number on the gauge when you hear the last beating sound.

9. After you have noted the last beating sound, loosen the screw more and allow the pressure in the cuff to be relieved completely.

10. Remove the cuff.

11. Record the date, time, and blood pressure.

When you write your blood pressure, remember to record the larger number (the systolic pressure) first in front of the slash mark. This number indicates the amount of pressure the blood forces against the arteries when the heart is pumping. It also indicates the pressure needed to move the blood through the arteries so that blood is distributed to all parts of the body.

Record the smaller number (the diastolic pressure) after the slash mark. This number indicates the amount of pressure the blood forces against the arteries between heartbeats, when the heart is relaxed and filling with more blood to pump. A high diastolic pressure indicates that the arteries are squeezed very tightly even when blood is not being pumped through them.

Use the following guidelines when taking your blood pressure at home. Your nurse will fill in the appropriate information before you leave the hospital. Be sure to bring your blood pressure record every time you visit your doctor.

Take your blood pressure (specify the frequency) _____

_____

in your _____ arm (specify right or left).

(continued)

According to your doctor, your blood pressure is controlled when it is:

_____

Call your doctor if your blood pressure is:

below _____ or above _____.

Write your doctor's name and number in the spaces below:

Doctor: _____

Phone: _____

Cardiac Anatomy and Physiology: Heart and Blood Vessels

TEACHING PLAN
Assessment
• Assess the patient's and family's understanding of cardiac anatomy and physiology as it applies to the patient's specific cardiovascular disease.

Materials needed
• Diagram or model of heart

Strategies to use
• Use group or individual teaching.
• Use model or diagram to clarify explanation.

Patient-teaching aid
See *Your heart and how it works,* page 266.

Evaluation method
• Have the patient and a family member explain, in their own words, the pertinent cardiac anatomy and physiology.

Interventions and outcome criteria
☑ Intervention 1
Using a model or diagram, describe the major points of general cardiac anatomy and physiology, including:
• basic anatomy of the heart
• role of the heart as a pump
• the need body tissues have for oxygen and how oxygen is supplied
• the way blood circulates through the heart into systemic circulation and back again.

Outcome criteria: The patient and family state that the heart is the muscle responsible for pumping blood that contains oxygen to all parts of the body. They state that all body tissues require oxygen to function correctly. They also state that blood, which contains oxygen, travels from the heart through the arteries to capillaries in all body tissues; blood returns back to the heart through the veins.

✓ Intervention 2

Describe the coronary circulation, including:
• the name and location of each coronary artery
• the part of the heart supplied by each coronary artery
• the role of coronary arteries in providing oxygen to the myocardium.

Outcome criteria: The patient and family state the names of major coronary arteries and the general part of the myocardium supplied by each artery. They also state that the coronary arteries supply the heart with the blood and oxygen it needs to work correctly.

✓ Intervention 3

Describe the structure and function of heart valves, including:
• the location of the aortic, mitral, tricuspid, and pulmonic valves (using a diagram)
• the function of valves in controlling blood flow through the heart.

Outcome criteria: The patient and family state the name and general location of major heart valves; they state that heart valves assist the blood to flow through the heart correctly.

✓ Intervention 4

Describe the role of the electrical conducting system of the heart.

Outcome criteria: The patient and family state that electrical stimulation is necessary for the heart to contract and pump blood throughout the body.

Your Heart and How It Works

Below is a brief explanation of the anatomy and physiology of the heart.

YOUR HEART

Your heart is located in the left side of the chest. It is about the size of your fist and consists of four chambers: the right atrium, right ventricle, left atrium, and left ventricle (see the accompanying illustration, *Heart structures*).

Your heart's job is to pump blood throughout the body; all parts of your body need an adequate supply of blood, which contains oxygen. Oxygen is essential for all parts of your body to work correctly. However, the amount of oxygen needed by any given part may vary. Tissues that need to work harder require more oxygen. For example, leg muscles have to work harder and need more oxygen when you are running than when you are sitting still. The body can supply more oxygen to a tissue by increasing the amount of blood going to it.

To understand how blood travels through your body, locate the left ventricle on the illustration. Blood is pumped out of the left ventricle into a large blood vessel called the aorta. From there, it travels to the other arteries in your body. From the arteries, the blood travels through smaller and smaller blood vessels. Finally, it reaches the capillaries, which are tiny blood vessels located in all tissues in the body.

In the capillaries, the oxygen moves from the blood into the tissues. Blood returns to the heart from the capillaries through veins. Eventually, all the blood flows into two major veins: the superior vena cava and inferior vena cava. From these major veins, the blood flows first into the right atrium, then to the right ventricle. After leaving the right ventricle, the blood travels to the lungs, where it picks up oxygen. From the lungs, the blood flows into the left atrium and then into the left ventricle, where it again is pumped throughout your body.

CORONARY CIRCULATION

Like any muscle, your heart needs an adequate supply of oxygen to work properly. The oxygen is carried to your heart through special vessels called coronary arteries. The coronary arteries lie on the outside of your heart.

Two major coronary arteries—the right coronary artery and left coronary artery—normally supply all the oxygen-rich blood your heart needs to work correctly. The right coronary artery supplies the right side of your heart. The left coronary artery, which supplies the left side of your heart, splits into two major branches: the left anterior descending and the left circumflex. You can find these arteries on the illustration titled *Coronary arteries*.

(continued)

HEART VALVES

Your heart contains valves—specialized pieces of tissue that keep blood flowing through the heart. The four major valves are discussed below; you can find these on the illustration titled *Heart structures*.
• The tricuspid valve is located between the right atrium and right ventricle.
• The pulmonic valve is between the right ventricle and the artery that carries blood from the heart to the lungs to get oxygen.
• The mitral valve lies between the left atrium and left ventricle.
• The aortic valve lies between the left ventricle and the aorta.

Electrical conducting system of the heart

Your heart also contains special cells that make your heart beat. These cells produce an electrical impulse that travels through your heart; this impulse stimulates the heart muscle to contract and pump blood to the rest of your body.

HEART STRUCTURES

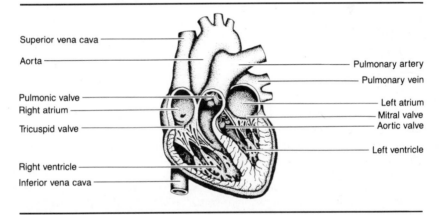

Superior vena cava
Aorta
Pulmonary artery
Pulmonary vein
Pulmonic valve
Right atrium
Left atrium
Mitral valve
Aortic valve
Tricuspid valve
Left ventricle
Right ventricle
Inferior vena cava

CORONARY ARTERIES

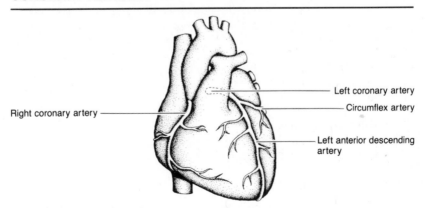

Left coronary artery
Circumflex artery
Right coronary artery
Left anterior descending artery

Cardiovascular Disease Risk Factors: Cigarette Smoking

TEACHING PLAN
Assessment
• Determine the amount that the patient smokes.
• Determine whether family members or significant others smoke.
• Determine the patient's and family's knowledge about the effects of smoking on cardiovascular functioning.
• Determine whether the patient has attempted to quit smoking before and what happened.
• Determine whether the patient desires to quit smoking.

Materials needed
• Written materials explaining the effects of smoking on the heart and cardiovascular function and how these effects accelerate cardiovascular disease
• Written list of quit-smoking resources

Strategies to use
• If the patient and his family do not know the effects of smoking on cardiovascular function and the accompanying increased risk of cardiovascular disease, present factual information, allowing opportunities for questions and answers.
• If the patient desires to quit smoking, help him develop an acceptable strategy. Have the patient problem-solve how to handle situations that stimulate his desire to smoke.
• If the patient does not wish to quit smoking, make sure that he understands the consequences of continuing to smoke. Then, determine whether he will consider reducing smoking. If he is agreeable, help him develop an acceptable reduction strategy. Help him problem-solve situations that stimulate his desire to smoke.
• If the patient understands the consequences and does not want to quit or reduce smoking, provide a written list of resources in case he changes his mind. Respect the patient's decision.

Patient-teaching aids
See *Smoking and your heart and blood vessels*, page 271; *How to stop smoking*, page 272; and *Reducing smoking*, page 275.

Interventions and outcome criteria
☑ **Intervention 1**
Explain the detrimental effects of smoking on the cardiovascular system, including how it:
• increases the heart's work load by increasing the pulse rate and blood pressure
• accelerates atherosclerosis and increases the risk of angina, myocardial infarction, cerebrovascular accident, and occlusive arterial disease
• decreases the oxygen supply to tissues by causing vasoconstriction and replacing oxygen in the bloodstream with carbon monoxide
• increases the risk of clot formation secondary to platelet adhesiveness.

Outcome criteria: The patient and family state that smoking increases the risk of angina, stroke, myocardial infarction, and occlusive arterial disease.

☑ **Intervention 2**
Discuss why changing to low-tar or low-nicotine cigarettes is ineffective in decreasing the risk of vascular disease, including these reasons:
• People frequently smoke an increased number of cigarettes when they switch.
• People usually inhale more deeply with these brands.

Outcome criteria: The patient and family state that changing to low-tar or low-nicotine cigarettes is ineffective in decreasing the risk of vascular disease.

☑ **Intervention 3**
Discuss the patient's plans for quitting or not quitting smoking.

Outcome criteria: The patient decides whether or not to quit or reduce smoking.

☑ **Intervention 4**
If the patient desires to quit, review major strategies, including:
• quitting cold turkey
• reducing the number of cigarettes smoked each day over a period of several days until he has completely quit
• delaying the time to start smoking each day by several hours until the target quit day is reached.

Outcome criteria: The patient who wishes to quit chooses a strategy for quitting.

☑ **Intervention 5**
If the patient does not want to stop but is interested in reducing smoking, present the following strategies:
• Suggest that he reduce the total number of cigarettes smoked each day.
• Have him determine how many fewer cigarettes he will smoke.

Outcome criteria: The patient who wishes to reduce smoking chooses a strategy for doing so.

☑ Intervention 6

Review methods the patient may use in situations that stimulate his desire to smoke.

Outcome criteria: The patient states methods to use when he is in a situation that stimulates his desire to smoke.

☑ Intervention 7

Provide a list of written resources.

Outcome criteria: The patient states what community resources are available to help him quit smoking.

Smoking and Your Heart and Blood Vessels

Understanding the effects of smoking on your heart and blood vessels is important. When you smoke, you inhale several chemicals into your lungs that can hurt your heart and blood vessels. As blood travels through your lungs to pick up oxygen, it also picks up these chemicals.

Nicotine is one of the major chemicals you inhale while smoking. Once it gets into your bloodstream, it makes your heart beat faster and your blood pressure rise. This increases the work of the heart. Eventually, your heart can become damaged from the extra work.

Nicotine also speeds up atherosclerosis, a disease in which fatty substances stick to the inside of one or more arteries. The arteries become narrowed, resulting in less blood and oxygen traveling through them to the tissue. If enough fatty substances build up in the coronary arteries (on the outside of the heart), angina or heart attack (myocardial infarction) may result. Your heart can be permanently damaged.

Fatty substances can also build up in other arteries. If the arteries transporting blood and oxygen to the brain are narrowed too much, a stroke may result. Fatty substances can also build up in the arteries transporting blood to your legs and feet. Narrowing of the arteries supplying blood to the feet can cause pain in the legs with activity or at rest. It may lead to loss of a leg or foot if the arteries become too narrowed and too much blood supply is lost.

Nicotine also increases the risk of clot formation in the bloodstream. This increases your chances of having a heart attack or myocardial infarction. Remember that a heart attack can occur when a clot totally blocks an artery on the outside of your heart.

Carbon monoxide is another chemical inhaled with smoking. Nicotine and carbon monoxide together decrease the amount of oxygen supplied to your tissues. Nicotine causes your blood vessels to narrow (constrict). This allows less blood to travel through them. Carbon monoxide replaces the oxygen normally carried by your blood. As a result, the amount of oxygen supplied to the various parts of your body can drop below the amount needed. Permanent damage can result.

If you are wondering whether low-tar or low-nicotine cigarettes are better for your heart, the answer is NO. Studies have shown that changing over to this type of cigarette results in smoking more cigarettes per day. It also results in a tendency to inhale more deeply when smoking. As a result, harmful amounts of nicotine and carbon monoxide are still inhaled.

How to Stop Smoking

Congratulations! You are thinking about quitting smoking or you have already made the decision to quit.

Although quitting smoking is not easy, you can do several things to make it easier on yourself. Different methods work better for different people. You may decide to use one or a combination of all of the methods presented in this patient-teaching aid.

QUITTING COLD TURKEY

With this method, choose a specific day on which to stop smoking. On that day, stop smoking entirely. Get rid of any cigarettes, matches, and lighters. Clean up the ashtrays and put them away. Most people who quit successfully use this method.

TAPERING OFF

This method allows you to stop smoking gradually. Over a period of several days (not weeks) decrease the number of cigarettes you smoke each day. To do so, first count the number of cigarettes you normally smoke each day. Then, make specific plans for reducing the number smoked by a set amount each day. For instance, if you normally smoke 20 cigarettes each day, you might smoke 15 cigarettes on the 1st day of tapering, 10 on the 2nd, 5 on the 3rd, and none on the 4th.

POSTPONING SMOKING

Another method of stopping gradually over a period of days (not weeks) allows you to delay the time you start smoking each day by a set number of hours. For example, on the 1st day, you might not start to smoke until 10 a.m.; on the 2nd day, you might wait until 1 p.m. This continues until you reach the day that you have decided to quit completely.

HANDLING THE DESIRE TO SMOKE

Once you have decided on a method to use to quit smoking, you need to plan what to do when you find yourself wanting a cigarette. People smoke for various reasons. Determining why you smoke will help you choose ways of handling your desire to smoke.

(continued)

Listed below are common reasons why people smoke. Read through each one and place a check mark by those that best describe why you smoke.*

☐ I smoke because I feel it gives me more energy, especially when I am tired.

☐ I smoke because it relaxes me.

☐ I smoke because I like it; it gives me a lot of pleasure.

☐ I smoke when I am angry or unhappy. Whenever I have had a bad day or have faced a hard situation, I smoke.

☐ I smoke when I feel lonely. I am never alone if I can smoke.

☐ I smoke because I don't think that I can go without smoking. I often have an intense hunger for cigarettes. I usually cannot last even a few hours without smoking a cigarette.

☐ I smoke out of habit. Certain times and places trigger me to light up automatically, sometimes without realizing that I am doing so.

Here are some suggestions for ways to handle your desire to smoke. Place a check mark by those you think would be helpful to you.*

☐ Take a brisk walk or do some other form of exercise when you want to smoke (you may need to discuss the amount and type of exercise with your doctor).

☐ Engage in regular physical activity (consult your doctor for the type and amount).

☐ Substitute a phone call or visit to a friend for a cigarette when you are feeling upset.

☐ Use another relaxation technique instead of a cigarette.

☐ Change your smoking habits. Put your cigarettes in a place that is harder to get to.

☐ Keep a record of each cigarette you smoke. Think about each one and decide if you really wanted or needed it.

☐ Tell your family and friends that you are quitting.

☐ Get nonsmoking or quit-smoking buttons or other items from the American Cancer Society. Display these where you will see them readily.

(continued)

*This list is adapted from the *Quitter's Guide,* published by the American Cancer Society.

☐ Talk to yourself about the harmful effects of smoking and the positive benefits of stopping.

☐ Carry low-calorie snacks with you to eat when you feel the desire to smoke.

☐ Put aside the money you would have spent on cigarettes. Use that money to buy something to reward yourself.

You may decide to quit smoking successfully by yourself, or you may want some help. Listed below are the addresses and phone numbers for some resources in your area that you can contact.

Local chapter of the American Cancer Society:

_____

_____

_____

_____

Stop-smoking programs at local wellness centers:

_____

_____

_____

Other:

_____

_____

_____

PATIENT-TEACHING AID

Reducing Smoking

Congratulations! You have decided to cut down on the number of cigarettes you smoke.

The best way to cut down on the amount you smoke is to reduce your smoking by a set number of cigarettes each day. Start by counting how many cigarettes you normally smoke in a day's time. Then decide how many cigarettes you will cut back to. You may find that, at first, you will want to smoke more than the amount you have allotted yourself. However, do not let yourself smoke even one cigarette more than your goal number each day.

People smoke for various reasons. Understanding why you smoke can help you find ways of handling your desire to smoke more.

Listed below are common reasons why people smoke. Read through each one and place a check mark by those that best describe your desire to smoke.*

☐ I smoke because I feel it gives me more energy, especially when I am tired.

☐ I smoke because it relaxes me.

☐ I smoke because I like it; it gives me a lot of pleasure.

☐ I smoke when I am angry or unhappy. Whenever I have had a bad day or have faced a hard situation, I smoke.

☐ I smoke when I feel lonely. I am never alone if I can smoke.

☐ I smoke because I don't think that I can go without smoking. I often have an intense hunger for cigarettes. I usually cannot last even a few hours without smoking a cigarette.

☐ I smoke out of habit. Certain times and places trigger me to light up automatically, sometimes without realizing that I am doing so.

Here are some suggestions for ways to handle your desire to smoke. Place a check mark by those you think would be helpful to you.*

☐ Take a brisk walk or do some other form of exercise when you want to smoke (you may need to discuss the amount and type of exercise with your doctor).

(continued)

*These lists are adapted from the *Quitter's Guide,* published by the American Cancer Society.

☐ Engage in regular physical activity (consult your doctor for the type and amount).

☐ Substitute a phone call or a visit to a friend for a cigarette when you are feeling upset.

☐ Use another relaxation technique instead of a cigarette.

☐ Change your smoking habits. Put your cigarettes in a place that is harder to get to.

☐ Keep a record of each cigarette that you smoke. Think about each one and decide if you really wanted or needed it.

☐ Tell your family and friends that you are reducing the amount you smoke.

☐ Carry low-calorie snacks with you to eat when you feel a desire for an extra cigarette.

☐ Put aside the money you would have spent on the extra cigarettes. Spend it on something to reward yourself.

Cardiovascular Disease Risk Factors: Diabetes Mellitus and Atherosclerosis

TEACHING PLAN

An extensive and exhaustive plan for teaching diabetic self-management to patients exceeds the scope of this book. The purpose of the material provided below is to describe the relationship between atherosclerosis and diabetes, to provide suggestions for assessing how well the patient and his family manage diabetic care at home, and to provide a general overview of content to cover when teaching diabetic self-care.

Assessment

• Determine whether the patient has diabetes mellitus.
• Assess the patient's and family's knowledge about self-management of diabetes.
• Assess the patient's and family's knowledge about the relationship between diabetes and atherosclerosis.
• Collaborate with the doctor about the patient's prescribed regimen, including diet, medications, and glucose self-monitoring.
• Identify any previous problems the patient and his family have encountered in managing diabetes.
• Assess how well the patient's diabetes has been controlled in the past. Factors to assess might include:
—determining how many times in the last year the patient has been admitted with uncontrolled blood glucose levels or ketoacidosis
—assessing the patient's most recent glycosylated hemoglobin or hemoglobin A level
—reviewing the patient's blood glucose levels over a period of time.
• Assess the patient's and family's performance of pertinent psychomotor skills, including insulin administration and self-monitoring of glucose levels.

Materials needed

• Written materials on diabetic exchange diet
• Written materials or diagrams illustrating proper insulin administration
• Written list of resources for diabetic self-management
• Insulin syringe, insulin, and glucose monitoring equipment

Strategies to use

• Stimulate interest in the topic by explaining to the patient and family that diabetes is a risk factor for atherosclerosis.

• Individualize teaching by addressing areas of diabetic self-management the patient identifies as a problem or discuss an area that the patient or his family is not managing correctly.

Patient-teaching aid
See *Your diabetes and atherosclerosis,* page 280.

Evaluation method
• Have the patient and family explain, in their own words, the role of diabetes in atherosclerosis.
• Have the patient and family demonstrate pertinent aspects of diabetic self-management, including planning 2 or 3 days of meals using a diabetic exchange diet correctly, administering insulin in the hospital setting, and performing self-monitoring of glucose levels in the hospital setting.

Interventions and outcome criteria
☑ **Intervention 1**
Review atherosclerosis, if necessary (see "Atherosclerosis: Disease Process and Risk Factors" in this section).

☑ **Intervention 2**
Explain the relationship between diabetes mellitus and atherosclerosis, including the following:
• the increased risk of atherosclerotic plaque formation secondary to elevated blood glucose and blood lipid levels seen in diabetes
• the positive benefits of strict control of diabetes in reducing the risk for atherosclerosis.

Outcome criteria: The patient and family state that diabetes can increase the risk of atherosclerosis by increasing the level of fatty acids circulating in the bloodstream; they state that tight control of diabetes decreases the risk that it will accelerate atherosclerosis.

☑ **Intervention 3**
Review the patient's prescribed regimen, including:
• dietary restrictions
• medications, including:
—insulin administration
—use of oral agents
• self-monitoring of glucose levels
• any problems encountered by the patient while trying to control diabetes at home
• use or need for outside resources or referrals, including:
—dietitian
—local chapter of the American Diabetes Association.

Outcome criteria: The patient and family correctly plan meals within the prescribed diet. They also correctly administer prescribed medication to control diabetes and correctly demonstrate the prescribed method for self-monitoring of glucose levels.

☑ **Intervention 4**
Explain the cumulative effects of risk factors in relation to the patient's overall risk for developing atherosclerosis.

Outcome criteria: The patient and family state that controlling other risk factors reduces the patient's overall risk for atherosclerosis.

☑ **Intervention 5**
Assist the patient and family to identify modifiable risk factors.

Outcome criteria: The patient and family identify personal risk factors.

Your Diabetes and Atherosclerosis

Because you have diabetes, you are at greater risk for developing athero-sclerosis and heart disease. You can help to decrease this risk by controlling your diabetes as strictly as possible.

DIABETES AS A RISK FACTOR
As you may know, poorly controlled diabetes increases the amount of sugar and fatty substances in your bloodstream. This increases the chance that fatty substances will stick to the inside of your arteries. The deposit of fatty substances narrows the arteries and decreases the amount of blood and oxygen traveling to various parts of your body. When the amount of oxygen traveling to any part of your body drops below the amount that it needs, permanent damage can result.

Controlling your diabetes involves sticking to your prescribed diet, taking your prescribed medication, and checking your blood glucose levels fre-quently. Think about how you have been managing your diabetes at home. Are you having any problems? Do you have any questions?

In the spaces below, write down any questions you may have about managing your diabetes at home. Your nurse will be glad to answer your questions and provide you with additional information.

_____

_____

_____

_____

_____

_____

_____

_____

_____

(continued)

OTHER RISK FACTORS

Because you have diabetes, it is important for you to find out what other risk factors for atherosclerosis you have. Your chances of getting heart disease increase with each risk factor you have. Reducing these factors will help reduce your chance of having angina, a heart attack, a stroke, or problems with the circulation to your feet.

Common risk factors that you can change or reduce include:
• smoking
• hypertension, or high blood pressure
• excessive levels of fatty substances circulating in the bloodstream
• obesity (overweight)
• excessive tension or stress
• lack of exercise.

Which of the above risk factors apply to you? You may want to list them in the spaces below. The nurse will provide you with more information about each risk factor you list.

_____

_____

_____

_____

_____

_____

_____

_____

Cardiovascular Disease Risk Factors: Dietary Measures to Control Hyperlipidemia

TEACHING PLAN
Assessment
• Assess the patient's and family's normal dietary patterns (including use of fast foods and restaurant meals).
• Assess the patient's and family's knowledge about dietary measures that help control hyperlipidemia.
• Assess the patient's and family's past experiences with limiting dietary intake of saturated fats and cholesterol; identify areas that previously have posed a problem for the patient and family.
• Identify which family members routinely buy the groceries and prepare the food.
• Assess the patient's and family's willingness to change dietary habits.
• Collaborate with the doctor to determine the patient's specific diet order after discharge.
• Collaborate with the dietitian to determine what other dietary teaching the patient will receive; coordinate teaching to provide consistency and reinforcement for the patient and family.

Materials needed
• Written list of resources, including cookbooks available in local bookstores and the name, address, and telephone number of the local chapter of the American Heart Association
• Written information summarizing a prudent diet for controlling heart disease, including a list of foods high in saturated fats or cholesterol as well as appropriate substitutes

Strategies to use
• Stimulate interest in the topic by explaining the role of diet in accelerating atherosclerosis.
• Help the patient and family to decide which eating patterns they should change to decrease their consumption of saturated fats and cholesterol.

Patient-teaching aids
See *Your diet and your heart*, page 284; *Guidelines for limiting cholesterol and saturated fats in your diet*, page 285; and *Personal diet work sheet*, page 286.

Evaluation method
• Have the patient and family:
—describe, in their own words, the role of diet in atherosclerosis
—plan 2 to 3 days' meals using guidelines presented for a prudent diet for the heart
—set one or more specific goals for limiting intake of saturated fats and cholesterol.

Interventions and outcome criteria
☑ **Intervention 1**
Review the process of how atherosclerosis develops, if necessary.

☑ **Intervention 2**
Discuss the role of cholesterol in the development of atherosclerosis, including information that:
• cholesterol is a major component of atherosclerotic plaque
• high levels of cholesterol circulating in the bloodstream accelerate atherosclerosis.

Outcome criteria: The patient and family state that high levels of cholesterol can accelerate atherosclerosis.

☑ **Intervention 3**
Describe the sources of cholesterol, including:
• the amount manufactured by the body
• the amount obtained from eating foods high in cholesterol and saturated fats.

Outcome criteria: The patient and family state that eating foods high in cholesterol and saturated fats can increase blood cholesterol levels.

☑ **Intervention 4**
Describe the means to lower saturated fat and cholesterol intake.

☑ **Intervention 5**
Help the patient and family to make realistic plans for dietary changes, including:
• assessing their current patterns by keeping a food diary or using a questionnaire
• identifying the major sources of cholesterol and saturated fats in their diet
• setting specific and realistic plans to decrease their intake of cholesterol and saturated fats.

Outcome criteria: The patient and family develop specific, realistic plans for reducing their intake of saturated fats and cholesterol.

☑ **Intervention 6**
Provide a list of written resources and a summary of dietary instructions for home use.

Your Diet and Your Heart

What you eat can increase your chances of developing atherosclerosis. Specifically, eating foods that are high in fat causes high levels of fatty substances to circulate in your bloodstream. The higher the levels, the greater your chances of developing atherosclerosis.

Cholesterol, one of the main fatty substances in the bloodstream, is needed in small amounts for the body to work correctly. It is manufactured by the body as well as supplied by the food you eat. Although you cannot control the amount of cholesterol your body makes, you can decrease the amount of cholesterol in your diet. Cholesterol is found in such animal products as egg yolks, whole milk and whole milk products, meats, poultry, fish, organ meats, and shrimp.

Foods high in saturated fats also increase the amount of cholesterol in your bloodstream. Saturated fats are usually hard at room temperature. They can come from such animal products as beef, pork, lamb, ham, butter, cream, and cheeses made from whole milk. They can also come from vegetable sources, such as the solid shortenings used in store-bought cakes, pies, cookies, candy, and fried foods.

Foods containing polyunsaturated fats help to lower the amount of cholesterol in your bloodstream. Found in the oils of vegetable products (corn oil, safflower oil, sunflower oil, and soybean oil), polyunsaturated fats are usually liquid at room temperature.

Changing your diet is an individual matter. The next few pages contain some guidelines and activities to help you plan ways to limit the amount of cholesterol and saturated fats in your diet.

Guidelines for Limiting Cholesterol and Saturated Fats in Your Diet

Follow these simple guidelines to limit the amount of cholesterol and saturated fats in your diet:
• Read the labels on foods you buy. Choose salad dressings and cooking oils that have a higher percentage of polyunsaturated fats than saturated fats. Do not use dressings or oils that are high in saturated fats.
• Avoid store-bought foods containing saturated fats. Read the labels carefully on bakery products and nondairy milk products.
• Limit the amount of meat, fish, and poultry that you eat to 5 to 7 ounces each day.
• Steam or broil your food. Limit the amount of food that you fry.
• Limit the amount of fats and oils that you use in cooking and baking or as dressings to 5 to 8 teaspoons per day.
• When buying beef, choose lean cuts of meat. Trim off all extra fat before cooking.
• Substitute chicken or turkey frequently for other meats in your meals. Remove the skin before eating.
• Have at least two meatless meals as your main meals each week. (Recipes are available in cookbooks.)
• Do not eat more than two egg yolks per week, including those used in baking.
• Substitute low-fat dairy products (such as low-fat milk, cheese, or yogurt) for whole-milk dairy products.
• Substitute reduced-fat products for ones with regular fat levels when possible. Many foods, such as mayonnaise and salad dressings, are available in a reduced-fat form.

Personal Diet Work Sheet

The decision to change your diet is yours. If you decide to cut down on the amount of saturated fats and cholesterol that you eat, you may find the following work sheet helpful in developing specific plans for changing.

Start by identifying which foods you frequently eat that are high in saturated fats and cholesterol. You can do this in several ways.

• Write down on a sheet of paper what you usually eat at each meal at home. To do this, you might want to think specifically about what you ate at home for 2 or 3 days before coming into the hospital (if you had been eating normally) and write down the foods you ate and how they were prepared.

• Using your list, fill out the form below to determine the major sources of cholesterol and saturated fats in your diet.

• Check off which of the following foods you eat and how many times you eat them each week.

DIET WORK SHEET

Foods eaten	Times per week				
	More than 7	5 to 7	2 to 4	1	Less than 1
Eggs as part of meal					
Eggs used in baking or cooking					
Butter on food					
Butter used in cooking/frying					
Whole milk as beverage					
Whole milk in cooking/baking					
Sour cream					
Hard cheeses					
Bacon as part of meal					
Bacon drippings as seasoning					
Pork					

(continued)

DIET WORK SHEET *(continued)*

Foods eaten	Times per week				
	More than 7	5 to 7	2 to 4	1	Less than 1
Fatty cuts of beef					
Ham hocks/lard/salt pork					
Organ meats					
Meat drippings in cooking					
Luncheon meats					
Sausage					
Bakery cakes, cookies, or pies					
Nondairy cream substitute					
Hydrogenated shortenings					
Regular mayonnaise					
Salad dressings					
"Fast Foods" (specify)					
"Fast Foods" (specify)					
"Fast Foods" (specify)					

Keep in mind that this list is incomplete. You or your nurse or dietitian may identify other foods that you eat regularly that are high in saturated fats or cholesterol. List these in the spaces provided below.

Foods eaten	Times per week				
	More than 7	5 to 7	2 to 4	1	Less than 1

(continued)

DIET WORK SHEET *(continued)*

Foods eaten	Times per week				
	More than 7	5 to 7	2 to 4	1	Less than 1

(continued)

Next, looking at your chart, pick out the foods you eat most often and list them in the spaces provided below.

_____

_____

_____

_____

_____

Now, pick out some eating habits you think you will change, writing down how you plan to change each one. For example, if you eat eggs every morning for breakfast, a plan for change might read as follows: "I will eat eggs for breakfast 3 mornings a week instead of 7. Instead of eggs on the other 4 mornings, I will eat cooked cereal."

Use the list of resources that the nurse or dietitian has given you to help choose foods that you like as substitutes for less healthy foods.

Your plans:

1. _____

_____

_____

_____

_____

2. _____

_____

_____

_____

_____

(continued)

3. _____

_____

_____

_____

_____

4. _____

_____

_____

_____

_____

When you get home, try out these plans. They may need to be changed slightly. Use the written resources provided by the nurse or dietitian for help.

Once these changes become a comfortable part of your eating habits, you may want to make additional changes to further reduce the saturated fat and cholesterol in your diet. Use your chart, the written materials, and a cookbook to plan a reduced-fat, low-cholesterol diet.

Congestive Heart Failure: Disease Process and Home Care

TEACHING PLAN
Assessment
• Collaborate with the doctor to determine the patient's discharge orders.
• Assess the patient's and family's knowledge of congestive heart failure (CHF) and its signs and symptoms.
• Assess the patient's and family's knowledge of home management of CHF, including medication administration, diet, fluid restrictions, activity, and use of oxygen at home.
• Assess the patient's and family's previous experience with managing CHF at home.
• Determine whether the patient and family have any special concerns.

Strategies to use
• Stimulate interest in the topic by beginning with patient or family concerns about how to manage the patient's CHF at home.
• Assist the patient and family to problem-solve the following:
 —limiting the patient's sodium intake as prescribed
 —limiting the patient's fluid if indicated
 —pacing the patient's activity to limit fatigue and dyspnea
 —taking and recording daily weights
 —obtaining additional medical care appropriately.

Patient-teaching aid
See *How to manage your congestive heart failure at home*, page 294.

Evaluation method
Have the patient and a family member:
• describe in their own words home management of CHF
• state plans for when and how to obtain medical care appropriately
• state plans for limiting fluids, limiting sodium, and monitoring daily weights.

Interventions and outcome criteria
☑ **Intervention 1**
Briefly review the normal role of the heart, as necessary.

☑ Intervention 2
Explain the pathophysiology of CHF.

Outcome criteria: The patient and family state that CHF occurs when the heart is not pumping effectively enough to meet the body's needs.

☑ Intervention 3
Discuss measures to control CHF and its symptoms, including:
• prescribed medications
• a sodium-restricted diet
• fluid restrictions and fluid plans
• general principles of activity management for patients with CHF, such as:
—alternating periods of activity with periods of rest
—considering activities of daily living as "activities" when planning a rest-activity schedule
—stopping the patient's activity when he becomes fatigued or short of breath
—performing all activities at a slow to moderate pace
—using the patient's response to activity in the hospital as a guideline for making specific recommendations for home activity.
Also, help the patient and family to manage the patient's activity in the hospital.

Outcome criteria: The patient and family state major ways of limiting CHF and its symptoms; they state the general principles of activity for patients with CHF and develop realistic plans for managing the patient's activity at home.

☑ Intervention 4
Instruct the patient and his family in the appropriate procedure for taking and recording daily weights.

Outcome criteria: The patient and family state the correct way to monitor daily weights at home.

☑ Intervention 5
Assist the patient and family in how to use oxygen correctly at home, if indicated.

☑ Intervention 6
Describe common factors that can precipitate acute episodes, including:
• failure to take prescribed medications
• failure to follow prescribed fluid and sodium restrictions
• any form of excessive physical or emotional stress, such as that associated with:
—systemic infection
—tachycardia
—excessive activity
• any particular risk factors that can be identified from the patient's history.

Outcome criteria: The patient and family state major factors that can precipitate acute episodes of CHF.

☑ Intervention 7

Describe signs and symptoms that indicate worsening CHF, including:
• increased dyspnea with activity or at rest
• severe dyspnea at rest
• increased fatigue without increased activity
• weight gain of 2 lb or more in 24 hours
• edema in the hands and feet
• development of cough (may be nonproductive or productive of large amounts of pink, frothy sputum)
• feeling of suffocation
• cold, clammy skin.

Outcome criteria: The patient and family state signs and symptoms of increased CHF as listed above.

☑ Intervention 8

Instruct the patient and family to seek immediate medical help if the above symptoms occur; help them to determine how they will obtain medical assistance.

Outcome criteria: The patient and family state they should get medical help if any of the above symptoms occur and identify specific plans for obtaining that help.

How to Manage Your Congestive Heart Failure at Home

Your doctor has told you that you have congestive heart failure (CHF). CHF is the medical term for the condition in which the heart is not working well enough as a pump to meet the body's needs for blood and oxygen. Your doctor has ordered some medications and other treatments to help your heart pump more effectively. It is important that you follow these orders carefully.

CONTROLLING CHF AT HOME

To control your condition, you will need to follow the doctor's orders carefully. Remember to do the following:
• Take all your medications as the doctor has ordered. These medications help your heart pump better. They also help decrease such symptoms as shortness of breath and swelling in your hands and feet. The nurse will give you additional information for each of the medications you will be taking at home.
• Limit the amount of sodium (salt) you eat, as ordered by your doctor. Your nurse will give you additional information on this.
• Limit the amount of fluid you drink, as ordered by your doctor. Your nurse will give you additional information on fluid plans.
• Limit your activity, as ordered by your doctor.

The specific amount of activity your doctor wants you to do at home is:

_____

_____

_____

MANAGING YOUR ACTIVITY

It is important for you to get enough rest during the day. To ensure that you get the proper amount, you might want to follow these general guidelines:
• Space out your activities during the day. Do not perform numerous activities all at one time without resting in between.
• Consider your normal daily activities (such as bathing, shaving, eating, and dressing) as "activities," and rest in between them.
• Do your activities at a slow to moderate pace. Do not hurry.
• Remember that resting does not always mean sleeping. You can rest by sitting quietly in a chair for 20 to 30 minutes.
• Stop any activity when you first begin to feel tired or more short of breath.

(continued)

Based on the amount of activity you can do in the hospital, you or your nurse may want to add additional guidelines to follow at home. Write these in the spaces provided below.

_____

_____

_____

_____

TAKING YOUR DAILY WEIGHT

Weighing yourself each day is important. To weigh yourself correctly, be sure to:
• weigh yourself at the same time each morning using the same scale
• weigh yourself after you urinate in the morning and before you eat breakfast
• record the date and your weight
• notify the doctor if you gain 2 lb or more overnight.

USING OXYGEN

Your doctor may want you to use oxygen at home. Using oxygen helps decrease some patients' shortness of breath. If you are supposed to use oxygen at home, your nurse will give you additional information.

WORSENING CHF

Your CHF may get worse; if it does you will have more symptoms. CHF can worsen for several reasons, including:
• not taking your medications as the doctor has ordered
• eating too many high-sodium foods or adding too much salt to your food
• drinking more water or other fluids than allowed
• fever and infections
• too much activity
• a very rapid or irregular heartbeat
• strong emotions, such as fear, excitement, and anxiety.
You will know that your CHF is getting worse if you develop any of the following warning signs:
• you become more short of breath than usual (with activity or at rest)
• you become extremely, severely short of breath at rest
• you become more tired than usual with your typical day's activities
• you notice that your shoes have become too tight or that your feet and ankles are swollen
• you develop a cough without any flulike symptoms
• you notice that your hands are swollen or that your rings are too tight
• you or a family member notices that you have swelling in your lower back or hips (if you spend most of your day in bed)
• you gain 2 lb or more overnight
• you feel very anxious
• your skin is cold to touch, and you are in a cold sweat.

(continued)

You may have had worsening CHF at home before. Think about how you felt. List the symptoms you had in the spaces below.

_____

_____

_____

If you have any symptoms of worsening CHF, you need to get immediate medical help. In the spaces provided, list how you will get additional medical care if you should need it.

Who to call (include name and telephone number):

during the day: _____

on the weekend: _____

at night: _____

How I will get to the doctor's office/clinic/hospital (include telephone numbers if needed):

during the day: _____

on the weekend: _____

at night: _____

I will keep my emergency numbers: _____

You may have other questions about managing CHF at home. Write any additional questions you have in the spaces below, and discuss these questions with the nurse.

_____

_____

_____

_____

_____

Coronary Artery Bypass Grafting Surgery: Home Care

TEACHING PLAN

Assessment
• Collaborate with the doctor about the patient's discharge orders.
• Assess the patient's and family's knowledge of home care after coronary artery bypass grafting (CABG) surgery, including medications, activity, diet, and possible complications.
• Determine the patient's and family's specific areas of concern about home care.

Strategies to use
• Stimulate interest in the topic by beginning with the patient's and family's concerns.
• Assist the patient and his family to problem-solve the following:
—managing the patient's activity at home
—decreasing the risk of common complications
—recognizing complications and knowing what to do if they occur
—managing postoperative pain
—identifying risk factors for recurrent coronary artery disease (CAD) and knowing how to modify them.

Patient-teaching aid
See *Home care after coronary artery bypass grafting surgery,* page 300.

Evaluation method
• Have the patient and family explain, in their own words, home care measures and their specific plans for implementing each measure.

Interventions and outcome criteria
☑ **Intervention 1**
Discuss all prescribed medications.

Outcome criteria: Use the outcome criteria from "Medication Guidelines" in this section.

☑ **Intervention 2**
Discuss the patient's activity at home, including:
• activities of daily living
• pacing activities
• need for sleep and rest
• visitors and phone calls
• how to increase activity
• warning signs of overexertion.

Outcome criteria: The patient and family state appropriate plans for managing the patient's activity at home.

☑ Intervention 3
Discuss the resumption of sexual activity at home.

Outcome criteria: The patient and family state guidelines for resuming sexual activity.

☑ Intervention 4
Discuss home management of incisional pain.

Outcome criteria: The patient and family state how to manage the patient's pain at home.

☑ Intervention 5
Discuss care of the incision lines and sternum, including:
• daily care of incisions
• daily inspection for signs of infection
• precautions to use until the sternum heals, such as
—no driving
—limited lifting (less than 10 lb)
—avoidance of activities that involve pushing or pulling heavy objects.

Outcome criteria: The patient and family state how to care for the patient's sternum and incision lines.

☑ Intervention 6
If a saphenous vein graft was taken, discuss care of the donor leg, including:
• daily inspection of incision lines
• use of elastic stockings or support hose, if prescribed
• daily observation for edema
• measures to reduce edema.

Outcome criteria: The patient and family state appropriate care of the donor leg.

☑ Intervention 7
Discuss typical emotions experienced by the patient after CABG surgery.

Outcome criteria: Use the outcome criteria from "Stress Management" in this section.

☑ Intervention 8
Discuss a low-cholesterol, low-saturated-fat diet.

Outcome criteria: Use the outcome criteria from "Dietary Measures to Control Hyperlipidemia" in this section.

☑ Intervention 9
Describe how to take and record daily weights.

Outcome criteria: The patient and family state how to take and record daily weights.

☑ Intervention 10
Identify the patient's specific risk factors for recurrent CAD.

Outcome criteria: Use the outcome criteria from "Atherosclerosis: Disease Process and Risk Factors" in this section.

☑ Intervention 11
Discuss modification of the patient's individual risk factors as indicated, including:
• following a low-saturated-fat and low-cholesterol diet
• stopping smoking
• control of hypertension
• control of diabetes
• exercise.

Outcome criteria: The patient and family state plans for modifying the patient's individual risk factors.

☑ Intervention 12
Discuss possible complications and how to obtain appropriate medical care if any should occur. Cover these complications:
• pericarditis and its characteristic pain
• dysrhythmias, including:
—changes in pulse rate and rhythm
—signs of decreased cardiac output
• deep vein thrombosis, including:
—pain and swelling
—preventive measures.

Outcome criteria: The patient and family state signs of complications; they state plans for obtaining medical care when needed.

☑ Intervention 13
Discuss follow-up care.

Outcome criteria: The patient and family state prescribed follow-up care.

Home Care after Coronary Artery Bypass Grafting Surgery

Congratulations! You will soon be going home. Like many patients who have had coronary artery bypass surgery, you may have questions about your care at home. This patient-teaching aid will answer some common questions you or your family may have. If you have other questions that are not answered in this aid, be sure to ask your nurse or doctor.

MEDICATIONS
Remember that it is important for you to take all of your medications exactly as your doctor has ordered. Your nurse will give you more information about each medication you will be taking at home.

ACTIVITY
When you first get home, do about the same amount of activity at the same pace as you did in the hospital. Continue this level of activity for the first couple of weeks. Gradually, you will increase your activity. How fast varies from patient to patient.

Follow these general guidelines for your activity:
• Shower or bathe, as desired. If you shower, you might want to put a stool in the shower to sit on. If you bathe, you may need some help to get in and out of the tub for the first few days. Avoid using extremely hot water in either the tub or shower. Shaving is permitted.
• Plan to get enough rest. Remember that rest does not always mean sleeping. It may include sitting quietly for 20 to 30 minutes. Be sure to rest in between activities.
• Plan to get enough sleep. It is a good idea for you to take one or two brief naps during the day. However, be careful. If you sleep too much during the day, you will not sleep well at night. Plan to get 8 to 10 hours of sleep at night.
• Stop any activity when you begin to feel tired. Do not let yourself become overtired.
• Stop any activity immediately if you feel short of breath, experience palpitations, feel faint or dizzy, break out in a cold sweat, or experience angina-like chest pain.
• Pace your activities. Spread them out during the day; do not try to do too many things all at one time. Also, do not rush through any activity. When you first get home, your activities will include bathing, eating, walking, talking on the telephone, and visiting with friends. A slow pace and plenty of rest are important.
• Unless your doctor tells you differently, you can climb stairs. Take them at a slow pace. If you feel short of breath or tired, sit down and rest. Plan your day to avoid extra trips up and down the stairs.

(continued)

• Limit visits from friends to two or three per day. If you feel tired during a visit, do not hesitate to leave the room and rest in another part of your home or to ask your visitors to leave.

Think about your usual level of activity at home. Do you have any questions or concerns about when to resume any specific activity? If so, write down your questions below and discuss them with your nurse or doctor.

_____

_____

_____

_____

EXERCISING
Exercise is an important part of your recovery after open-heart surgery. Your nurse will give you more information on how and when to exercise. You might also want to consider participating in an outpatient cardiac rehabilitation program. Discuss this with your doctor.

SEXUAL ACTIVITY
Many patients are concerned that resuming sexual activity will damage their heart. Sexual activity puts about the same amount of stress on your heart as walking up a flight of stairs quickly or walking one or two blocks at a brisk pace. Your nurse will give you some guidelines on how to safely resume sex at home after open-heart surgery.

CARING FOR YOUR STERNUM
As you probably know, your sternum (breastbone) was cut in half during surgery. It is now being held together by wires; these wires will not come out. Your sternum will heal completely in 4 to 12 weeks. While it is healing, you may hear a slight clicking sound when you take a breath or turn. This is normal and will go away when your sternum is completely healed.

While your sternum is healing, you need to be careful to avoid putting too much strain on it. This means you should:
• avoid any activities that involve lifting more than 10 lb. This may include carrying children, lifting or carrying bags of groceries, or carrying suitcases.
• avoid any activities that involve pushing or pulling of heavy objects. Examples include mowing the grass, vacuuming, opening and closing heavy doors, and moving furniture.
• avoid driving or riding a bicycle, motorcycle, horse, or lawn mower. An accident involving any of these could damage your sternum and slow its healing.

Your surgeon wants you to follow the above precautions for _____ weeks.

(continued)

CARING FOR YOUR INCISION LINES

Gently wash the incision lines with mild soap and warm water each day. Avoid scrubbing them vigorously with a washcloth. Pat them dry gently. Do not put any lotions, creams, or powders on the incision lines unless prescribed by your doctor.

Take a good look at your incision lines each day. You may need to use a mirror to see your chest incision well. Eventually, you will notice your incisions begin to look better. You may notice a touch of redness around the edges or a small area of swelling at the top of your chest incision. These are normal. Also, expect your incisions to itch somewhat as they heal.

Look at your incision lines each day for any of the following trouble signs:
• increasing tenderness of the incision line
• increasing redness around the edges of the incision line
• increasing swelling around the edges of the incision line
• any drainage from the incision line.

If any of the above trouble signs occur, call your doctor right away. You may be developing an infection.

CARING FOR YOUR DONOR LEG

Read through this section if your bypass surgery was done using a vein from your leg.

Follow these guidelines:
• Care for your leg incision as described above; look at it daily for any signs of infection.
• Check your leg daily for any signs of swelling. If you notice swelling, put your feet up when sitting. If your doctor has recommended that you use support hose or elastic stockings, wear them as directed. The nurse will show you how to put them on and will give you more written information on their use.
• Avoid crossing your legs, as this impairs circulation to your lower legs.
• Avoid sitting in one position or standing for long periods of time.
• If you continue to have swelling in your donor leg, talk with your doctor.

MANAGING INCISIONAL PAIN

When you get home, you will probably have some pain from your incision just like you have had in the hospital. You may notice this pain more when you take a deep breath, turn, or move. You may also notice it more at night when you are trying to fall asleep.

To decrease your pain, your doctor has prescribed that you take:

You may take _____ tablets every _____ hours as needed.

(continued)

Medication guidelines

Here are some suggestions for taking your pain medication:
• Take the medication at night just before you try to fall asleep. Do not substitute sleeping pills for pain medication. If you are hurting, the sleeping pill will not work. The pain medication will relieve your pain and help you sleep at the same time.
• Take one tablet in the morning before you begin your day's activities.
• Take your medication often enough during the day to allow you to complete your planned activities comfortably. (Remember, you can only take your medication every _____ hours.)
• If you find that you are sleeping frequently during the day, you may be taking too much pain medication. If you are taking two tablets, try taking only one. Or wait longer between taking each dose.
• Try using distraction techniques to decrease your pain. These may include watching television, listening to the radio, visiting with friends or family, or engaging in some other activity.
• Participate in your prescribed exercise and activity program to help decrease your incisional pain.

DIET

Your doctor has prescribed a _____
diet for you. The nurse and dietitian will be giving you more information about this diet and how to use it at home.

DAILY WEIGHTS

Weighing yourself each day is important. To obtain accurate weights, be sure to:
• weigh yourself at the same time each morning using the same scale
• weigh yourself before you eat breakfast and after you urinate in the morning
• record the date and your weight
• notify your doctor if you gain 2 lb or more overnight.

PREVENTING ATHEROSCLEROSIS

Your surgery did not cure your atherosclerotic disease. If you do not take measures to slow or prevent atherosclerosis, you will again develop blockages in your arteries. These blockages can lead to angina, heart attack, stroke, or problems with the circulation in your legs.

The nurse will give you more information on risk factors for atherosclerosis and how to change them. After reading the material, list your individual risk factors in the spaces below.

_____

_____

_____

(continued)

WARNING SIGNS

Some patients develop problems after coronary artery bypass surgery. Knowing the warning signs allows you to recognize the problems quickly and get appropriate medical care.

Problems with heart rhythm

Notify your doctor immediately if you develop any of the following signs:
• pulse rhythm changing from regular or slightly irregular to extremely irregular
• feelings of palpitations in your chest
• dizziness, faintness, or breaking out in a cold sweat.
The above signs are warnings that your heartbeat has become so irregular that your body is not getting enough blood and oxygen to meet its needs.

Pericarditis

Pericarditis is another common problem that can develop. Your heart is covered by a thin lining called the pericardium. This lining can become inflamed after heart surgery. This inflammation is called pericarditis. The major sign that you might notice is pain that gets worse when you take a deep breath, swallow, or bend over. This pain may be mild to severe; you may feel it in your chest, shoulder, or neck. This is not an emergency; however, you do need to notify your doctor.

Deep vein thrombosis

Deep vein thrombosis, a serious problem that can occur after bypass surgery, is most likely to happen while your activity is still limited. Its signs include:
• pain in one leg (other than pain from a leg incision). Some people describe this pain as a feeling of tenderness that will not go away. It also may feel like a heaviness or aching. This pain may be lessened when you sit down and put your feet up.
• swelling or edema in one leg. You might notice that the calf or thigh of one leg is bigger than the calf or thigh of the other leg.
    If these signs develop, call your doctor immediately. Because deep vein thrombosis can be serious, prevention is very important. Your nurse will give you additional information on how to reduce your risk of developing this complication.

Plan now how you will get additional medical care if any of the above problems develop. In the spaces below, list pertinent names and telephone numbers.

Surgeon:_____

Phone:_____

Address:_____

(continued)

Cardiologist:_____

Phone:_____

Address: _____

Family doctor: _____

Phone: _____

Address: _____

Hospital: _____

Phone: _____

Address: _____

FOLLOW-UP
Finally, keeping all follow-up appointments is extremely important. Your first appointment is:

Doctor: _____

Phone: _____

Address: _____

Date and time: _____

Deep Vein Thrombosis: Disease Process and Prevention

TEACHING PLAN
Assessment
• Assess the patient's and family's knowledge of deep vein thrombosis (DVT), its signs and symptoms, and how to prevent recurrent episodes.
• Assess the patient's and family's past experience in recognizing deep vein thrombosis.
• Assess the patient's risk factors for deep vein thrombosis.
• Collaborate with the doctor regarding the patient's discharge orders (anticoagulant therapy, use of antiembolism stockings).

Materials needed
• Antiembolism stockings, if applicable
• Sample of prescribed anticoagulant medication

Strategies to use
• Stimulate interest in the topic by explaining to the patient and his family that he has an increased chance of developing DVT; explain that complications from DVT can be quite serious and that prevention and early detection are critical.
• Present the information, using demonstration and return demonstration for use of antiembolism stockings when applicable.
• Have the patient and family problem-solve the following:
  —what risk factors the patient has and how to modify them
  —when additional medical care is needed and how that care will be obtained.

Patient-teaching aids
See *Managing deep vein thrombosis at home*, page 309; and *Preventing deep vein thrombosis: Antiembolism stockings*, page 311.

Evaluation method
• Have the patient and family explain, using their own words, deep vein thrombosis and its signs and symptoms.
• Have the patient and family state plans for modifying the patient's specific risk factors.
• Have the patient and family state when and how to obtain additional medical care.

Interventions and outcome criteria

☑ **Intervention 1**

Using a diagram, review the normal anatomy and physiology of veins, if needed.

☑ **Intervention 2**

Describe what occurs in deep vein thrombosis.

Outcome criteria: The patient and family state that a clot forms in a vein.

☑ **Intervention 3**

Describe the major signs and symptoms associated with deep vein thrombosis, including:
• pain (often described as a heavy, aching sensation in the leg that may be relieved or lessened when leg is elevated and that is not precipitated by exercise)
• edema in one leg (may occur in the calf or thigh; may be recognized by comparing one thigh or calf to the other).

Outcome criteria: The patient and family state that pain and swelling in one leg are major signs of deep vein thrombosis.

☑ **Intervention 4**

Instruct the patient and family to notify the doctor if any symptoms develop.

Outcome criteria: The patient and family state that presence of pain and edema in one leg are signs that additional medical care should be obtained.

☑ **Intervention 5**

Have the patient and family develop specific plans for obtaining additional medical care if needed.

Outcome criteria: The patient and family plan how and when to obtain medical care if needed.

☑ **Intervention 6**

Explain that preventing deep vein thrombosis is important to decrease the risk of emboli and permanent damage to the vein.

Outcome criteria: The patient and family state that prevention of deep vein thrombosis is important.

☑ **Intervention 7**

Discuss the risk factors for deep vein thrombosis, including:
• immobility
• varicose veins
• prolonged standing or sitting in one position
• obesity
• other risk factors specifically related to the patient.

Outcome criteria: The patient and family identify risk factors specific to the patient.

☑ Intervention 8

Explain preventive measures, including:
• use of prescribed anticoagulants
• use of antiembolism stockings or elastic or support hose
• other measures to prevent venous stasis, including:
  —changing positions
  —leg and foot exercises
  —planned walking program (or other exercise)
  —avoiding constrictive clothing.

Outcome criteria: The patient and family state plans to modify the patient's risk factors for deep vein thrombosis.

PATIENT-TEACHING AID

Managing Deep Vein Thrombosis at Home

Deep vein thrombosis is the medical term for a blood clot that forms in one of the large veins deep inside the body. You may remember that veins are the vessels that pick up blood from the capillary beds in your body and return the blood back to your heart.

SYMPTOMS

With deep vein thrombosis, the first symptom you may notice is pain that occurs in usually only one leg. Sometimes, this pain is described as a feeling of tenderness that will not go away. It is also described as a feeling of heaviness or aching. The pain may lessen when you sit down and put your feet up.

Swelling or edema in one leg is another symptom you may have. You may notice that the calf or thigh of one leg is bigger than the calf or thigh of your other leg.

If any of these symptoms develop, you need to seek medical care. Prompt treatment can help prevent additional problems.

In the spaces provided below, write down pertinent information concerning where you will get medical care.

Name: _____

Address: _____

Telephone number: _____

IMPORTANCE OF PREVENTION

Preventing deep vein thrombosis is very important. The clot that forms in the vein can damage the inside of the vein. This damage increases the chance that you could develop deep vein thrombosis or a clot again.

Also, small pieces of the clot can break off in the vein. These pieces travel through your body in your blood vessels. They can get stuck in a small vessel in your heart, lungs, or brain. When these pieces get stuck in a vessel, they completely block the vessel. No blood is able to travel past the piece. Permanent damage, including severe breathing problems, a heart attack, or a stroke can occur.

RISK FACTORS

Listed below are common factors that can lead to deep vein thrombosis. Check which factors apply to you:

☐ varicose veins

(continued)

☐ prolonged sitting or standing in one position

☐ being confined to bed for a long time (such as after surgery)

☐ being overweight

☐ pregnancy.

Some patients have additional risk factors. Your nurse will list any other factors that increase your chance of developing deep vein thrombosis in the spaces below.

_____

_____

Each of these risk factors can cause blood flow through your veins to slow down. Whenever blood flow through the veins slows down too much, clots can form.

PREVENTIVE MEASURES

You can do several things to decrease your chance of forming blood clots, including the following:
• Avoid sitting or standing in one position for long periods of time. If your job requires you to sit or stand in one place, do leg exercises for about 5 minutes every 1 to 2 hours. Easy leg exercises include:
　—bouncing up and down on the tips of your toes (your nurse can show you how to do this)
　—walking around at a slow to moderate pace for 5 minutes every 1 or 2 hours (if your job permits)
　—when traveling, walking for 5 to 10 minutes every 1 to 2 hours. (You can walk in the aisles of a plane or get out of your car and walk around.)
• Elevate your feet when sitting down. Putting your feet up whenever you sit down helps the blood travel back to the heart.
• Wear support hose. Your doctor may have ordered a specific type of elastic stocking for you. If your doctor has not ordered anything, it is probably a good idea for you to wear support hose during the day when you are up and about. You can buy support hose in the hosiery section of most department stores.
• Actively exercise your feet and legs every day. Ask your nurse to show you some simple exercises.
• Develop a plan for physical exercise. Walking at a moderate pace is always a good exercise. Talk with your doctor about the amount and type of exercise you should do.
• Avoid putting any pressure on your thighs, backs of your knees, or calves. Do not cross your feet or ankles. Avoid clothing that is tight around your legs. Do not sit or lie down with pressure against the backs of your knees.

PATIENT-TEACHING AID

Preventing Deep Vein Thrombosis: Antiembolism Stockings

Your doctor has suggested that you wear antiembolism stockings at home. These stockings help the blood travel back from your legs to your heart and will help prevent clots from forming in your legs.

USING ANTIEMBOLISM STOCKINGS

Your nurse will show you the easiest way to put these stockings on. Begin by lightly dusting your foot and leg with powder. This will help the stockings go on more easily. Make sure that you pull the stockings up all the way and that they contain no wrinkles. Check your stockings frequently to make sure that they stay smooth.

Your doctor wants you to wear these stockings:

☐ day and night

☐ only during the day (you may remove them at night).

If you are to wear the stockings day and night, you may remove them once in the morning and once at night for 15 to 30 minutes. If you are to wear them only during the day, make sure that you put the stockings on before you get out of bed in the morning and take them off after you get in bed at night. You may also take them off to bathe or shower.

Wash your legs each day and carefully look at the skin under your stockings for any reddened areas. Redness is often caused by wrinkles in your stockings. Make sure your stockings stay smooth. If they will not stay smooth and snug, talk with your doctor or pharmacist about getting a different pair.

Endocarditis, Infectious: Disease Process and Prevention

TEACHING PLAN
Assessment
• Assess the patient's and family's understanding about the pathophysiology of infectious endocarditis.
• Assess the patient's and family's knowledge and past experience with prevention of infectious endocarditis.
• Identify specific risk factors the patient has for infectious endocarditis.

Strategies to use
• Stimulate interest in the topic by explaining to the patient and his family that the patient is at risk for developing infectious endocarditis.
• Explain that prevention is important because infectious endocarditis can result in serious complications.

Patient-teaching aid
See *Recognizing and preventing infectious endocarditis*, page 314.

Evaluation method
• Have the patient and family explain, using their own words, what occurs in infectious endocarditis.
• Have the patient and family state when prophylactic measures should be used and how these measures should be implemented.

Interventions and outcome criteria
☑ **Intervention 1**
Briefly define infectious endocarditis.

Outcome criteria: The patient and family state that infectious endocarditis is an infection that can develop on the inside lining of the heart.

☑ **Intervention 2**
Explain the effects of infectious endocarditis on the heart and body functioning, including:
• development of vegetation
• permanent damage to heart valves
• risk of emboli formation.

Outcome criteria: The patient and family state that the infection causes growth of vegetation on the heart valves, that natural and artificial valves can be permanently damaged by the infection, and that pieces of vegetation can break off and cause damage to other parts of the body.

☑ Intervention 3
Have the patient and family identify the patient's risk factors from the major ones listed below:
- history of congenital heart disease
- history of valvular heart disease
- presence of a prosthetic valve
- abuse of I.V. drugs
- previous history of infectious endocarditis.

Outcome criteria: The patient and family identify the patient's specific risk factors.

☑ Intervention 4
Describe the use of prophylactic antibiotics, including:
- the need to notify all doctors and dentists about the risk of bacterial endocarditis
- the types of procedures requiring prophylactic antibiotics
- how to take antibiotics correctly
- the importance of good oral hygiene and regular dental care.

Outcome criteria: The patient and family state that all doctors and dentists that the patient sees should be told of the patient's high risk for infectious endocarditis. They also state that the patient will need to take antibiotics before many surgical and invasive diagnostic procedures and that they should be taken exactly as prescribed. They also state the importance of good oral hygiene.

☑ Intervention 5
Discuss how to recognize signs and symptoms of infectious endocarditis, which may be insidious or have a rapid onset, including:
- fever
- chills and night sweats
- flulike symptoms
- malaise and weight loss.

Outcome criteria: The patient and family state major signs and symptoms of infectious endocarditis.

☑ Intervention 6
Have the patient and family plan how they will obtain medical care if signs and symptoms of infectious endocarditis develop.

Outcome criteria: The patient and family state plans for obtaining medical care, if needed.

Recognizing and Preventing Infectious Endocarditis

Infectious endocarditis is a medical term for a type of infection that can develop on the inside lining of your heart. This infection causes vegetation to grow on one or more of the valves in your heart. This vegetation is made up of the bacteria that causes the infection, as well as some other cells and substances in your bloodstream.

Such vegetation can damage valves so that they no longer work properly. When the valves don't work correctly, problems develop with blood flow through your heart. Your heart has to work harder to pump the blood out to the body and becomes damaged by the extra work. Sometimes the valves become so badly damaged that they must be removed and replaced surgically. Artificial valves can be easily damaged by this type of infection.

Pieces of vegetation can also break off and travel in your bloodstream. Eventually, these pieces get stuck in a small vessel and keep blood from getting to the surrounding tissue. This could cause permanent damage to the heart, lungs, or brain.

RISK FACTORS

Although anyone can develop infectious endocarditis, your chances of developing it increase if you have:
• a history of congenital heart disease
• a history of heart valve disease
• an artificial heart valve in your heart
• had infectious endocarditis previously
• used I.V. drugs at home that are not prescribed by a doctor.

List your specific risk factors in the spaces provided below.

_____

_____

_____

PREVENTION

To lessen your chances of developing infectious endocarditis, take the following measures:
• Be sure to tell every doctor or dentist you see that you are at high risk for getting infectious endocarditis. Also tell them what your specific risk factor is.

(continued)

• Take good care of your teeth and gums. Brush and floss as directed by your dentist. See your dentist regularly for checkups.
• Certain diagnostic tests and surgical procedures can increase your chances of developing infectious endocarditis. Your doctor or dentist will prescribe antibiotics for you to take before, during, or after the procedure. Sometimes, the doctor may order this medication to be given intravenously. Other times, you may need to take the medication in tablet or capsule form. If tablets or capsules are ordered, be sure to take the medication exactly as ordered.
• Expect that you will have to take antibiotic medication before any of the following procedures:
— most dental procedures
— procedures involving the ear, nose, or throat
— procedures involving the trachea and bronchi (breathing tubes) or lungs that require the insertion of any instrument or tube
— procedures involving the lower gastrointestinal tract that require the insertion of any instrument
— procedures involving the gallbladder or its ducts (tubes) that require the insertion of any instrument
— procedures involving the bladder, kidneys, or other parts of the genito-urinary system that require the insertion of any instrument.
    If you have any questions about whether you should be taking antibiotics for any procedure, ask either the doctor performing the procedure or your family doctor.

WARNING SIGNS
Warning signs of infectious endocarditis include:
• fever
• chills and night sweats
• flulike symptoms (feeling achy or hurting all over)
• feeling more tired than usual
• weight loss
• loss of appetite.
These warning signs can develop slowly over time or very quickly. If you notice any of these symptoms, contact your doctor.

Plan now how to get medical care if any of these symptoms develop. Write any pertinent information below.

Doctor: _____

Address: _____

Phone: _____

Exercising after Myocardial Infarction or Heart Surgery

TEACHING PLAN
Assessment
• Assess the patient's level of activity in the hospital.
• Collaborate with the doctor to determine a recommended rate of activity progression and pulse rate limits (see Nurse's notes: Exercise prescriptions).
• Assess the patient's and family's knowledge of how activity should progress at home.

Strategies to use
• Have the patient perform the prescribed exercises and walking program, including monitoring his own pulse rate and his response to activity (under a nurse's supervision).
• Have the patient and family problem-solve the following:
—determining the best place and time for the patient to exercise at home
—using the patient's individual response to guide the amount of exercise performed.

Patient-teaching aids
See How to exercise at home, page 319; and Exercise prescription, page 321.

Evaluation method
• Have the patient demonstrate the prescribed walking and exercise program without assistance from the nurse.
• Have the patient and a family member state warning signs that indicate activity should be stopped.
• Have the patient and a family member state plans for how and when the patient will exercise, including plans for reducing exercise if indicated by the patient's response.

Interventions and outcome criteria
☑ Intervention 1
Teach the patient to count and record his radial pulse. Have him count his pulse for 10 seconds, then multiply by six for an exercise check.

Outcome criteria: The patient and family counts the patient's radial pulse for 10 seconds and multiplies correctly (see also the appropriate outcome criteria in "Radial Pulse Measurement"in this section).

NURSE'S NOTES: EXERCISE PRESCRIPTIONS

Exercise prescriptions should be carefully individualized for each specific patient based on the patient's response to activity in the hospital. Many doctors are ordering low-level exercise stress tests before the patient is discharged; the results of such tests are used to plan the patient's exercise program.

Determining the patient's pulse rate limit
Three methods are currently in use for determining the patient's pulse rate limit for exercise:
• Taking the patient's resting heart rate and adding 20 beats/minute.
• Setting the limit at a maximum of 120 beats/minute.
• Basing the limit on the results of the patient's individual exercise stress test.
   Of the three methods, determining the pulse rate limit based on the patient's exercise stress test is the most individualized.

Increasing the patient's exercise limit
Developing a standard exercise prescription that can be applied to any patient is difficult, if not impossible. However, here are some examples of how walking might be increased.
• If the patient can walk ¼ mile without presenting symptoms of activity intolerance (as with an uncomplicated myocardial infarction) before discharge from the hospital, have him walk:
   —¼ mile in 15 minutes for 1 to 2 weeks
   —¼ mile in 5 to 10 minutes for 1 to 2 weeks
   —½ mile in 20 to 25 minutes for 1 to 2 weeks
   —½ mile in 10 to 15 minutes for 1 to 2 weeks.
Note: Have the patient continue this pattern of increasing the distance by ¼ to ½ mile followed by increasing the pace.
• If the patient can walk 1 mile without presenting symptoms of activity intolerance (as with an uncomplicated coronary artery bypass grafting) before discharge from the hospital, have him walk:
   —1 mile in 30 minutes for 1 to 2 weeks
   —1 mile in 20 to 25 minutes for 1 to 2 weeks
   —1½ miles in 30 to 35 minutes for 1 to 2 weeks
   —1½ miles in 20 to 25 minutes for 1 to 2 weeks.
Note: Have the patient continue this pattern of increasing the distance followed by increasing the pace.

☑ **Intervention 2**
Discuss the exercise prescription, including:
• warm-up exercises
• a home walking program
• cool-down exercises
• a plan for increasing the amount of exercise performed.

Outcome criteria: The patient and family state a specific activity prescription for the patient.

☑ **Intervention 3**
Review the warning signs that indicate the patient should stop or reduce activity.

Outcome criteria: The patient and family state warning signs that indicate activity should be stopped or reduced.

☑ Intervention 4

Discuss appropriate management for symptoms discussed in Intervention 3, including:
• when to notify the doctor before resuming exercising
• how to reduce the amount of exercise performed when indicated.

☑ Intervention 5

Have the patient perform the prescribed exercise program and, under a nurse's supervision, monitor his own response.

Outcome criteria: The patient correctly demonstrates the exercise program (initial level) and correctly monitors his own pulse and response to activity (with his family's assistance, if needed).

How to Exercise at Home

Attached to this patient-teaching aid is your exercise prescription. Follow this prescription to gradually increase the amount of exercise you perform at home.

WARM-UP EXERCISES

Begin your exercises each time with a warm-up. Warm-up exercises help your heart and muscles get ready for more strenuous exercise.

For warm-up exercises, use the same stretching exercises you used in the hospital before walking. Do not hold your breath while doing these stretching exercises; instead, use the rhythmic breathing technique your nurse has taught you. Count your pulse rate before, halfway through, and after your stretching exercises.

WALKING

After your warm-up, begin your walk. Walk at a moderate pace, for the time or distance indicated on your exercise prescription.

Begin walking on a flat, level surface. Count your pulse rate before, halfway through, and after completing your prescribed walk.

Think about the best place and time for you to walk. The temperature should be comfortable. If needed, a family member may drive you to a place away from home for your walk, such as a shopping mall.

COOL-DOWN EXERCISES

After you have finished your prescribed walking, begin your cool-down. Cool-down exercises let your heart, blood pressure, and breathing gradually return to their normal resting rates. The best cool-down exercise is to walk slowly for a few minutes.

LENGTH OF EXERCISE PERIOD

Begin with about the same amount of exercise that you were doing in the hospital. You can continue to increase the amount of exercise you do as long as your pulse rate stays less than _____ beats/minute and you do not have any of the warning signs listed below.

WARNING SIGNS

Warning signs are clues that the amount of exercise you are doing is too stressful for your heart. Stop any exercise immediately if:
• your heart rate exceeds _____ beats/minute during the exercise
• your heart rate suddenly becomes very slow
• your heart rate suddenly becomes very rapid
• your heart rhythm becomes irregular
• you have any chest pain
• you feel dizzy, light-headed, or break out in a cold sweat.

(continued)

If you develop any of these warning signs, you may need to completely stop exercising or reduce the amount of exercise you are doing. See the guidelines listed below for help.

GUIDELINES FOR STOPPING OR REDUCING EXERCISE

If you have any of the following warning signs during exercise, stop your exercise program immediately. Check with your doctor before starting to exercise again.

• Your pulse rate suddenly becomes extremely slow or extremely fast.
• Your pulse rhythm becomes very irregular.
• You feel dizzy, light-headed, or faint, or you break out in a cold sweat.
• You have chest pain that is more severe or unusual for you.
• Your pulse rate exceeds _____ beats/minute for several days (even with a decreased amount of exercise).

If you have any of the following warning signs, you may continue your exercise program; however, you should reduce the amount of exercise that you are doing.

• Your pulse rate exceeds _____ beats/minute during the exercise.
• Your pulse rate exceeds _____ beats/minute for 10 or more minutes after you stop exercising.
• Your shortness of breath lasts 10 or more minutes after you stop exercising.
• You have insomnia (when you normally do not).
• You are more tired than usual for a day or more after the exercise.
• You have chest pain that is "usual" for you when you have done too much activity.
• Other (related to specific patient): _____

_____

_____

REDUCING YOUR EXERCISE

If you need to reduce the amount of exercise you are doing, use one of the following suggestions:

• Do the exercise at a slower pace (for instance, you could walk at a slow pace rather than a moderate one).
• Do the exercise for a shorter period of time. Reduce the time spent on each part of your exercise prescription, but don't completely skip any part.
• Do fewer repetitions of your stretching exercises. You may want to reduce the number of times you do each exercise by one or two.
• Walk for a shorter distance.
• Decrease the number of times you do your exercises each day (for instance, you could exercise only once each day instead of twice).
• Look at the amount of overall activity that you are doing. You may need to cut back on the amount (for instance, you may need to see fewer visitors or do fewer tasks or chores around the house).

Exercise Prescription

Your doctor has prescribed the following exercises for you to do at home. Be sure to ask the nurse to explain any part of the prescription you do not understand.

Heart rate limit: _____ beats/minute

Perform these exercises _____ times/day.

WARM-UP EXERCISES

Length of time: _____

Number of repetitions: _____

Exercises to use:

1. _____

2. _____

3. _____

4. _____

5. _____

6. _____

7. _____

8. _____

Increase repetitions by _____ times every _____ weeks

TRAINING EXERCISE

Type: _____

Length of time: _____

Distance: _____

(continued)

Increase walking by

_____ distance in _____ minutes for _____ weeks

_____ distance in _____ minutes for _____ weeks

_____ distance in _____ minutes for _____ weeks

_____ distance in _____ minutes for _____ weeks

_____ distance in _____ minutes for _____ weeks

_____ distance in _____ minutes for _____ weeks

_____ distance in _____ minutes for _____ weeks

COOL-DOWN EXERCISES

Type: _____

Length of time: _____

Fluid Plans

TEACHING PLAN
Assessment
• Collaborate with the doctor about the patient's fluid limit and diet restrictions to follow at home.
• Assess the patient's and family's knowledge of the prescribed fluid limit and how to manage a fluid limit at home.
• Assess the patient's current fluid intake (that is, does the patient drink consistently less than the prescribed amount of fluid? Does the patient consistently try to exceed the prescribed amount?).

Materials needed
• Sample chart of intake for home use
• Cup or glass to use for measuring

Strategies to use
• Stimulate interest in the topic by explaining to the patient and family that excessive fluid intake can precipitate an acute episode of congestive heart failure.
• Present the information using didactic teaching and problem-solving.
• Have the patient and his family problem-solve the following:
—which fluids the patient prefers that are permitted on the diet
—how the patient and family will keep a record of those fluids
—a general plan of when the patient will drink fluids (such as how much he will drink with meals or taking medications) and how the patient and family will measure fluids.

Patient-teaching aid
See *Managing your fluid limit at home*, page 325.

Evaluation method
• Have the patient and family manage and record the patient's fluid intake in the hospital setting under a nurse's supervision.

Interventions and outcome criteria
☑ **Intervention 1**
Explain the purpose of the prescribed fluid limit to the patient and family.

Outcome criteria: The patient and family state that limiting fluids decreases the work of the heart and helps the heart to pump more effectively.

☑ **Intervention 2**
Explain to the patient and his family how much the patient will be permitted to drink every 24 hours, explaining in terms of cups or ounces. Provide the patient with a glass marked in ounces.

Outcome criteria: The patient and family state the patient's prescribed fluid limit in measurable terms.

☑ Intervention 3
Have the patient and family develop a fluid plan, including:
• how much the patient will drink with each meal
• how much the patient will drink with medications
• other times that the patient would like to have fluids and how much he will drink at each time.

Outcome criteria: The patient and family develop a fluid plan correctly.

☑ Intervention 4
Write down the fluid plan; have the patient and his family develop a means of keeping track of fluid intake.

Outcome criteria: The patient and family develop a method of monitoring the patient's fluid intake.

☑ Intervention 5
Have the patient and family manage the patient's fluid intake and record it on the form they will use at home (under a nurse's supervision).

Outcome criteria: The patient and family correctly manage and record the patient's fluid intake under the nurse's supervision.

Managing Your Fluid Limit at Home

Because you have congestive heart failure, your heart is not pumping well enough to meet your body's demands for blood and oxygen. To help your heart pump better, your doctor wants you to limit the amount of fluid that you drink. If you drink too much fluid, your heart failure will worsen and you will have more symptoms.

Your fluid limit is _____ milliliters, which is equal to _____ ounces or _____ glasses (using a pre-measured glass). You may drink only this amount of fluid each day.

You may find it difficult to avoid drinking more fluid than you are permitted. To help you stay within your fluid limit, you may want to plan how and when you will drink most of the fluid that you may have.

The chart below lists some common times when you may want to drink something. Fill in the times that you plan to drink, and write down how much you will drink at each time. Also write down what fluid you will drink; remember that the type of fluid must be allowed on your diet restrictions. You'll also find blank spaces at the end of the list for you to fill in additional times.

The amount of fluid you decide to drink at each time should add up to _____ (the amount that your doctor has prescribed).

FLUID SCHEDULE

Times	Amount and type of fluid
At breakfast	_____
With morning medications	_____
At lunch	_____
With noon medications	_____
With afternoon medications	_____
At dinner	_____

(continued)

FLUID SCHEDULE *(continued)*

Times	Amount and type of fluid
With late afternoon or evening medications	_____
With nighttime medications	_____
Just before bed	_____
	_____
	_____
	_____
Other times	_____
Total amount of fluid/day	_____

To help you stick to your fluid limit, you may find it helpful to write down how much you drink each day. You can do this easily on a sheet of paper or in a notebook. For each day, write down the specific amount each time you have something to drink. Your sample page might look like this:

Monday, July 14:
3 ounces of water for breakfast

2 ounces of juice with medications

4 ounces of coffee for lunch

6 ounces of water for dinner and with medications

2 ounces of juice at bedtime

Total amount of fluid = 17 ounces (Limit = 20 ounces/day)

(continued)

You may want to use a check sheet instead. You can use your fluid schedule and simply check off each amount of fluid as you drink it each day.

Time	Amount	Checked
At breakfast	½ glass	☐
With medications	1 glass	☐
At lunch	1 glass	☐
In the afternoon	½ glass	☐
At dinner	½ glass	☐
At bedtime	1 glass	☐

Throughout the day, you may have times when you feel especially thirsty. However, this does not mean you should drink extra fluids. To satisfy your thirst without drinking more, you can:
• suck on hard, sugar-free candy
• suck on ice (1 ounce of crushed ice equals about ½ ounce of fluid on your fluid limit)
• drink small amounts of fluids frequently instead of large amounts less frequently
• sip each drink slowly; don't gulp it down.

Hypertension, Essential: Disease Process and Risk Factors

TEACHING PLAN
Assessment
• Assess the patient's and family's understanding of hypertension and its effects on the body.
• Assess the patient's and family's understanding of factors that increase the risk of developing hypertension.
• Assess the patient's and family's previous experience in modifying risk factors, and identify their areas of concern.

Materials needed
See Nurse's notes: Suggestions for audiovisual aids for materials to use.

Strategies to use
• Stimulate interest in the topic by explaining that hypertension can damage the body without the patient's knowledge until the damage leads to blindness, stroke, other problems, or death. Explain that modifying risk factors can facilitate lowering blood pressure and, in some instances, can control hypertension without using medications.
• Assist the patient and his family to problem-solve the following:
  —specific risk factors the patient and family have for hypertension
  —how to modify individual risk factors to control blood pressure.

Patient-teaching aids
See Basic reminders about hypertension, page 333; Hypertension: Controlling disease and reducing risk factors, page 335; Controlling hypertension by weight reduction, page 338; Exercising regularly, page 342; and Drinking alcoholic beverages in moderation, page 344.

Evaluation method
• Have the patient and family describe, in their own words, hypertension and its effects on the body.
• Have the patient and family identify their specific risk factors.
• Have the patient and family state specific plans for modifying each risk factor.

**NURSE'S NOTES: SUGGESTIONS FOR
AUDIOVISUAL AIDS**

Here are some suggestions for audiovisual aids to use in teaching patients and
their families about hypertension.

Modifying risk factors
Develop a chart with pictures illustrating modifiable risk factors and desired
changes, such as:
• an obese person contrasted with a person of normal weight
• a person sitting in a lawn chair contrasted with a person walking or jogging
• a person sitting before a table full of foods that are high in calories and
saturated fat, adding salt to his food, contrasted with a person sitting before a
table full of more healthful foods, refusing the salt shaker and foods high in
saturated fats and calories
• several cigarettes and different types of alcoholic beverages contrasted with
fewer cigarettes and alcoholic beverages
• a person with gestures and facial expression indicating stress contrasted with
a person with a calm, relaxed expression
• a person with a perplexed expression looking at a medicine bottle contrasted
with a person talking to a doctor.

Effects of hypertension on the body
Develop a chart illustrating normal arteries connecting the heart, brain, kidneys,
and eyes and extending into the arms and legs. Also include an artery tapering
into arterioles, then capillaries.
    Contrast the illustration above with one depicting a damaged heart connected
to arteries that constrict at damaged kidneys, eyes, and brain. Also include an
artery tapering into constricted arterioles, then constricted capillaries.

Interventions and outcome criteria

☑ Intervention 1
Review normal cardiac circulation and the role of blood in normal body
functioning.

Outcome criteria: Use the outcome criteria from "Cardiac Anatomy and
Physiology: Heart and Blood Vessels" in this section.

☑ Intervention 2
Explain the damage that occurs when blood supply is insufficient.

Outcome criteria: The patient and family state that body parts become
injured and eventually stop working if not enough blood reaches them.

☑ Intervention 3
Explain the pathophysiology of hypertension, including the following in-
formation:
• Arterioles are constricted in hypertension.
• The heart must pump harder to force blood into systemic circulation
through constricted arterioles.
• Insufficient blood supply reaches major organs, resulting in damage to
the organs.

Outcome criteria: The patient and family state that hypertension causes injury to body parts because it decreases the amount of blood that reaches those parts of the body. They also state that hypertension injures the heart by making it work harder until it does not pump blood well to other parts of the body.

☑ Intervention 4
Explain that major signs may not be noticed until some damage has occurred to parts of the body.

Outcome criteria: The patient and family state that a hypertensive person may have no signs until he has had the disease for some time and damage has occurred.

☑ Intervention 5
Describe the major signs and symptoms associated with damage to major organs and relate them to the patient's specific symptoms. Major organs include:
• heart
• brain
• kidneys
• eyes.

Outcome criteria: The patient and family state signs that indicate damage has occurred from hypertension.

☑ Intervention 6
Describe the possible consequences of prolonged, untreated hypertension, including:
• heart failure
• myocardial infarction
• cerebrovascular accident
• renal failure
• blindness
• death.

Outcome criteria: The patient and family state disorders and consequences that can occur with uncontrolled hypertension.

☑ Intervention 7
Explain that medications are the main means used in controlling hypertension.

Outcome criteria: The patient and family state that taking medications is the main means for controlling hypertension.

☑ Intervention 8
Explain that certain risk factors can have the following effects on hypertension control:
• tendency for increased risk of developing hypertension
• hindering the effectiveness of medications prescribed to control hypertension.

Outcome criteria: The patient and family state that some risk factors can increase hypertension and interfere with the ability of medications to control hypertension.

☑ **Intervention 9**
Discuss modifiable risk factors, including:
• obesity
• sedentary life-style
• high-sodium diet
• high-saturated-fat and high-cholesterol diet
• heavy alcohol intake
• cigarette smoking
• increased stress (emotional and psychosocial)
• other medical conditions that are uncontrolled, such as:
—diabetes
—gout
—kidney stones.

Outcome criteria: The patient and family identify risk factors that can be changed to control hypertension.

☑ **Intervention 10**
Have the patient and family identify their own risk factors.

Outcome criteria: The patient and family state their own risk factors that will need to be changed to control hypertension.

☑ **Intervention 11**
Explain that changing certain practices and habits can decrease the patient's risk of developing hypertension. Identify measures to use, including:
• gradual weight reduction
• regular isotonic exercise
• moderate sodium-restricted diet
• reduced saturated-fat and cholesterol diet
• alcohol intake reduced to moderate (or less)
• reducing or quitting cigarette smoking
• stress reduction
• following a prescribed treatment to control other medical conditions.

Outcome criteria: The patient and family state measures that can reduce risk factors and control hypertension.

☑ **Intervention 12**
Have the patient and his family develop specific plans for modifying their individual risk factors.

Outcome criteria: The patient and family develop specific, realistic plans for modifying individual risk factors.

☑ Intervention 13

Discuss nonmodifiable risk factors. Have the patient and family identify individual risk factors regarding:
• heredity
• age
• sex
• race.

Outcome criteria: The patient and family identify individual nonmodifiable risk factors.

☑ Intervention 14

Explain the importance of regular blood pressure screenings and physical examinations for those with nonmodifiable risk factors.

Outcome criteria: The patient and family state the importance of regular blood pressure screening and physical examinations.

☑ Intervention 15

Explain that having a combination of risk factors increases the risk of developing hypertension.

Outcome criteria: The patient and family state that the more risk factors they have, the greater their risk of developing hypertension.

☑ Intervention 16

Emphasize that controlling hypertension continually for life is dependent on modifying risk factors for the rest of one's life.

Outcome criteria: The patient and family state that life-style changes must be maintained for life.

Basic Reminders about Hypertension

Hypertension, or high blood pressure, is a life-threatening disease. Having hypertension means that your blood pressure is high (above normal) all the time. This is determined by a series of consistently high blood pressure readings, not just one reading that is high. However, if you have had a high blood pressure reading, it is important for you to have your blood pressure checked regularly by your doctor.

You are considered hypertensive if your blood pressure is 160/95 mm Hg or greater at age 50 or older, or if your blood pressure is 140/90 mm Hg or greater and you are under age 50.

CAUSES OF HYPERTENSION

Hypertension is sometimes caused by other medical problems that can be treated and cured with medications and surgery. However, this type of hypertension occurs only in a small number of cases. Most of the time (over 90%), the cause is unknown. This is the type of hypertension you have.

Although the cause of hypertension is unknown, it is important for you to know what happens when you have this disease.

You already know that the heart pumps blood to all parts of the body. Blood carries the oxygen and food that the parts of the body need to work well and thrive. In hypertension, for some unknown reason, the smaller arteries are squeezed tightly and therefore do not allow enough blood to reach some parts of the body. When this occurs, the parts stop working and eventually die. The heart has to pump harder as it tries to force more blood through the squeezed arteries. Over time, the heart becomes damaged until it does not pump well enough to supply enough blood to all parts of the body.

SIGNS OF DAMAGE

Some signs indicating that the heart has become damaged include:
• fast or irregular heartbeats
• difficulty breathing when walking or performing activities that previously caused no difficulty
• waking up from sleep feeling extremely short of breath
• swelling of the ankles or hands
• chest pain
• heart attack.

Hypertension can cause other damage. When the smaller arteries are squeezed and do not allow enough blood to get to parts of your body, other signs of injury become apparent. Hypertension can ultimately lead to blindness, kidney failure, stroke, and death.

(continued)

Signs indicating damage to the eyes include:
• blurry vision
• blindness.
Signs indicating damage to the kidneys include:
• waking up more than once at night to urinate
• difficulty urinating
• blood in the urine
• kidney failure.
Signs indicating damage to the brain include:
• headaches on awakening and rising in the morning, particularly headaches in the back of the head
• migraine headaches (occur sometimes)
• weakness, on and off again, in various parts of the body or on one side of the body
• stroke.

Hypertension also speeds up the process of atherosclerosis. In atherosclerosis, fatty deposits build up on the inside of arteries. This narrows the arteries and decreases the amount of blood and oxygen getting through to the tissues. Atherosclerosis can damage any artery in your body, including those which supply blood to your heart, brain, and legs.

Frequently, people with hypertension do not feel any different or notice any problems for years, until enough damage has occurred and parts of the body stop working well.

Although it cannot be cured, hypertension can be controlled by lowering high blood pressure. However, because it has no cure, this disease must be controlled lifelong. Even though you may feel better, you must continue with your treatment. Remember, you feel better because you are controlling your hypertension and the problems it can cause.

PATIENT-TEACHING AID

Hypertension: Controlling Disease and Reducing Risk Factors

Lowering your blood pressure is important so that your body does not suffer damage that can lead to heart problems, kidney failure, stroke, or death. By keeping your blood pressure lowered, you control your hypertension.

Taking your medication daily is the major way you can control your hypertension. However, you will also need to make other changes in habits, practices, and life-style—your risk factors—to help your medicine work effectively. Modifiable risk factors for hypertension refer to any of the changeable habits or practices that tend to make your blood pressure rise. Nonmodifiable risk factors refer to unchangeable factors such as heredity, age, sex, and race.

MODIFIABLE RISK FACTORS

Although you may not be able to change all of your risk factors, you can modify many of them to help control your hypertension. As you read the factors listed below, check the ones that are risks for you.

☐ Overweight

☐ Drinking large amounts of alcohol (2 oz or more of 100-proof whiskey a day, 8 oz or more of wine a day, or 24 oz or more of beer a day)

☐ Performing activities that do not include regular exercise

☐ Eating foods high in sodium (for example, adding salt to foods or eating canned foods, luncheon meats, bacon, hot dogs, ham, cheese, pickles, salted crackers, or meat tenderizers)

☐ Working or living in situations in which you feel that you are under a lot of pressure or that worry or upset you most of the time

☐ Smoking cigarettes

☐ Eating foods that are high in saturated fats and cholesterol (for example, fried foods, egg yolks, beef, pork, and whole milk)

☐ Having other medical conditions (such as diabetes, gout, or kidney stones) that are not well controlled

(continued)

NONMODIFIABLE RISK FACTORS

Now, take a look at the risk factors you cannot change—your nonmodifiable risk factors. Check the factors that apply from the following list:

☐ Heredity (Having a parent or blood relative with hypertension; this increases your risk of having hypertension and increases your children's risk for developing the disease.)

☐ Age (Being between ages 30 and 50 or older; hypertension usually develops in those between ages 30 and 50 and is seen more in elderly persons.)

☐ Sex (With males, hypertension occurs earlier in life; with females, hypertension may occur after the onset of menopause.)

☐ Race (Being a black American; hypertension occurs more frequently and with more severity in black Americans.)

REDUCING YOUR RISK FACTORS

Count the total number of checks you have made and place the number of risk factors in this space: _____. This reflects the number of risk factors that you have that tend to make your blood pressure high.

The more risk factors you have, the greater your chances of not being able to control your blood pressure. Therefore, as you can see, it is important to reduce your risk factors to control your hypertension.

To help control your hypertension, your doctor and nurses have advised you to make the following changes:

☐ Reducing your weight

☐ Reducing alcohol intake

☐ Increasing regular isotonic exercises (walking, jogging, swimming, or aerobics)

☐ Reducing your intake of foods high in sodium

☐ Avoiding stressful situations in your life

☐ Stopping cigarette smoking

☐ Reducing your intake of saturated fats and cholesterol

☐ Controlling other medical conditions, such as diabetes, gout, and kidney stones, by following your doctor's advice

(continued)

Identify from the preceding list of modifiable risk factors those which you will try to change to help control your hypertension. Your doctor will recommend the best way for you to make *gradual* changes in reducing these factors. By following his instructions closely, you can help prevent any harm that quick changes may cause.

Your nurse will review with you some general information about hypertension and risk factors; this will help to reinforce your doctor's advice and instructions.

Remember: To help control your hypertension, you'll need to make these changes in habit and life-style a permanent part of your life.

Controlling Hypertension by Weight Reduction

Research has shown that hypertension can be controlled by weight loss in persons who are overweight. Gradual weight reduction, by decreasing the amount of calories in foods eaten, often results in a significant decrease in blood pressure.

LOSING WEIGHT GRADUALLY
An acceptable measure for losing weight gradually and safely is losing 1 to 2 lb each week until you reach your desired and appropriate weight.

Your doctor may recommend that you lose weight by:
• reducing your daily total intake of calories
• following suggested meal plans made with a dietitian or nutritionist
• increasing your activities and exercising regularly
• joining a weight reduction group and following the suggested plan for weight loss.

Your doctor has recommended that you reduce your weight by:

_____

_____

PLANS FOR REDUCING WEIGHT
Below are some helpful tips on weight reduction:
• Eat three balanced meals a day. Let breakfast be your largest meal; supper, the smallest. Try to plan your meals ahead of time—before you are hungry. Also, keep a diary or list of the type and amounts of foods eaten at each meal. Include foods from the following basic food groups to help nourish your body:

Meat group
—Lean meat, fish, poultry, eggs (limit to three per week)
—Can substitute with: dried peas, dried beans, low-fat cottage cheese, plain low-fat yogurt

Milk group
—Skim milk, ice milk, low-fat yogurt, low-fat cottage cheese

Fruit-vegetable group
—Dark green, leafy, or orange vegetables and fruit (three to four times per week)
—Citrus fruit or fruit juice (each day)

(continued)

Grain group
   —Whole grain and enriched grain products
   —Fortified grain products, such as breads, rice, pasta, and cereals
   —Can substitute with: white potato, dried peas, beans.

• Boil, broil, bake, roast, or stew foods (avoid frying foods).
• Eat slowly and chew foods thoroughly.
• Reduce the amount of foods eaten.
• If you usually have snacks, save some of the food from your meals that are low in calories to eat as snacks.
• Make your meals more appealing by adding color and variety to your meals.
• Avoid distractions when eating (such as watching television, working, or reading the paper).
• Eat out at restaurants that provide salads and foods that are baked or broiled.
• Cut down on the amounts until you can avoid foods that contain high amounts of sugar, such as most desserts, some carbonated beverages (canned or bottled soft drinks), alcoholic beverages (beer, whiskey, wine).
• Drink six to eight glasses of water daily unless you have been advised by your doctor not to drink this amount.
• Try to eat your evening snack 3 to 4 hours before going to bed and perform some activity (such as a taking a brisk walk) about 1 to 2 hours after eating.

Place a check mark beside some of the changes you can make from the list below to help you lose weight:

☐ Eat three balanced meals a day.

☐ Let breakfast be the largest meal and supper the smallest.

☐ Plan meals ahead of time, before you get hungry.

☐ Keep a diary or list of the type and amounts of foods eaten at each meal.

☐ Eat foods from the basic food groups at mealtimes.

☐ Boil, broil, bake, roast, or stew foods (avoid frying foods).

☐ Eat slowly and chew foods thoroughly.

☐ Reduce the amount of foods eaten.

☐ Save some food from meals that are low in calories to eat as snacks.

☐ Make meals more appealing by adding color and variety to them.

(continued)

☐ Do not eat while being distracted with watching television, working, or reading the paper.

☐ Eat at restaurants that provide salads and foods that are baked and broiled.

☐ Cut down on the amounts of foods that contain high amounts of sugar until eating these foods can be avoided.

☐ Cut down on desserts.

☐ Cut down on carbonated beverages (canned or bottled soft drinks) that are high in calories.

☐ Cut down on alcoholic beverages (beer, whiskey, and wine).

☐ Drink at least six to eight glasses of water each day, unless the doctor has advised against it.

OTHER HELPFUL TIPS

• If your eating habits are different on the weekends than during the week, be sure to include this in your meal planning.
• Do not be discouraged and stop trying to reduce your weight if you go on a binge, eat a large amount of food, or eat foods that are high in calories. Instead, try to resume eating the proper amounts and types of food at your next meal.
• Try to weigh yourself no more than once a week. If you begin gaining weight, look at your list of meals that you have eaten to see what may have caused your weight gain.
• Concentrate on forming new eating habits to which you can adjust your life so that, when you have lost weight, you can continue to keep the weight off.

MEAL PLANNING

Use this chart for daily meal planning, incorporating some of the changes you plan to use to lose weight.

Breakfast

Meat group: _____

Grain group: _____

Fruit-vegetable group: _____

Milk group: _____

Food you will save from above for a snack: _____

_____

(continued)

Lunch

Meat group: _____

Grain group: _____

Fruit-vegetable group: _____

Milk group: _____

Food you will save from above for a snack: _____

_____

Dinner

Meat group: _____

Grain group: _____

Fruit-vegetable group: _____

Milk group: _____

Food you will save from above for a snack: _____

_____

Exercising Regularly

Performing isotonic exercises on a regular basis can help control hypertension by lowering your blood pressure. Isotonic exercises include activities in which the muscles move naturally over and over again, such as with walking, aerobic exercises, jogging, swimming, and dancing. Doing them on a regular basis (at least every other day) increases your activity and helps make exercising a normal part of your life-style.

Performing exercises that involve lifting, squeezing, and pressing any muscles of the body against some form of resistance can actually be harmful if you have hypertension. These types of exercises, such as weight lifting and pushing or squeezing against heavy equipment, can raise the blood pressure.

A sedentary life-style, one in which your activities or job result in your getting little or no exercise, does not help to lower your blood pressure.

BENEFITS OF EXERCISE

Increasing your activities (exercising) on a regular basis can help you in several ways, including:
• improving blood circulation to all parts of your body
• helping to keep your high blood pressure lowered and therefore under control
• helping in weight reduction when you follow a proper diet
• helping to handle stress by relieving tension and increasing relaxation.

GETTING STARTED

Remember that you should increase your activities *gradually*. Check with your doctor before beginning a regular exercise program. He will advise you about the type of activities you should start doing and how often you should do them. He may even suggest an exercise group for you to join or advise you to follow an exercise program designed by a physiatrist or physical therapist.

Don't be discouraged if, at certain times, you prefer not to exercise. This is a natural feeling shared by many people. However, when planning your exercising with your doctor, try to pick activities that you like to do so that you'll be encouraged to exercise.

Read the list below and place a check mark beside activities that you can do and beside those you enjoy doing; you may check off both boxes for the same activity.

(continued)

	Can Do	**Enjoy Doing**
Walking for 20 to 30 minutes each day or every other day	☐	☐
Briskly walking for 20 to 30 minutes each day or every other day	☐	☐
Jogging for 20 to 30 minutes each day or every other day	☐	☐
Doing exercises at home for 20 to 30 minutes each day or every other day (such as sit-ups, waist-bends, running in place, or aerobics)	☐	☐
Doing exercises with others for 20 to 30 minutes each day or every other day (such as sit-ups, waist-bends, running in place, or aerobics)	☐	☐
Playing active sports every other day or at least 3 times a week (such as tennis, racquetball, or swimming)	☐	☐
Others (please list)	☐	☐

_____

_____

_____

_____

SPECIAL CONSIDERATIONS
When exercising, be sure to wear comfortable, proper-fitting shoes and comfortable, loose-fitting clothing. If you begin to have discomfort or pain in your chest or other areas for which you have been advised to stop exercising, immediately stop and notify the doctor.
Remember: Increasing your activity level and exercising should become a lifelong part of your normal life-style and habits.

Your doctor has recommended that you increase your activities and exercise more by:

_____

_____

Drinking Alcoholic Beverages in Moderation

Because you have hypertension, you need to be careful about the amount of alcoholic beverages you consume. Drinking large amounts of alcohol is associated with increased blood pressure. Therefore, to help control your blood pressure, you should drink in only moderate amounts.

Drinking large amounts of alcohol may be particularly harmful if consumed over a short period of time, such as binging or drinking large amounts over the weekend, at a social event, or all in 1 day. Heavy intake refers to drinking:
• more than 2 oz (shot) of 100-proof whiskey per day
• more than 8 oz of wine per day (1 average wine glass will hold about 8 oz)
• more than 24 oz of beer per day (2 cans or bottles of beer equal about 24 ounces).

Consuming alcohol in moderation is considered safer for hypertensive individuals who drink. Moderate intake refers to drinking:
• less than 2 oz of 100-proof whiskey per day
• less than 8 oz of wine per day
• less than 24 oz of beer per day.

YOUR ALCOHOL INTAKE
To help determine how much and what types of alcohol you typically consume, place a check in the appropriate boxes:

Amount

☐ None

☐ 1 or 2 drinks per month

☐ 1 or 2 drinks on the weekends only

☐ 1 or 2 drinks per day

☐ More than 2 drinks on the weekends only

☐ More than 2 drinks per day

(continued)

Type

☐ Beer

☐ Wine

☐ Cocktail (such as whiskey, gin, rum, or vodka)

Now, indicate some of the reasons you may drink alcoholic beverages by placing a check in the appropriate boxes:

☐ To be sociable

☐ To help relieve tension and stress

☐ A habit I enjoy

☐ Other reasons (please list):

_____

_____

_____

If you indicated that you drink to be sociable, you might want to try the following suggestions to help you to drink moderately when you socialize:
• Substitute any additional drinks with soda or water with a twist of lime.
• Ask for other beverages, such as juice, a soft drink, coffee, or tea.

If you indicated that you drink to help relieve tension and stress, try any of the following ways to help you deal more effectively with stress:
• Participate in another form of activity, such as some form of exercise for 20 to 30 minutes, rather than having a drink. (Remember, though, to limit your exercises to only those which you have previously discussed with your doctor.)
• Use other forms of stress reduction.

If you indicated that you drink because it is a habit you find enjoyable, try the following suggestions to help you to reduce your alcohol intake:
• Buy smaller quantities of alcoholic beverages.
• Limit how much you drink to the recommended intake for moderate amounts discussed above.
• Substitute beer or wine for whiskey; this allows you to have a larger volume.
• Drink low-calorie beer.

(continued)

In the spaces below, write down how you specifically plan to reduce your alcohol consumption.

_____

_____

_____

_____

_____

YOUR DOCTOR'S RECOMMENDATION
If you find it hard to reduce your alcohol intake, discuss with your doctor other ways or programs that may be helpful.

Your doctor has recommended that you reduce your alcohol intake by:

☐ Continuing to drink alcoholic beverages in moderation

☐ Starting to drink alcoholic beverages in moderation

☐ Following a prescribed program that will help you to stop drinking alcoholic beverages

☐ Joining a program with others who are trying to stop drinking alcoholic beverages

It is important for you to concentrate on forming new drinking habits to better control your hypertension. _Remember:_ Following these plans should become a lifelong habit; it will help control your hypertension for the rest of your life.

Medication Guidelines

TEACHING PLAN
Assessment
• Assess the patient's and family's knowledge of prescribed medications, including:
—which medications should be taken at home
—what each medication does
—pertinent side effects and precautions
—what each medication looks like
—how often each medication should be taken
—what times the medication will be taken.
• Collaborate with the doctor to determine what medications will be prescribed for the patient to take at home.
• Determine if prescriptions will be filled with generic medications.
• Assess the ability of the patient, family, or caregiver to read and tell time.

Materials needed
• Examples or pictures of prescribed medications
• Written summary of medications
• Samples of medication reminder charts for home use
(See *Nurse's notes: Visual aids for medication administration,* page 348.)

Strategies to use
• Assist the patient and family to problem-solve the following:
—an appropriate medication schedule for home use
—measures that the patient and family will use to make sure that medications are taken as prescribed
—how medications will be obtained
—how to estimate when refill prescriptions should be obtained
—when to notify the doctor secondary to side effects.

Patient-teaching aids
See *Medication prescription: Guidelines to follow,* page 350; *Taking anticoagulants,* page 351; *Taking antiarrhythmic medications,* page 353; *Taking antihypertensive medications,* page 354; *Taking antiplatelet medications,* page 355; *Taking cardiac glycosides,* page 356; *Taking coronary vasodilators,* page 357; and *Taking diuretics,* page 358.

Evaluation method
• Have the patient and family explain the action, pertinent side effects, route of administration, and times and frequency of administration for each prescribed medication.
• Have the patient and family develop and write down a medication administration schedule for home use.

**NURSE'S NOTES: VISUAL AIDS FOR
MEDICATION ADMINISTRATION**

To help your patient remember when to take his medication, devise a visual aid like any of the ones suggested here.

1. Create a chart using the following format. Tell him to check the appropriate box after he has taken the medication.

Time of day	Medications to take	Taken
8 a.m.	_____	☐
9 a.m.	_____	☐

2. Draw two pictures of clocks, one for the morning and one for the evening. Then, paste or tape a sample of each prescribed medication on the time that it is to be taken.

3. Using envelopes or small cups, label one for each time that medications should be taken. Then, fill the envelopes or cups with the appropriate medications to be taken for 1 day's use. Instruct the patient to refill the cups or envelopes each morning. (Or have the patient label and fill several envelopes or cups, enough to last for 1 week; each group should be clearly labeled with the correct day of the week.)

4. Using an empty egg carton, label each crevice with a time that medication is to be taken. Then, fill each space with the appropriate medication. Have the patient refill the crevices each day.
Note: Commercial containers that hold a week's supply of medication separated by day may be purchased from a local pharmacy.

Interventions and outcome criteria

☑ **Intervention 1**
Review each prescribed medication with the patient and family, including:
• what the medication looks like
• what the medication does
• the medication's side effects and when to notify the doctor secondary to side effects
• how the medication should be taken
• how often the medication should be taken.

Outcome criteria: The patient and family correctly identify each prescribed medication, stating its action, pertinent side effects, and frequency and route of administration. They also state when the doctor should be called.

☑ **Intervention 2**
Assist the patient and family to develop an appropriate medication administration plan for home use. Consider the following:
• the frequency of administration of each prescribed medication
• the patient and his family's usual habits, such as:
—normal times for getting up and going to bed
—the patient's usual daily schedule at home.

Outcome criteria: The patient and family develop an appropriate medication schedule for use at home.

☑ **Intervention 3**
Have the patient and family plan how they will remember the prescribed medication schedule; suggestions may include:
• setting up a day's medication in separately labeled containers
• setting up a week's medication in separately labeled or colored containers
• using a sheet to check off each medication when taken.

Outcome criteria: The patient and family state how they will remember to take or give the prescribed medications.

☑ **Intervention 4**
Have the patient and family plan how to handle refills, including:
• where and how to obtain the refills
• how to estimate when refills should be obtained to prevent running out of prescribed medications
• how to pay for the refills.

Outcome criteria: The patient and family state how and when they will obtain refills.

Medication Prescription: Guidelines to Follow

Your doctor wants you to take the following medication at home.

Medication: _____

Description of medication: _____

_____

What the medication does: _____

_____

Any side effects to watch for: _____

_____

How the medication should be taken: _____

_____

How often the medication should be taken: _____

_____

When the medication should be taken: _____

_____

Paste sample medication here:

Name and telephone number of local pharmacy: _____

_____

(*Note:* Repeat this information for each medication, as needed.)

PATIENT-TEACHING AID

Taking Anticoagulants

Your doctor has prescribed _____
for you to take at home. This medication slows down the normal clotting of your blood. It will help to prevent clots from forming in your bloodstream.

DIRECTIONS FOR USE
For this medication to work correctly, you must take it exactly as your doctor has ordered. Be sure to take your anticoagulant tablet once a day and at the same time each day. You may take it with a meal or between meals. Do not skip doses and do not take extra or double doses.

As long as you are taking this medication, you will need to have frequent blood tests. Blood tests are ordered to ensure that you are taking the right amount of medication. In the spaces below, your nurse will write down where you are to go for these tests and when your first appointment will be. Be sure to keep your appointments for your blood tests; serious problems can result if you are taking the wrong amount of medication.

Where to go for blood test: _____

_____

_____

_____

Telephone number: _____

First appointment (date and time): _____

_____

SPECIAL CONSIDERATIONS
• Do not stop taking this medication for any reason without your doctor's approval.
• Notify your doctor if you have any of the following signs and symptoms:
—dark brown or red-tinged urine
—dark or tarry-colored stools
—large bruised areas that result from only small injuries (like bumping into a piece of furniture)
—nosebleeds
—a longer or heavier menstrual flow than usual.

(continued)

DO'S AND DON'TS

• As long as you are taking this medication, you should follow these general rules:

—DO tell every doctor and dentist you see that you are taking this medication.

—DO shave with an electric razor.

—DO use a soft toothbrush if you notice any bleeding from your gums.

—DO carry a Medic Alert bracelet or necklace that says you are taking this medication.

—DO check with your doctor about how to take this medication before traveling out of town.

—DO use safety measures to avoid injury, such as always wearing shoes, using gloves when working outside, and handling sharp objects carefully.

—DO store your tablets in a tightly closed container.

—DON'T take aspirin or any drugs containing aspirin (acetylsalicylic acid) unless specifically directed to do so by your doctor.

—DON'T take any over-the-counter medications (including cold and flu remedies) without first asking your doctor.

—DON'T allow your prescription to run out. Get a refill at least a week before your current bottle runs out.

—DON'T eat large amounts of foods high in vitamin K, such as liver, green leafy vegetables, cheese, egg yolks, and the fat from beef.

—DON'T drink large amounts of alcohol. Even as little as 2 to 3 oz can slow the clotting time of your blood too much so that you bleed too easily.

—DON'T skip doses. However, if you happen to forget to take a tablet on a given day, don't bother taking one to make up for it. If you forget to take your tablet on 2 consecutive days, call your doctor.

To obtain a Medic Alert bracelet or necklace, write to:

_____

_____

_____

or call: _____

_____

Taking Antiarrhythmic Medications

Your doctor has prescribed _____
for you to take at home. This type of medication is given to slow your heart rate or to keep your heartbeat regular.

DIRECTIONS FOR USE

Be sure to take this medication exactly as your doctor has prescribed. Do not skip doses or take double doses. If you happen to forget to take a dose, simply omit that dose. Do not take two doses the next time.

It is important that you not take certain medications at the same time you take your antiarrhythmic medication; doing so could cause drug interactions and possible side effects. Medications to avoid include:

_____

_____

_____

Also, before taking any over-the-counter medication, be sure to talk with your doctor first.

SPECIAL CONSIDERATIONS

Be sure to take your medication (your nurse will check which one applies to you):

☐ With food or meals

☐ In between meals

☐ Either between meals or with meals.

• Count your pulse rate _____ (frequency).
• Notify your doctor if your pulse rate goes above _____ or drops below _____.
• Call your doctor if you notice any of the following:
   —an extremely irregular pulse rate
   —dizziness or light-headedness
   —blurred vision
   —continued constipation or diarrhea.

Taking Antihypertensive Medications

Your doctor has prescribed _____
for you to take. This type of medication is given to help lower your blood
pressure.

DIRECTIONS FOR USE
Take this medication exactly as your doctor has prescribed, either with
meals or between meals. Do not skip doses, and do not take double doses.
If you happen to forget a dose, simply omit that dose; do not take 2 doses
the next time.
   Continue taking this medication until your doctor tells you to stop.

SPECIAL CONSIDERATIONS
• Check your blood pressure _____ (frequency) at home.
• Notify the doctor if your blood pressure is higher than _____ or lower
than _____.
• Do not stand up quickly from either a lying or a sitting position. Always
change positions slowly. If you are lying down, sit up first; then stand up.
• Do not take a hot shower or bath. This can make your blood pressure
drop too low and make you feel dizzy.
• Take special care when driving or operating heavy equipment for 2 hours
after taking this medication. Antihypertensives may cause drowsiness when
you first begin taking them; however, this effect usually stops after you
have been taking the medication for several weeks.
• If you feel dizzy or faint, stop what you are doing and lie down or sit with
your head down.
• If you begin to develop any side effects, notify your doctor but continue
taking the medication.

Taking Antiplatelet Medications

Your doctor has prescribed _____ for you to take at home. The reason you are taking this medication is (your nurse will check the reason you are taking this medication):

☐ to prevent blood clots from forming

☐ to decrease your chance of having a heart attack (myocardial infarction)

☐ to keep the new grafts in your artery working well.

DIRECTIONS FOR USE
Take this medication exactly as your doctor has prescribed, at the same time each day. Do not skip doses; do not take extra doses. Continue taking this medication until your doctor tells you to stop.

SPECIAL CONSIDERATIONS
• Tell any doctor or dentist you see that you are taking this medication.
• Notify your doctor if you notice any of the following:
   —dark or tarry-colored stools
   —blood in the stools
   —dizziness or light-headedness.

Taking Cardiac Glycosides

Your doctor has prescribed _____ for you to take at home. This medication was prescribed (your nurse will check the reason you are taking this medication):

☐ to help your heart pump more effectively

☐ to slow your heart rate or keep your heartbeat regular.

DIRECTIONS FOR USE

Take this medication exactly as your doctor has prescribed, at about the same time each day. You may take it with or between meals. Do not skip doses; do not take extra doses. If you happen to forget to take your medication on a given day, simply omit that dose. Do not take an extra dose the next day. Continue taking this medication until your doctor tells you to stop.

SPECIAL CONSIDERATIONS

• Count your pulse _____ (frequency). Notify your doctor if your pulse rate is greater than _____ or less than _____.
• Let every doctor you see know that you are taking this medication. Consult your doctor before taking any other medications, including all over-the-counter medications.
• Avoid taking antacids, medications for diarrhea, or laxatives 2 hours before or 2 hours after taking this medication.
• Notify your doctor if you develop any of the following:
—nausea and vomiting
—changes in your usual appetite
—increased tiredness with your normal activity
—blurred or double vision
—drop in your pulse rate below the limit listed above
—pulse rhythm changes from regular or slightly irregular to extremely irregular
—a rise in your pulse rate above the limit listed above.

Taking Coronary Vasodilators

Your doctor has prescribed _____ for you to take at home. This type of medication helps decrease your angina by increasing the amount of oxygen to your heart or decreasing the amount of oxygen that your heart needs.

DIRECTIONS FOR USE

Take this medication exactly as your doctor has prescribed, either with or between meals. Do not skip doses; do not take double doses. Continue taking this medication until your doctor tells you to stop.

If you are using the nitroglycerin paste:

—Squeeze the prescribed amount onto the special paper included with the medication (squeezing the medication tube like a tube of toothpaste).

—Spread the medication all over the paper in a thin layer (use the paper to spread it; do not use your fingers). Your nurse will help you practice this.

—Take off the old paper and carefully wash and dry that area.

—Put the new paper (medication-side down) on a different place on your body.

Note: You may put plastic wrap over the paper to protect your clothes if you wish.

SPECIAL CONSIDERATIONS

• If you have frequent, severe headaches after taking this medication, talk with your doctor. Do not stop taking the medication.

• If you feel dizzy or faint after taking this medication, sit down and lower your head.

• Tell any doctor or dentist that you see that you are taking this medication.

Taking Diuretics

Your doctor has prescribed _____ for you to take at home. This type of medication is prescribed (your nurse will check the reason you are taking this medication):

☐ to help lower your blood pressure

☐ to limit your symptoms of congestive heart failure.

DIRECTIONS FOR USE
Take this medication exactly as your doctor has ordered. Do not skip doses; do not take extra doses. Continue taking this medication until your doctor tells you to stop.

SPECIAL CONSIDERATIONS
• Because you will have to urinate frequently for 8 or more hours after taking the medication, think about the best time of day for you to take this medication. Discuss this with your nurse.
• Weigh yourself daily. Using the same scale each time, weigh yourself before breakfast and after urinating. Keep a record of your weights for your doctor.
• If you are taking a diuretic that causes an excessive loss of potassium from your body:
  —be sure to take any potassium your doctor may prescribe, and take it exactly as prescribed.
  —make sure you include foods high in potassium in your diet every day. Common foods include bananas, orange juice, dried apricots, baked potatoes, raisins, yellow squash, and peaches.

Myocardial Infarction: Disease Process and Home Care

TEACHING PLAN
Assessment
• Assess the patient's and family's knowledge of myocardial infarction (MI), its causes, and its symptoms.
• Assess the patient's and family's knowledge of home care after MI, including medications, diet, activity, and complications.
• Determine the presence of complications and extent of damage to the patient's heart, including results of low-level exercise stress testing and left ventricular function and ejection fraction, if known.
• Assess the patient's and family's previous experience with MI and determine areas of concern.
• Collaborate with the doctor to determine the patient's discharge orders.

Materials needed
• Model or diagram of heart and coronary circulation

Strategies to use
• Stimulate interest in the topic by beginning with the patient's and family's areas of concern.
• Help the patient and family to problem-solve the following:
  —how to manage the patient's activity at home
  —how to manage the patient's diet at home
  —how to modify risk factors for atherosclerosis
  —how to recognize complications and what to do if they occur.

Patient-teaching aid
See *Caring for yourself at home after a heart attack*, page 363.

Evaluation method
• Have the patient and a family member describe, using their own words, what occurs in a myocardial infarction.
• Have the patient and a family member describe home care measures and their plans for implementing each measure.

Interventions and outcome criteria
☑ **Intervention 1**
Briefly review normal heart function, need for oxygen, and coronary blood flow (see "Cardiac Anatomy and Physiology: Heart and Blood Vessels" in this section).

Outcome criteria: Use the outcome criteria from "Cardiac Anatomy and Physiology: Heart and Blood Vessels" in this section.

☑ Intervention 2
Explain about MI, covering:
• loss of blood flow to the myocardium, including:
 —the role of atherosclerosis
 —thrombus formation and occlusion of the coronary artery
 —tissue damage secondary to loss of blood supply
• signs and symptoms associated with infarction, including
 —chest pain
 —associated symptoms
 —atypical presentation
• how the heart heals.

Outcome criteria: The patient and family state that MI occurs when the oxygen supply to part of the heart is completely cut off by occlusion of a vessel by atherosclerosis and blood clot formation resulting in permanent tissue damage. They also state the major warning signs of MI and that the heart heals slowly over time.

☑ Intervention 3
Discuss the medications prescribed for discharge (see "Medication Guidelines" in this section).

Outcome criteria: Use the outcome criteria from "Medication Guidelines" in this section.

☑ Intervention 4
Discuss the prescribed diet, including:
• limiting saturated fats and cholesterol
• limiting caffeine
• limiting alcoholic beverages
• avoiding overeating
• limiting sodium, as ordered.

Outcome criteria: The patient and family state the patient's dietary restrictions and plans for implementing such restrictions at home.

☑ Intervention 5
Discuss the patient's home activities, including:
• pacing of activities
• managing activities of daily living
• the need for sleep and rest
• limiting visitors and phone calls
• plans for gradually becoming more active
• warning signs of overexertion.

Outcome criteria: The patient and family state plans for managing the patient's activities at home.

☑ Intervention 6

Discuss the patient's resumption of sexual activity at home (see "Sexual Activity and Heart Disease" in this section).

Outcome criteria: Use the outcome criteria from "Sexual Activity and Heart Disease" in this section.

☑ Intervention 7

Discuss how to count and record a radial pulse (see "Radial Pulse Measurement" in this section).

Outcome criteria: The patient and family demonstrate correctly how to count and record a radial pulse.

☑ Intervention 8

Discuss how to take and record daily weights.

Outcome criteria: The patient and family state the correct way to take and record daily weights.

☑ Intervention 9

Discuss common emotional reactions to MI (see "Stress Management" in this section).

Outcome criteria: Use the outcome criteria from "Stress Management" in this section.

☑ Intervention 10

Discuss common complications after MI and warning signs, including:
• recurrence of angina, including a discussion of:
  —chest pain and its associated symptoms
  —management of an acute attack
• reinfarction, including:
  —chest pain and its associated symptoms
  —atypical presentation
  —obtaining medical care
• congestive heart failure (CHF), including:
  —increased dyspnea, fatigue, cough, dependent edema, and weight gain of 2 lb or more in 24 hours
  —obtaining medical care
• dysrhythmias, including:
  —changes in pulse rate and rhythm
  —symptoms of decreased cardiac output
  —obtaining medical care.

Outcome criteria: The patient and family state the warning signs of complications and state their plans for obtaining appropriate medical care.

☑ Intervention 11

Discuss modification of risk factors for atherosclerosis.

• Have the patient and his family identify specific risk factors.

• Have the patient and his family develop specific plans for modifying individual risk factors.

Outcome criteria: The patient and family state plans for modifying the patient's specific risk factors.

☑ Intervention 12

Discuss follow-up care.

Outcome criteria: The patient and family state the importance of follow-up care.

Caring for Yourself at Home after a Heart Attack

As you will soon be going home from the hospital, you may have certain questions about how to care for youself at home. This patient-teaching aid discusses some common questions that patients and families have. If you have other questions not answered in this aid, be sure to ask your nurse or doctor.

MYOCARDIAL INFARCTION

You remember that your heart is a muscle. Like other muscles in your body, it requires oxygen to work correctly. When the oxygen supply is cut off to a part of the heart, the heart can become permanently damaged. This damage is called a myocardial infarction (MI).

Often, several things working together cause part of the heart to get too little oxygen. First, the coronary arteries are often narrowed by fatty deposits (caused by atherosclerosis) so that less blood and oxygen can get to part of the heart. Also, a blood clot can form in the narrowed artery. This clot can totally block the artery so that no blood or oxygen can get through to that part of the heart. When this occurs, the part of the heart supplied by that artery is permanently damaged.

SIGNS AND SYMPTOMS

Most people experience chest pain when they have an MI. This chest pain is usually described as crushing, viselike, sharp, or stabbing. It is not relieved by rest or nitroglycerin. Often located in the left side of the chest, the pain may travel down your left or right arm or up the left or right side of your neck.

Other signs and symptoms that go with the chest pain include shortness of breath, dizziness, restlessness or anxiety, cold sweat, and feelings of palpitations.

Some people do not have chest pain with an MI. Older people and people with diabetes are more likely not to have chest pain. Instead, they may become very short of breath. Their skin may feel cold to touch, and they may break out in a cold sweat. They may also feel very tired, appear very confused, or complain of feeling sick to the stomach.

HOW THE HEART HEALS

After an MI, your heart gradually heals by replacing the damaged tissue with other cells called scar tissue. It takes time for your heart to heal completely. How quickly you recover and how much you will be able to do depends on how much of your heart was damaged by your MI and whether or not you have had any major complications.

(continued)

HOME CARE

Follow these guidelines for caring for yourself at home after an MI.

Medication

Be sure to take all of your medications exactly as your doctor has ordered. Your nurse will give you more information about each of the medications you will be taking at home.

Diet

Follow your doctor's orders for your diet. Your doctor wants you to use the following diet at home:

_____

_____

Your nurse and dietitian will be giving you more information about this diet and how to use it at home.

Also follow these guidelines:
• Limit the amount of caffeine you have each day. Caffeine is found in tea, coffee, chocolate, many soft drinks, and some over-the-counter medications. Caffeine is a stimulant that makes your heart work harder. Limiting your caffeine intake is important in decreasing the work of your heart.
• Limit the amount of alcoholic beverages you drink to 2 to 3 oz per day.
• Don't overeat, as this increases the stress on your heart. You may want to eat three or four smaller meals a day instead of eating fewer, larger meals.

Activity

When you first get home, do about the same amount of activity at the same pace as you were doing in the hospital. Continue this level of activity for the first 1 to 2 weeks that you are home.

Keep in mind that you will gradually increase your activity. How fast you return to your usual level of activity will depend on how much of your heart was damaged and whether or not you had any complications.

Follow these general guidelines concerning your activity:
• Shower or bathe, depending on your preference. If you shower, you might want to put a stool in the shower to sit on. Avoid using extremely hot or cold water. Don't take prolonged showers or baths; however, don't hurry unnecessarily.
• Limit the amount of things that you do with your arms above your head. Try to plan to do most activities with your arms at no more than waist level.
• Plan to get enough rest. Remember that resting does not always mean sleeping. It may include sitting quietly for 20 to 30 minutes. Be sure to rest after activities.
• Plan to get enough sleep, preferably 8 to 10 hours per night. You may want to take one or two brief naps during the day; however, be careful not to get too much sleep during the day, because you will not sleep well at night.

(continued)

• Stop any activity when you first begin to become tired. Don't let yourself become overtired.

• Stop any activity immediately if you have chest pain, feel short of breath, have palpitations, feel faint or dizzy, or break out in a cold sweat.

• Pace your activities, spreading them out during the day. Don't try to do too many things all at one time or to rush through any activity. When you first get home, "activities" include bathing, eating, walking, talking on the phone, and visiting with friends. A slow pace and plenty of rest are important.

• Limit your stair climbing to _____ times per day. When you climb stairs, take them at a slow pace. If you get short of breath or tired, sit down and rest.

• Limit visitors to two to three short visits per day. If you become tired during someone's visit, don't hesitate to leave the room and rest in another part of your home or to ask your visitor to leave.

Exercise
Exercise is important for your recovery. The nurse will give you additional information on how and when to exercise.

Sexual activity
You may be concerned that resuming sexual activity will hurt your heart. Sexual activity puts about the same amount of stress on your heart as walking up a flight of stairs quickly or walking 1 to 2 blocks at a brisk pace. Your nurse will give you some guidelines on how to safely resume sex at home.

Pulse rate and daily weight
Remember to weigh yourself each day. To do so correctly, you should:

• weigh yourself at the same time each morning using the same scale
• weigh yourself before breakfast and after urinating each morning
• record the date and your weight
• notify your doctor if you gain 2 lb or more overnight.

    You may also need to count your radial pulse each day. Your nurse will give you additional information on how to do this.

Warning signs
Because you may develop problems after an MI, knowing the warning signs lets you recognize the problems quickly and get appropriate medical care.

Angina
You may experience some chest pain after your heart attack at rest or with activity. This type of pain is frequently described as a feeling of tightness or pressure in the chest and is often felt on the left side of the chest. You may also feel dizzy, perspire heavily, or feel weak or short of breath.

(continued)

If you have experienced angina in the past, think back to one of your attacks. In the spaces below, list the symptoms you had.

_____

_____

_____

_____

_____

When you first notice any symptoms of chest pain, immediately:
• Stop what you are doing and sit down.
• Take your sublingual nitroglycerin. Place one tablet under your tongue and let it dissolve. If your chest pain is unrelieved in 5 minutes, take a second tablet. You may take one tablet every 5 minutes up to a total of _____ tablets or until your pain is relieved. (*Note:* If you have never used sublingual nitroglycerin before, your nurse will give you additional information on how to store and carry it.)
• If your chest pain is unrelieved after you have taken _____ tablets, seek medical help. You may be having another heart attack or MI.

If you develop angina, let your doctor know. He will want to know how often you have attacks, what seems to bring them on, and how much nitroglycerin you have to take to relieve them.

Another MI
There is a possibility that you may have a second heart attack or MI. If you develop any of the signs and symptoms that you had with your first MI (or any of the symptoms mentioned earlier in this aid) get to the hospital immediately.

Heart failure
Heart failure develops when the heart is not pumping well enough to meet the body's needs for blood and oxygen. Notify your doctor immediately if:
• you become more short of breath than usual (with activity or at rest)
• you become more tired than usual with your typical day's activities
• you notice that rings or shoes have become too tight or that your feet and ankles are swollen
• you or someone in your family notices swelling in your lower back or hips (this is associated with patients who spend most of the day in bed)
• you develop a cough without flulike symptoms
• you gain 2 lb or more overnight.

Problems with heart rhythm
Notify your doctor immediately if:
• your pulse rate drops below _____ beats/minute or rises above _____ beats/minute
• your pulse rhythm changes from regular or slightly irregular to extremely irregular

(continued)

• you feel dizzy, faint, or tired with any of the above changes in your pulse rate or rhythm.

These are warning signs that your heartbeat has become so irregular that your body is not getting enough blood and oxygen to meet its needs.

Plan now how you will get additional medical care if problems develop. In the spaces below, record pertinent names and numbers.

Doctor: _____

Phone: _____

Address: _____

Hospital: _____

Phone: _____

Address: _____

Ambulance: _____

Phone: _____

How I will get medical care:

During the day: _____

On the weekend: _____

At night: _____

I will keep my emergency numbers (specify where):

_____

_____

PREVENTION

If you do not take measures to slow or prevent more atherosclerosis from developing, you will develop additional blockages in other arteries. You may even have another heart attack or stroke or develop problems with the circulation in your feet.

The nurse will give you more information on risk factors for atherosclerosis and how to change them.

(continued)

After reading the material, list your individual risk factors in the spaces below.

_____

_____

_____

_____

_____

FOLLOW-UP

Keeping your doctor's appointments is extremely important. Your first appointment is:

Doctor: _____

Phone: _____

Address: _____

Date: _____

Time: _____

Occlusive Arterial Disease: Disease Process and Home Care

TEACHING PLAN
Assessment
• Assess the patient's and family's understanding of home management of occlusive disease, including foot care, management of complications, modification of risk factors, and walking program.
• Collaborate with the doctor about the patient's readiness and ability to engage in planned walking.

Materials needed
• Diagram showing a normal artery, a diseased artery, and major vessels affected by atherosclerosis for the individual patient
• Basin, towel, lotion, and cornstarch

Strategies to use
• Present the information on foot care and exercise using demonstration and return demonstration.
• Have the patient and family problem-solve the following:
  —when and how to obtain additional medical care if needed
  —how to manage the patient's walking program at home.

Patient-teaching aids
See *Understanding occlusive arterial disease,* page 372; *Foot care: Guidelines to follow at home,* page 373; and *Planned walking program,* page 376.

Evaluation method
• Have the patient and a family member state, in their own words, major points of home management.
• Have the patient perform the walking program without the nurse's assistance.
• Have the patient and a family member demonstrate, without the nurse's assistance, proper foot care; have the patient and a family member state other major principles of good foot care.

Interventions and outcome criteria
☑ **Intervention 1**
Briefly review peripheral circulation, if necessary.

☑ Intervention 2
Explain the role of atherosclerosis in the development of occlusive arterial disease.

Outcome criteria: The patient and family state that atherosclerosis narrows arteries and decreases the amount of oxygen-enriched blood that reaches tissues.

☑ Intervention 3
Describe major signs and symptoms associated with occlusive arterial disease, including:
• intermittent claudication
• rest pain
• sensation of cold feet
• diminished or absent pulses.

Outcome criteria: The patient and family state major signs and symptoms of occlusive arterial disease.

☑ Intervention 4
Teach the patient and family appropriate foot care, including:
• demonstration on daily foot care routine, including:
—how to wash and dry feet
—use of lotion and cornstarch
—proper toenail care
• demonstration on daily foot inspection, including:
—observing for areas of redness, injury, blisters, or breakdown
—observing for corns, calluses, or bruises
• return demonstration by the patient and family, under the nurse's supervision, on performing foot care and inspection
• management of the following problems:
—corns and calluses
—blisters
—areas of redness
—areas of injury
—infection
• when to notify the doctor
• measures to prevent injury, including:
—use of properly fitting shoes and socks
—ways to keep the feet warm.

Outcome criteria: The patient and family demonstrate, without assistance from the nurse, proper foot care and inspection techniques. They state how to prevent injury to the legs and feet and when to seek additional medical care.

☑ Intervention 5
Teach the patient and family to use a walking program.
• Explain that the patient should:
—walk at a slow to moderate pace on a level surface
—walk until intermittent claudication occurs
—stop walking when pain occurs until the pain stops

—resume walking when the pain is gone and continue walking until it returns
—repeat the process for the prescribed length of the exercise.
• Have the patient demonstrate the walking program under the nurse's supervision.

Outcome criteria: The patient demonstrates the walking program correctly without assistance from the nurse.

☑ Intervention 6
Discuss the role of atherosclerosis in occlusive arterial disease (see "Atherosclerosis: Disease Process and Risk Factors" in this section).

Outcome criteria: Use the outcome criteria from "Atherosclerosis: Disease Process and Risk Factors" in this section.

☑ Intervention 7
Discuss modification of risk factors; assist the patient and family to plan how to alter individual risk factors, including:
• stopping smoking (see "Cardiovascular Disease Risk Factors: Cigarette Smoking" in this section)
• reducing dietary intake of saturated fats and cholesterol (see "Cardiovascular Disease Risk Factors: Dietary Measures to Control Hyperlipidemia" in this section)
• controlling diabetes mellitus (see "Cardiovascular Disease Risk Factors: Diabetes Mellitus and Atherosclerosis" in this section)
• controlling hypertension (see "Hypertension, Essential: Disease Process and Risk Factors" in this section).

Outcome criteria: Use the outcome criteria from the specific teaching plans mentioned in this intervention.

Understanding Occlusive Arterial Disease

Occlusive arterial disease is the medical term for narrowing or blockage of the arteries that supply the arms, legs, and feet with blood and oxygen. The most common cause of these blockages is atherosclerosis; your nurse will give you another teaching aid on atherosclerosis.

SIGNS AND SYMPTOMS
When the arteries in your legs become too narrowed, symptoms usually develop. Such symptoms include:
• pain in the calf that occurs with activity and is lessened or relieved with rest; this is usually one of the first symptoms noticed.
• severe pain in the leg or foot, even at rest, which may be lessened by sitting up and putting the feet on the floor. This pain occurs because, as the arteries become more narrowed, they are unable to supply the needs of your feet and legs even at rest.
• feet that feel cold, even when the rest of your body is warm.

RISK FACTORS
To help slow the growth of the blockages in your arteries, you may need to make some changes in your life-style. Read through the teaching aid on atherosclerosis and identify any risk factors that you may have for this disease. Your nurse will give you additional information on each of the specific risk factors you identify.

PATIENT-TEACHING AID

Foot Care: Guidelines to Follow at Home

Because you have occlusive arterial disease, you must take proper care of your feet at home. As you know, with this disease, the vessels carrying blood and oxygen to your feet and legs are narrowed, resulting in less blood getting through to your feet. Consequently, your feet may become easily damaged. If they become damaged or injured, they may not heal well and permanent damage could result.

WASHING AND DRYING FEET
Be sure to wash your feet every day in warm, never hot, water; using hot water can damage your feet. Carefully check the water temperature with your hand or wrist before putting your feet in the water. If it feels hot to your hand or wrist, it is too hot for your feet. Add more cool water.

Carefully wash your feet with a mild soap. Be sure to wash between each of your toes. Then, dry each foot gently, using a clean, soft towel. Avoid rubbing your feet hard with the towel; pat them dry instead. Also, remember to gently dry between the toes.

APPLYING LOTION OR POWDER
After your feet are dry, you may apply some lotion gently to your skin. Be sure to use a lotion that contains lanolin. *Note:* Never apply lotion between the toes.

If your feet tend to sweat, you may want to use foot powder or cornstarch. Dust a small amount of powder over your feet with your fingers. Do not let the powder cake on your feet.

CUTTING TOENAILS
You need to be especially careful with your toenails. Cut them only after soaking and washing your feet and in adequate light. Make sure you cut each nail straight across, then file each nail carefully to eliminate any rough edges. If your nails are too thick or crack when you cut them, have a podiatrist cut them for you. Attached is a list of podiatrists in your area.

DAILY INSPECTION
Each day after washing and drying your feet, inspect them carefully for any signs of damage or injury. Look for any of the signs listed below.

Redness
Redness is usually caused by too much pressure on a particular part of your foot. Check your shoes for proper fit. Also check your socks; wrinkles or seams in socks can put too much pressure on your skin. Replace shoes or socks, as necessary.

(continued)

Sitting or lying in bed with your feet always in the same position can cause redness as well. Change the position of your feet every 1 or 2 hours.

Blisters

Blisters can be caused by burns from bath water that is too hot. They may also be caused by ill-fitting shoes or wrinkled socks. Make sure that you check the water carefully before washing your feet. Also check the fit of your shoes and be sure to keep your socks smooth.

Avoid popping blisters on your feet. Instead, pad the area with some gauze or a bandage. Check the area frequently to make sure it does not become infected.

Corns or calluses

Calluses may be caused by ill-fitting shoes. Check the fit of your shoes and wear another pair, if needed. Talk to your doctor if you have recurring problems with corns or calluses.

Gently rub corns and calluses with lotion containing lanolin. Pad them with soft pads. Avoid using over-the-counter treatments or medications for corns and calluses. Also, do not cut them with a razor or a knife.

Breaks in the skin

To treat breaks in the skin of your foot, wash the area well using warm or cool (never hot) water and mild soap. Cover the area with a dry, sterile dressing (you can get these from your drugstore or grocery store). Change the dressing once a day. Watch the area closely for any signs of infection.

Signs of infection

Signs that indicate an injury is becoming infected include:
• redness around the injured area
• swelling at the injured area
• warmth at the injured area
• drainage or fluid oozing from the injured area.
If you see any signs of infection, call your doctor at once.

COMPLICATIONS

Because injuries have the potential of causing permanent damage to your legs and feet, be sure to notify your doctor immediately if you develop any of the following:
• slow healing of an injured foot or leg, especially if the injury does not appear to be better within 3 days
• signs of infection developing from a cut, sore, or other injury
• increased pain in the calf when performing your usual amount of activity
• pain in the calf or foot while at rest
• sudden coldness of the foot or part of the leg (the skin suddenly feels colder to the touch farther down your leg).

(continued)

Write in the spaces below where and how to obtain additional medical care, if needed.

Who to call: _____

Phone: _____

Address: _____

How to get to the hospital/doctor/clinic: _____

_____

_____

_____

_____

PREVENTION

Preventing damage to your feet is extremely important. Follow these guidelines:
• Always wear well-fitting shoes. Shoes should have a closed heel and a closed toe; they should fit comfortably and give good support.
• Change into clean socks, preferably cotton or wool, daily.
• Begin breaking in new shoes slowly. Wear them only 30 minutes the 1st day, then 1 hour longer each subsequent day. Inspect your feet carefully for any signs of redness.
• Avoid walking barefoot.
• Never use a heating pad or hot water bottle directly on your feet.
• Wear socks or place extra covers on your feet if your feet feel cold.
• Wear warm socks when going outdoors in the winter.

Planned Walking Program

Because you have occlusive arterial disease, your doctor has recommended that you start a planned walking program at home. Walking is an important exercise. As you remember, the arteries carrying blood to your legs and feet are partially narrowed. Walking helps increase the collateral circulation—a fine network of tiny vessels carrying blood and oxygen to your legs and feet—near the area of the narrowed artery. With good collateral circulation, you may notice less pain in your legs; however, it will take some time for collateral circulation to grow.

Before you begin your walking program, make sure you have a sturdy pair of shoes and a flat, level place to walk. Then, start walking.

Beginning at a slow pace, continue walking until you start to feel pain in the calf of your leg. Then stop walking and rest without sitting. When the pain stops, resume walking. Continue walking until the pain returns. When you begin to feel pain in your calf again, stop and rest. Then, when the pain is gone, go back to walking.

Continue this exercise for _____ minutes.

Oxygen Use at Home

TEACHING PLAN
Assessment
• Collaborate with the doctor to determine whether the patient should use oxygen at home; determine the specific orders for oxygen administration.
• Collaborate with discharge planning services or social services to determine what company will supply oxygen for the patient at home.
• Assess the patient's and family's knowledge on use of the prescribed oxygen system.
• Assess the patient's and family's previous experiences with home use of the prescribed oxygen system; identify any past problems or concerns.

Materials needed
• Written summary of instructions
• Name and telephone number (including emergency service number) of company that will supply oxygen to the patient's home

Strategies to use
• Individualize your teaching by arranging for a company representative to demonstrate the prescribed oxygen system and its use to the patient and family before discharge.
• Assist the patient and his family to problem-solve the following:
 —where and how to obtain help 24 hours a day if problems develop with the oxygen system.
 —how to estimate the amount of oxygen left and how to obtain a new tank when needed.

Patient-teaching aid
See Guidelines for using oxygen at home, page 379.

Evaluation method
Have the patient and a family member describe, in their own words, appropriate use of oxygen at home.

Interventions and outcome criteria
☑ Intervention 1
Explain briefly why oxygen has been prescribed for home use.

Outcome criteria: The patient and family state the reasons for using oxygen.

☑ Intervention 2
Provide the patient and family with the name and telephone number of the company that will supply the home oxygen system.

Outcome criteria: The patient and family state the name and number of the company that will supply the oxygen system.

☑ Intervention 3
Assist the patient and family to contact the company and arrange for an instruction and demonstration session on the use of the prescribed system. Suggest that they listen carefully for the following information during the demonstration:
• how to set up the system
• how to turn the oxygen on and off (including how to correctly set the oxygen flow)
• common problems that may occur and ways of troubleshooting them
• how to obtain a replacement tank when needed
• how to obtain help if a problem arises with the system.

Outcome criteria: The patient and family demonstrate the correct setup and know the correct use of the prescribed oxygen system. They also state that they know how to troubleshoot common problems with the system, obtain a replacement tank, and obtain help for problems.

☑ Intervention 4
Instruct the patient and family on the use of a nasal cannula or face mask, as indicated.

Outcome criteria: The patient and family demonstrate how to correctly apply and remove the nasal cannula or face mask, as prescribed.

☑ Intervention 5
Review the general precautions the patient and family will need to take when oxygen is being used in the home, including the following:
• Do not smoke in the house.
• Notify the fire department that oxygen is being kept in the house.
• Keep an all-purpose fire extinguisher handy.
• Keep the oxygen supply at least 5′ from a heat source or electrical appliance.
• Do not use oxygen around stoves or space heaters.
• Do not put the oxygen tubing under rugs, furniture, or bed linens.
• Turn the oxygen on only when the patient is using it.

Outcome criteria: The patient and family state all of the general precautions listed above.

PATIENT-TEACHING AID

Guidelines for Using Oxygen at Home

Your doctor has ordered oxygen for you to use at home. Using oxygen helps to increase the amount of oxygen that gets to all parts of your body. It can help you feel less short of breath and may enable you to perform more activity.

Oxygen is given through either a face mask or a nasal cannula. Your nurse will show you how to put on and take off the type your doctor has ordered for you. She will also fill in the following spaces with specific information about the oxygen system you will use at home.

Amount of oxygen:————————————————————

Face mask or nasal cannula: ————————————————

Oxygen uses: ————————————————————————

Oxygen supply company: ————————————————————

Phone number: ————————————————————————

24-hour service number: ————————————————————

Keep this information near your telephone in case you need to contact the oxygen supply company for help. Your nurse or a social worker will help you to make arrangements for the company to supply your oxygen when you are discharged. She will also help with arranging for a representative of the company to show you how to set up and work your specific oxygen system before you go home.

During the demonstration by the company representative, pay particular attention to the following (use the spaces below to fill in the appropriate information).

How to set up the system: ————————————————

————————————————————————————————

————————————————————————————————

————————————————————————————————

————————————————————————————————

(continued)

How to tell when the tank is nearly empty and needs to be replaced:

_____

_____

How to set the correct oxygen flow: _____

_____

_____

How to turn the oxygen on and off: _____

_____

_____

Any special precautions: _____

_____

_____

_____

SPECIAL PRECAUTIONS

Oxygen must always be used with extreme care. It can make a fire burn harder or a smoldering object burst into flames. Oxygen under pressure (such as the oxygen in oxygen tanks) can explode if it becomes too hot.

To use oxygen safely, follow these guidelines:
• Do not allow anyone to smoke in the house.
• Keep the oxygen system out of children's reach.
• Be careful of the oxygen tubing. Do not run it under rugs, furniture, or sheets or bed linens.
• Do not use oxygen near a stove or a space heater.
• Do not put the oxygen system within 5' of any heat source or electrical appliance.
• Alert your local fire department that you are keeping oxygen in the house.
• Keep an all-purpose fire extinguisher in the house handy for emergency use.
• If any problems develop with your oxygen system, notify the company immediately.

Pacemaker, Permanent: Home Care

TEACHING PLAN
Assessment
• Assess the patient's and family's knowledge of home management after permanent pacemaker insertion.
• Assess the patient's and family's previous experience with pacemakers and identify their areas of concern.
• Collaborate with the doctor to determine the patient's discharge orders, including medications, activity, and acceptable pulse rate limits.
• Review the manufacturer's written materials on the patient's specific pacemaker.

Materials needed
• Written information on the type of pacemaker, pacemaker settings, and manufacturer
• Information on how to obtain a pacemaker identification card

Strategies to use
• Stimulate interest in the topic by beginning with the patient's and family's specific concerns.
• Assist the patient and his family to problem-solve the following:
  —when, how, and where to obtain appropriate medical help if needed
  —where information related to the pacemaker's programming, model number, manufacturer will be kept.

Patient-teaching aid
See *Permanent pacemaker: Home care and precautions*, page 384.

Evaluation method
• Have the patient and a family member explain, in their own words, home care measures.
• Have the patient and family describe, in their own words, the warning signs of various complications.
• Have the patient and family develop plans for obtaining appropriate medical care for each of the problems discussed.

Interventions and outcome criteria
☑ **Intervention 1**
Explain how the pacemaker works, including:
• a brief description of the pacemaker's major parts
• how the pacemaker stimulates the heart to contract
• the specific reason the patient needed a permanent pacemaker.

Outcome criteria: The patient and family state that the pacemaker produces an electrical impulse that causes the heart to pump blood throughout the body.

☑ Intervention 2
Teach the patient and family to monitor the patient's pulse as follows:
• Take and record the pulse rate daily.
• Note the rhythm while checking the rate.
• Notify the doctor if the pulse rate exceeds the preset parameters (provide specific parameters for each individual patient).

Outcome criteria: The patient and family state the specific parameters for the patient's pulse rate and when the doctor should be notified.

☑ Intervention 3
Describe the home care measures the patient and family will need to follow after pacemaker insertion, including:
• caring for the patient's affected arm. Instruct the patient that he:
  —may perform routine range-of-motion exercises when soreness has completely disappeared.
  —may gradually resume lifting when soreness has completely disappeared; advise him to limit lifting to 5 to 10 lb during the first few weeks.
  —should avoid strenuous activity with the affected arm for the first few weeks.
• showering and bathing as desired
• resuming sexual activity when desired
• taking all medications as prescribed
• following the prescribed diet (based on the patient's overall condition)
• how to handle activity (based on the patient's overall condition).

Outcome criteria: The patient and family state general measures of home management.

☑ Intervention 4
Describe the general precautions the patient should take when wearing a permanent pacemaker, including:
• always carrying a pacemaker identification card that includes information on the pacemaker type, manufacturer, programming, and current pacemaker settings
• notifying all health professionals, such as dentists and other doctors, that he is wearing a permanent pacemaker
• avoiding the following:
  —letting the pacemaker's generator come in close contact with a large car or boat motor
  —standing near high tension wires, large magnets, or arc welding machines
  —contact sports that may cause blunt trauma over the pacemaker generator

• standing near microwave ovens. Make sure the patient understands that:
—newer pacemakers are well shielded and are unaffected by microwaves
—if he is concerned about microwaves, he should stand 3' to 5' away
from the operating oven to ensure no contact with his pacemaker
• letting security guards at airports know he has a pacemaker before going
through security screening.

Outcome criteria: The patient and family state general precautions the
patient should take as listed above.

☑ Intervention 5
Explain appropriate follow-up measures, including:
• keeping doctor's appointments
• transtelephone monitoring of pacemaker functioning (including its purpose, procedure, and frequency)
• use of a pacemaker surveillance clinic (if applicable).

Outcome criteria: The patient and family state specific follow-up measures
that have been prescribed for the patient.

☑ Intervention 6
Discuss the warning signs indicating the pacemaker's lifespan limit as well
as any major complications, including:
• end-of-life characteristics for the patient's specific pacemaker (review the
manufacturer's materials for specific information)
• pacemaker syndrome, which includes the following symptoms after pacemaker insertion:
—decreased activity tolerance
—dizziness and faintness
—persistent fatigue or malaise
—dyspnea
• pacemaker failure, indicated by:
—pulse rate that drops significantly below the lower rate limit
—pulse rate that exceeds the upper rate limit (as determined by the doctor)
—pulse rhythm that changes from regular to significantly irregular
—fainting
—recurrence of symptoms experienced before the pacemaker was inserted
• pacemaker pocket infection, as evidenced by:
—warmth, redness, or pain at the insertion site
—drainage from the insertion site
—systemic fever.

Outcome criteria: The patient and family state the warning signs indicating
the pacemaker's lifespan limit and of major complications, such as pacemaker syndrome, pacemaker failure, and infection.

☑ Intervention 7
Help the patient and family plan how to obtain medical help when needed.

Outcome criteria: The patient and family state that additional medical
help should be obtained if any of the above warning signs develop and
mention specific plans for how they will obtain that help.

Permanent Pacemaker: Home Care and Precautions

A pacemaker is a small device that produces an electrical impulse to make your heart beat and pump blood throughout your body. Normally, special cells in your heart produce this electrical impulse. However, sometimes these cells do not work right and a pacemaker becomes necessary to keep your heart beating properly.

Your pacemaker, which is permanently inserted, consists of two main parts: a generator containing a battery that produces the electrical impulse and tiny wires that take the impulse to your heart.

COUNTING YOUR PULSE RATE

Counting your pulse rate is an important part of your home care. Your pulse rate tells you how many times a minute your heart is beating. Counting your pulse rate each day tells you if your pacemaker is working correctly. Your nurse will help you learn to do this and will give you some additional information on counting and recording pulse rates.

CARING FOR YOUR AFFECTED ARM

When you get home from the hospital, you will need to be careful using your _____ arm (the arm closest to where your pacemaker generator was inserted). Avoid strenuous activity during the first few weeks. Twice a day, you may do gentle range-of-motion exercises (the same ones the nurse taught you in the hospital) with that arm. When the soreness is completely gone, you may start to lift objects with that arm; however, limit your lifting to 5 to 10 lb for the first few weeks.

OTHER CONCERNS

No special restrictions apply to resuming your bathing or sexual activity. Depending on your personal preference, you may shower or take a tub bath. You may resume sexual activity whenever you would like.

Your doctor will determine your diet and any other specific activity based on your overall health. In the spaces below, you or your nurse may write your specific diet and activity orders.

Diet:_____

_____

_____

(continued)

Activity: _____

_____

_____

PRECAUTIONS

You will need to take certain precautions now that you are wearing a pacemaker.

• Always carry a pacemaker identification card with you (your nurse will help you obtain a completed identification card before you leave the hospital). The following information should be listed somewhere on this card:

—pacemaker manufacturer and model number

—pacemaker mode of function

—programmable features and current settings (update whenever these settings are changed)

—type of leads

—date of implantation

—your doctor's name and telephone number.

• Notify any doctor or dentist you see that you are wearing a permanent pacemaker.

• Keep your pacemaker's generator from coming in close contact with large car or boat motors. Also, avoid standing near high tension wires, large magnets (such as those in car junkyards or magnetic resonance imaging machines), or arc welding machines. These items will not damage your pacemaker. However, they may temporarily affect the normal functioning of your pacemaker.

• Avoid any contact sports that may cause injury, such as pain or bruising, over the pacemaker generator site.

• If you travel by air, let the security guards at all airports know that you are wearing a permanent pacemaker before going through security screening. Although the screening will not hurt your pacemaker, your pacemaker may trigger the alarm.

• You may be concerned about using or standing near microwave ovens. Your pacemaker is well protected; it will not be affected by an operating microwave oven. However, if you are still concerned, stand 3' to 5' away from the oven while it is in use to eliminate the possibility of any problems.

You may have some questions about specific activities or precautions that have not been covered here. Write the questions down in the spaces provided and discuss them with your nurse or doctor.

_____

_____

_____

(continued)

FOLLOW-UP

An important part of your home care, follow-up care includes visits to your doctor or the pacemaker clinic and transtelephone monitoring.

Doctor's visits

Be sure to keep all scheduled appointments with your doctor or the pacemaker clinic. In the spaces below, you or your nurse should write the date, time, and location of your first appointment.

Date: _____

Time: _____

Location: _____

Transtelephone monitoring

This type of monitoring is done electronically by a pacemaker center over the telephone, so you don't have to go to the center for a checkup. If any problems with your pacemaker are detected, your doctor will contact you and instruct you to come into the office or the hospital for further evaluation.

Transtelephone monitoring is easy to do. First, you dial the number that your nurse will give you. Then, you place sensing devices (called electrodes) over your pacemaker site, following the specific instructions your nurse will provide. A tracing of your heart rate and rhythm is then transmitted over the telephone. From the tracing, your doctor can tell if your pacemaker is working correctly.

The center may want you to use a magnet during part of your heart tracing transmission. Your nurse will show you how to use a magnet for your specific pacemaker. Although the magnet will not hurt your pacemaker, you should be extremely careful to use it only when you are asked to do so and only as you were shown. In the spaces below, your nurse will write specific directions on how you should use your magnet:

_____

_____

_____

How frequently you should use transtelephone monitoring will depend on your doctor. Your doctor wants you to do this every _____.
Note: You may call the transtelephone monitoring center any time you are concerned about how your pacemaker is functioning.

(continued)

REPLACING YOUR PACEMAKER'S BATTERY

Eventually, your pacemaker's battery will wear out. However, it can be replaced. Different types of pacemakers give different signs to let you and your doctor know that the battery is wearing out. This information is available in the literature provided by the manufacturer of your particular model. Your nurse will give you a copy to read over, or you may want to write the specific signs in the spaces below.

_____

_____

_____

_____

_____

_____

_____

WARNING SIGNS

Notify your doctor immediately if you notice any of the following warning signs that your pacemaker is not functioning correctly:
• Your pulse rate drops suddenly and significantly below _____ beats/ minute.
• Your pulse rate drops below _____ beats/minute for _____ consecutive days.
• Your pulse rhythm changes from regular to extremely irregular.
• You feel dizzy or faint with changes in your pulse rate and rhythm.
• Your pulse rate exceeds _____ beats/minute.
• For a patient whose pacemaker has an upper rate limit: you become extremely short of breath, develop a cough without flulike symptoms, notice swelling in your feet and hands, and your pulse rate is more than _____ beats/minute.
• You notice the same symptoms that you had before your pacemaker was inserted. You can list these symptoms in the spaces provided below.

_____

_____

_____

_____

(continued)

Also contact your doctor if you notice that you:
• are more tired than usual with activity
• feel short of breath with activity or at rest
• feel dizzy or faint since your pacemaker was implanted.
These signs do not indicate an emergency; however, your doctor should know about them.

Check your incision line and the area around the pacemaker generator daily for signs of infection. If you notice any of the following signs, notify your doctor immediately:
• warmth, redness, or pain over the site where the pacemaker pocket is located
• drainage from the pacemaker pocket site.

Plan ahead how you will get additional medical care if you need it. Write any pertinent information in the spaces below.

Doctor: _____

Phone: _____

Address: _____

Pacemaker clinic: _____

Phone: _____

Address: _____

Transtelephone monitoring service: _____

Phone: _____

24-hour emergency number: _____

Hospital: _____

Phone: _____

Address: _____

Radial Pulse Measurement

TEACHING PLAN
Assessment
• Assess the patient's and family's knowledge about counting the radial pulse.
• Obtain rate settings (lower and upper rate limits) for the patient's pacemaker (when applicable).
• Collaborate with the doctor to determine the lowest pulse rate acceptable for a patient taking antiarrhythmic medications.
• Assess the patient's and family's ability to see and read a watch with a second hand.
• Assess the patient's and family's ability to palpate and sense the radial pulse.

Materials needed
• Diagram of the arm showing the radial artery and landmarks for finding the radial pulse
• Watch with a second hand

Strategies to use
• Stimulate interest in the topic by explaining why the patient and family need to learn to count the radial pulse.
• Present the information using demonstration and return demonstration.

Patient-teaching aid
See *How to count your radial pulse*, page 391.

Evaluation method
• Have the patient and a family member demonstrate how to count and record the radial pulse. Verify accuracy by simultaneously counting the pulse on the other arm.

Interventions and outcome criteria
☑ **Intervention 1**
Explain where the radial pulse is located on the wrist using a diagram for illustration.

☑ **Intervention 2**
Help the patient and family to locate the radial pulse on the patient's arm.
Outcome criteria: The patient and family correctly locate the radial pulse.

☑ **Intervention 3**
Explain that each impulse represents one heartbeat.

☑ Intervention 4

Instruct the patient and family to count the number of impulses or beats felt for 1 minute using the second hand of the watch for timing.

☑ Intervention 5

If the patient's pulse is to be checked during exercise, teach the patient and family to count the pulse for 10 seconds and to multiply by 6.

☑ Intervention 6

Have the patient and family practice counting the radial pulse several times before discharge (see interventions 4 and 5 above).

Outcome criteria: The patient and family correctly count the patient's radial pulse as verified by the nurse.

☑ Intervention 7

Have the patient and family record radial pulse rates on a chart.

Outcome criteria: The patient and family correctly record radial pulse rate.

☑ Intervention 8

Instruct the patient and family about when and how frequently the radial pulse should be counted.

Outcome criteria: The patient and family state when and how often the patient's pulse should be counted.

PATIENT-TEACHING AID

How to Count Your Radial Pulse

Counting your own heart rate is an important part of your home care. Specifically, you need to know your heart rate for the following reasons:

_____

_____

_____

You can find out how fast your heart is beating by learning to count your radial pulse. The radial pulse is located on the inside of your wrist, on the side closer to your thumb. It lies alongside the radius bone in your wrist.

FINDING YOUR PULSE

To locate your radial pulse, place the first three fingers of one hand over your wrist and gently feel for a pulse. It will feel like a steady beating against your fingertips. Your nurse will help you locate the pulse the first time; however, you should practice finding your radial pulse several times by yourself.

COUNTING YOUR PULSE RATE

To count your pulse rate, you will need a watch or clock with a second hand. You will need this to time the number of impulses or beats you feel over the course of 1 minute. The total number of beats that you count is your heart rate.

Begin by placing the watch or clock where you can see it comfortably. Then, find your radial pulse using the fingertips of your first three fingers. Once you have found your pulse, watch the second hand of the watch or clock closely. When the second hand reaches 12, begin counting each beat you feel; you might find it helpful to count out loud. Continue watching the second hand. When it gets to 12 again, stop counting. Then, write down the number of beats that you counted.

Your doctor may want you to count your pulse rate while you are exercising. To do this, begin counting the beats when the second hand reaches 12. Stop counting as soon as the second hand reaches 2. Then, multiply the number of beats felt by 6 to get your pulse rate.

The nurse will practice both of these methods with you the first few times. Practice on your own several times throughout the day.

(continued)

PULSE RHYTHM

When you count your pulse rate, notice if the rhythm is regular or irregular. With a regular rhythm, each beat is evenly spaced. With an irregular rhythm, the spacing between beats is uneven. You may find that the beats occur close together or that long pauses occur between each beat. If you notice any irregular beats, be sure to count your pulse rate for 1 full minute.

RECORDING YOUR RATE

Keeping a record of your pulse rate is important. Be sure to take this record with you when you see your doctor. On a sheet of paper, write down the date, time, and your pulse rate each time you count it. Also write down whether the pulse is regular or irregular.

NOTIFYING THE DOCTOR

Your doctor wants you to call if your heart rate:

☐ drops below _____ beats/minute for _____days

☐ goes above _____ beats/minute for _____days

☐ changes from a regular rhythm to an irregular rhythm

Remember to count your pulse rate _____times/day or week.

Sexual Activity and Heart Disease

TEACHING PLAN
Assessment
See "Sexual Dysfunction" in Section I for details.

Strategies to use
• Initiate a discussion of the topic by discussing, as part of your general teaching of managing activity at home, the patient's plans for resuming sexual activity.
• Alternatively, initiate the topic by responding to the patient's behavioral cues indicating his concern about resuming sexual activity.
• Discuss the topic and any concerns with the patient and his partner, both separately and jointly.

Patient-teaching aid
See *Sex and your heart*, page 394.

Evaluation method
• Have the patient and his partner state measures they will use to limit the patient's myocardial oxygen demand during sexual activity.
• Ask the patient and his partner if their concerns have been adequately addressed during discussions.

Interventions and outcome criteria
See "Sexual Dysfunction" in Section I for an outline of content to cover in your teaching.

PATIENT-TEACHING AID
Sex and Your Heart

Most people who have had a heart attack or open-heart surgery have questions about how and when they can safely resume sexual activity. Often, the partners of these patients also have questions and concerns.

This patient-teaching aid provides some basic guidelines on resuming sexual activity. If you or your partner have other questions not addressed in this aid, be sure to talk with your nurse or doctor.

WHEN TO RESUME SEXUAL ACTIVITY

One of the first questions most patients ask is "When can I have sexual intercourse again?" Because intercourse is a type of physical activity, the timing will vary from patient to patient.

Keep in mind that sexual intercouse puts about as much stress on your heart as climbing a flight of stairs rapidly, walking several blocks at a brisk pace, weeding your garden, or riding a bicycle at a moderate pace. When you can do these activities, you will be able to have sexual intercourse without hurting your heart.

Your doctor will make specific recommendations for when you may resume sexual intercourse. The nurse will check which of the following apply based on the doctor's recommendation.

Wait at least _____ weeks after discharge; at that time you may resume intercourse when you can:

☐ climb 20 steps in 10 seconds without experiencing shortness of breath, chest pain, excessive fatigue, dizziness, or palpitations

☐ walk two or three blocks at a brisk pace without having shortness of breath, chest pain, excessive fatigue, dizziness, or palpitations

☐ increase your pulse rate to 110 to 120 beats/minute with activity without having shortness of breath, chest pain, excessive fatigue, dizziness, or palpitations

☐ Other: _____

_____

_____

While you are waiting to resume full sexual activity, you may engage in other forms of sexual activity that are not stressful to your heart. These may include kissing, hugging, touching, caressing, and holding. You can begin these activities in the hospital if you wish.

(continued)

LIMITING STRESS DURING INTERCOURSE

Many patients and their partners are worried that sexual intercourse will hurt the heart by putting too much strain on it. You can take certain precautions to limit the stress on your heart during intercourse, such as the following:

• Resume sexual intercourse in a place that is familiar and comfortable for you. The room temperature should also be comfortable—not too hot or cold.

• Have intercourse with your usual partner.

• Have intercourse at a time when you are well rested.

• Use positions that are familiar and comfortable for you and your partner. (If you have had open-heart surgery, you may want to try slightly different positions if your usual ones make your chest incision hurt too much.)

• Wait at least 3 hours after eating a large meal or drinking alcoholic beverages before having intercourse.

• Avoid anal intercourse. (Anal intercourse can stimulate a major nerve in your body that can cause your heart rate to drop dangerously low.)

• Use foreplay to allow your heart rate, breathing, and blood pressure to rise gradually.

• Take a sublingual nitroglycerin tablet before engaging in intercourse if you are concerned that you might experience chest pain during intercourse.

WARNING SIGNS

Many patients wonder how they can tell if their sexual activity is too stressful for their heart. The following warning signs can serve as guidelines that your heart may be under too much stress during intercourse:

• frequent episodes of chest pain that occur during or after intercourse

• unusual shortness of breath during or after intercourse

• palpitations that occur for 10 or more minutes after orgasm

• unusual tiredness the day after having intercourse

• inability to sleep after having intercourse.

If you notice any of the signs above, do not have any more intercourse and notify your doctor.

SEXUAL PERFORMANCE

Some patients are concerned that they are not performing as well sexually as they did before their heart attack or heart surgery. Numerous things, including those mentioned below, can alter sexual performance.

Medications

Some heart medications can interfere with sexual desire and performance. Your nurse will discuss this further with you if you are taking one of these medications.

Emotions

Your feelings about yourself and your situation can affect your sexual performance. For example, you may be feeling depressed because of your recent heart attack or surgery and this could hurt your sexual performance or decrease your satisfaction with your sexual activity.

(continued)

Working through your depression should help. Your nurse will give you additional information on how to deal with your emotions effectively at home.

Fatigue
Whether you have had a heart attack or heart surgery, your body has undergone major stress; your body needs time to recover. During this recovery period, your sexual performance may be less than you would like it to be. However, keep in mind that as you recover, your sexual performance will also improve.

ADDITIONAL CONCERNS
You or your partner may have additional concerns or questions. List them in the spaces below and plan to discuss them with your nurse or doctor.

_____

_____

_____

_____

_____

_____

_____

_____

_____

_____

Sodium-Restricted Diet

TEACHING PLAN
Assessment
• Collaborate with the doctor regarding the patient's prescribed sodium-restricted diet for home use.
• Collaborate with the dietitian to ensure consistent teaching about the diet.
• Assess the patient's and family's knowledge about sodium-restricted diets.
• Assess the patient's and family's previous experience with sodium-restricted diets and determine any areas of concern or past problems.
• Assess the patient's and family's usual dietary practices, including use of "fast foods" and restaurant meals.

Materials needed
• Written summary of instructions
• List of commercially available cookbooks that have recipes appropriate for sodium-restricted diets
• Samples of food labels

Strategies to use
• Stimulate interest in the topic by relating the need for a sodium-restricted diet to the patient's specific health problem.
• Assist the patient and family to problem-solve the following:
—how much the patient and family plan to reduce their sodium intake
—what major sources of sodium are in their current diet
—how the patient and family plan to reduce their sodium intake (set specific goals)
—how to identify processed and pre-prepared foods that are high in sodium (use samples of labels to clarify).

Patient-teaching aids
See *Sodium and your heart,* page 399; and *Personal diet work sheet,* page 401.

Evaluation method
• Have the patient and family describe, in their own words, why sodium restriction is important for the patient.
• Have the patient and family state specific goals for reducing the patient's sodium intake.

Interventions and outcome criteria
☑ Intervention 1
Explain the role of sodium restriction in managing the patient's cardiovascular disease, specifically for:
• hypertension; limiting sodium can help reduce blood pressure

• congestive heart failure (CHF); limiting sodium decreases fluid retention and other symptoms.

Outcome criteria: The patient and family state that sodium restriction for hypertension helps to control elevated blood pressure. They also state that sodium restriction in CHF helps to decrease fluid retention and reduce other symptoms.

☑ Intervention 2
Describe general methods for limiting the patient's use of sodium, including the following:
• Do not add salt to food at the table.
• Do not add salt to food when cooking.
• Limit the use of foods naturally high in sodium.
• Limit the use of processed or pre-prepared foods with high sodium content. (Demonstrate how to read labels and provide a list of common names for sodium found in foods.)
• Use alternative seasonings to replace salt.

Outcome criteria: The patient and family state general means of reducing sodium intake as listed above. They also read sample food labels and accurately identify foods high in sodium.

☑ Intervention 3
Have the patient and family identify major sources of sodium in their current diet.

Outcome criteria: The patient and family identify major sources of sodium in their individual diets.

☑ Intervention 4
Have the patient and family set realistic goals for restricting and reducing sodium intake from their current level.

Outcome criteria: The patient and family set realistic goals for reducing their sodium intake.

☑ Intervention 5
Provide the patient and family with a written list of resources, including:
• commercial cookbooks that contain low-sodium recipes
• list of foods high in sodium.

Sodium and Your Heart

Your doctor wants you to limit the amount of sodium in your diet. Limiting your sodium intake is important to help control your heart disease.

If you have hypertension (high blood pressure), too much sodium can help keep your blood pressure too high. Limiting your sodium intake can help to lower your blood pressure, which could help you to avoid a stroke or heart attack.

If you have congestive heart failure, extra sodium makes your body retain excess fluid. This causes your heart to work harder and results in other symptoms of heart failure, including shortness of breath and swelling of your feet, ankles, or hands. Limiting your sodium helps your heart pump better and limits the symptoms you have.

Your doctor wants you to limit sodium in your diet to _____

_____

_____

REDUCING YOUR SODIUM INTAKE

Listed below are general guidelines for reducing your sodium intake. The nurse or dietitian will check the ones that apply to you.

☐ Do not add any salt to food when cooking. This includes adding table salt, any salty food such as ham or salt pork, or any type of seasoning salt to the food you are cooking. Salt is one of the major sources of sodium in your diet.

☐ Do not add any salt to your food at the table.

☐ Substitute other seasonings, such as lemon juice, pepper, or other spices, to replace salt in food.

☐ Use a salt substitute. Your doctor recommends that you use the following salt substitutes:

_____

_____

_____

(continued)

☐ Avoid or reduce the number of foods you eat that are naturally high in sodium.

☐ Reduce or avoid processed or pre-prepared foods that are high in sodium. Also, learn to read labels on all foods that you buy. Avoid foods that list any of the following as a major ingredient:
• soda (such as baking soda)
• sodium (sometimes abbreviated as "Na"; examples include sodium nitrite, sodium benzoate, and sodium alginate)
• monosodium glutamate (sometimes abbreviated as "MSG"; often found in restaurant cooking and many pre-prepared foods).

Personal Diet Work Sheet

Your doctor has recommended that you reduce the amount of sodium in your diet. However, the decision to change your eating habits is ultimately your own. If you decide to limit your daily intake of sodium, the work sheet included in this teaching aid may help you develop a specific plan.

IDENTIFYING MAJOR SOURCES OF SODIUM IN YOUR DIET
Start by thinking about what you normally eat each day. Then, check off which of the following statements apply to you.

I add salt to my food at the table:

☐ at every or almost every meal

☐ at about half my meals

☐ at fewer than three meals per week

I add salt to food when cooking:

☐ to almost every food I cook each day

☐ to about half the foods I cook each day

☐ to fewer than three foods I cook each week

Now, check off which of the following foods you eat and how often you eat them in an average week.

DIET WORK SHEET

Foods eaten	Times per week			
	5 to 7	2 to 4	1	0
Bacon				
Canned soups				
Processed cheeses				
Luncheon meats				

(continued)

DIET WORK SHEET (continued)

| | Times per week | | | |
Foods eaten	5 to 7	2 to 4	1	0
Salted popcorn				
Salted nuts				
Pickles/olives				
TV dinners				
Canned meats				
Ham				
Hot dogs				
Fast foods (specify)				
Fast foods (specify)				
Fast foods (specify)				
Fast foods (specify)				

Use the following spaces to write down any other foods you eat frequently that are high in sodium. Ask your nurse or dietitian to help.

| | Times per week | | | |
Foods eaten	5 to 7	2 to 4	1	0

(continued)

Now, review your lists. Identify the major sources of sodium in your diet. If you need help, ask your nurse or dietitian. Then, list the top four eating habits that add the most salt or sodium to your diet:

1. _____

2. _____

3. _____

4. _____

CHANGING YOUR EATING HABITS

Changing the eating habits you have already identified is a good place to start to limit the sodium in your diet. Plan how you can change those habits by reviewing the sample alternatives below.

For example, if you always add salt to your food when cooking, you might plan to stop using salt while cooking. Or you may decide to use other seasonings to add flavor to foods in place of salt.

If you eat bacon every morning, you might plan to eat bacon on only two mornings each week instead of every morning.

Use the following spaces to write down your specific plans.

1. _____

_____

_____

2. _____

_____

_____

3. _____

_____

_____

4. _____

_____

_____

Stress Management

TEACHING PLAN
Assessment
• Assess the patient's ability to describe his feelings.
• Assess patient-family interaction patterns. Does each listen to the other without interruption? What is the response of each to the other when feelings are expressed? Some possible reactions may include:
—silence
—belittling the feeling expressed; for example, ridiculing the other person in some way or making sarcastic remarks when a feeling is expressed
—questioning why the person has that particular feeling
—listening and responding with concern
—using gentle humor
—using touch.
• Assess the patient's and family's fears or concerns regarding home care.
• Assess the patient's and family's anticipated sources of stress, such as:
—change of residence
—change in family structure
—change in job after recovery
—possibility of not returning to work after recovery
—management of other illnesses.
• Assess the current state of the patient's feelings.
• Assess the feelings the patient and family experienced during this and previous hospitalizations.
• Assess the patient's and family's definition of stress.
• Assess the patient's and family's usual ways of coping with uncomfortable feelings and stress.

Strategies to use
• Stimulate interest in the topic by asking the patient and family what particular concerns they have about the patient's going home and what difficulties they expect to have. Explain that discussing their anticipated problems as well as your knowledge of others' experiences in similar situations may help make the transition easier.
• Use therapeutic communication techniques and a gentle, conversational style with the patient and family (see *Therapeutic communication techniques*, pages 17 to 19). Sit down and provide privacy. Use a combination of direct and indirect approaches.
• Begin your teaching several days before discharge as this material requires more than one discussion.
• Individualize the content of your teaching by focusing on the patient's previously expressed feelings and the reaction he and his family had to those feelings.

• Assist the patient and his family to problem-solve the following:
—methods to use to reduce discomfort of such unpleasant feelings as anxiety, anger, or depression
—methods the family can use to cope with the patient when he is experiencing anger, depression, or anxiety
—plans the patient and family have for resuming a productive or satisfying life
—support persons to call if methods used do not work to reduce discomfort
—methods the family will use when experiencing their own feelings in response to the patient's condition.

Patient-teaching aids
See *Normal feelings after hospitalization,* page 408; *Strategies for dealing with anxiety, depression, and other strong feelings,* page 413; and *Caregiver guidelines: Dealing with the patient's emotions at home,* page 418.

Evaluation method
• Have the patient list ways to overcome uncomfortable feelings, such as anxiety, depression, and anger.
• Have the family list means they will use when the patient is experiencing uncomfortable feelings.
• Have the family list means they will use to overcome their own uncomfortable feelings.
• Have the patient and family list persons who can serve as resources to them if needed.

Interventions and outcome criteria
☑ **Intervention 1**
Ask the patient and family what concerns each has about the patient returning home.

☑ **Intervention 2**
Using therapeutic communication techniques, assist the patient and family to be as specific as possible about their concerns (see *Therapeutic communication techniques,* pages 17 to 19). This may not be possible for all patients and family members to do; however, try to help them communicate in specific terms.

Outcome criteria: The patient and family state specific concerns. For example, they may state being frightened about the patient returning to work instead of just saying they are frightened about everything.

☑ **Intervention 3**
Discuss with the patient and family the feelings that are normal to have after experiencing a heart attack or heart surgery, including:
• depression
• irritability
• anger
• worry

- fear
- fatigue
- difficulty sleeping
- pain at incisional sites
- difficulty concentrating
- sadness or crying.

Outcome criteria: The patient and family state that the feelings listed above are normal upon returning home.

☑ Intervention 4
Ask the patient and his family if they anticipate having other feelings not mentioned in intervention 3.

☑ Intervention 5
Ask the patient and family what additional sources of stress each anticipates upon returning home, including:
- return to work or a change in occupation
- retirement (either voluntary or mandatory)
- birth, marriage, or some other event involving one or more of their children
- change in residence
- necessity to manage their own or others' illnesses other than cardiac
- plans for travel and other recreation.

Outcome criteria: The patient and family state what, if any, changes they anticipate in their usual pattern or style of living upon the patient's discharge.

☑ Intervention 6
Discuss the patient's and family's usual ways of managing the feelings mentioned in interventions 3 and 4.

Outcome criteria: The patient and family state what each usually does when experiencing the above feelings or when a family member is experiencing them.

☑ Intervention 7
Discuss plans the patient and family have for meeting the stresses mentioned in intervention 5.

Outcome criteria: The patient and family state what plans they have for each of the anticipated stresses.

☑ Intervention 8
Using your professional judgment and knowledge of the patient and family, evaluate whether various plans are realistic and discuss ways to make them more realistic, if necessary.

☑ Intervention 9

Ask the patient and family what community resources are available to them if anticipated plans prove inadequate, including:
• community social services located through their local health department
• a minister, priest, rabbi, or other religious counselor
• a psychologist or psychiatrist
• a psychiatric nurse specialist
• their family doctor
• a family counseling service.

Outcome criteria: The patient and family state resources they will use if they need assistance with their feelings or other stresses.

☑ Intervention 10

Ask the patient and family what social resources they have for friendship and support during times of stress.

Outcome criteria: The patient and family name groups to which they belong or on which they can call for friendship and social support.

Normal Feelings after Hospitalization

After being discharged from the hospital after a heart attack, open-heart surgery, or other serious illness, you can expect to experience a multitude of feelings. No doubt, you have experienced many of them already while still in the hospital. Now that you are preparing to go home, you are probably wondering what other feelings to anticipate.

Identifying and acknowledging your feelings are important to your health. Feelings create energy, which requires oxygen. Keeping feelings inside produces more stress on your body and heart; reducing feelings of stress is important.

Experiencing any of the following feelings after hospitalization is normal: depression, anger, anxiety, fear, irritability, fatigue, worry, discomfort, exhaustion, sadness, aggravation, helplessness, or uselessness. You may even feel somewhat down in the dumps, excessively tired, out of sorts, out of control, or unable to concentrate.

REASONS FOR FEELING THE WAY YOU DO
Understanding why you may be having some of the feelings mentioned above may help you to better manage your home care. For example, you may experience certain feelings because:
• you have just come through a life-threatening event and may have some leftover fear
• you are weak from spending so much time in bed; the longer the weakness continues, you feel depressed and worry that something is wrong with your heart
• you may have been told to change some of your habits and practices, and you are unsure whether you can or even want to
• your loved ones may be trying to help by doing things for you; this causes you to feel useless or powerless or as if you no longer control things as you once did.

Regardless of the source, such feelings are uncomfortable. Having them may cause you to feel angry, irritable, or out of control. If the feelings are more intense than usual or if they last longer than what you expect or are accustomed to, you may even begin to feel as though you are going crazy. *Remember:* These feelings are normal—you are not going crazy and you can regain your usual balance.

IDENTIFYING YOUR FEELINGS
Using the list below, put a check next to any words that apply to you:

☐ Depressed ☐ Uncomfortable ☐ Aggravated

☐ Angry ☐ In the dumps ☐ Helpless

(continued)

☐ Anxious   ☐ Low   ☐ Useless

☐ Scared   ☐ Excessively tired   ☐ Out of control

☐ Irritable   ☐ Exhausted   ☐ Constantly crying

☐ Fatigued   ☐ Sad   ☐ Unable to
                                                      concentrate
☐ Worried   ☐ Out of sorts

In the spaces below, list any additional feelings you remember experiencing as well as any feelings you fear you will experience in the near future.

_____

_____

IDENTIFYING SOURCES OF STRESS

Now, put a check next to any of the events below that may be a source of stress to you after discharge. Be sure to discuss them with your family or the nurse, and begin planning ways to reduce the stressful nature of such anticipated events.

☐ Retirement   ☐ Illness in the family

☐ Loneliness   ☐ Coping with own illness

☐ Living alone   ☐ Insomnia

☐ Loss of spouse   ☐ Reduced income

☐ Loss of friends   ☐ Anxiety

☐ Loss of relatives   ☐ Facing old age and death

☐ Spending time alone in   ☐ Having too much time on
  the evenings   your hands

☐ Not seeing children or grand-   ☐ Fear (for example, fear of dan-
  children   ger in the streets)

☐ Marriage of children or grand-   ☐ Feeling guilty about not doing
  children   what you should do

☐ Having grandchildren come to   ☐ Arguments with friends and
  visit   family

(continued)

☐ Changing lifelong health habits

☐ Change in physical ability

☐ Change in sexuality

☐ Making new friends

☐ New romance

☐ Traffic, crowds, and noise

☐ Moving

☐ Job responsibility

☐ Increasing self-awareness

☐ Lost opportunities

☐ Worrying about the weather

☐ Feeling new independence

☐ Feeling dependent

☐ Frustration

☐ Feeling inadequate

☐ Children leaving home

☐ Vacations

☐ Divorce or separation

☐ Holidays

☐ Having too many good things to do

List below any additional stresses you anticipate having after your discharge from the hospital.

_____

_____

Next, think about ways you expend the energy created by the feelings or events you have just checked or listed above. For example, think of what you usually do when you feel sad, are unable to sleep, or feel angry at your spouse or a friend. List some of those ways in the spaces below.

_____

_____

Identifying and discussing the feelings you have been experiencing or anticipate experiencing after leaving the hospital are important steps toward helping yourself feel better. Thinking of ways to reduce the stress associated with certain feelings and events will help you to better manage your recovery at home.

Remember: The feelings you have experienced or anticipate experiencing are normal, shared by most patients. The events you have identified as stress-producing happen to most people. How you choose to respond will determine how successful you are at controlling the stress.

(continued)

MANAGING DIFFICULT FEELINGS

Finding ways of managing your difficult feelings may seem impossible, especially if you don't understand their cause. Here are some possible causes for some of the feelings you may be experiencing as well as suggestions for how to deal with them.

Note: The usual length of time for these feelings to last after being discharged from the hospital is 6 to 8 weeks, rarely more than 3 months.

Depression

Depression may occur for several reasons, including the following:

• Having too-high expectations for yourself. Once home from the hospital, you may expect your energy level to be the same as before you became ill. You won't have the same amount of energy. In fact, many activities will cause you to feel tired and you may become discouraged. Try to be patient with yourself. Your energy level will return gradually after several weeks.

• Feeling that others expect too much of you. Your friends may remark how well you look or seem to be feeling, but you think you look bad and do not feel well. To deal with this type of situation, you'll need to begin trusting your own feelings and meeting your own realistic expectations, not expectations of family and friends.

• Realizing that you may need to make certain life-style changes but feeling that this will be too difficult to do. Try to keep in mind that changing your life-style and habits, although difficult, is not impossible to do. Deciding that you will make the changes because they will improve your health may help lessen the depression.

Anger

Anger frequently occurs under the following circumstances:

• You want something, but someone tells you that you can't have it.

• You want to be well and able to return to your usual activities and make your own decisions, yet your family wants to protect you from doing those things.

• You know you need to make changes, yet you don't want to.

• You are tired of having to take so many pills, adhere to a special diet, or do any of the other things your doctor asks you to do.

Sometimes, anger is expressed through frustration, irritability, or aggravation. It is a particularly difficult feeling for everyone involved—the person who is experiencing it as well as anyone around the person at that time. Keep in mind that you won't always be able to have what you want or have it as soon as you want it. However, you can help yourself by at least stating what it is you want, even if you can't get it.

Anxiety, fear, and worry

Anxiety, fear, and worry may develop from the following:

• The threat of having had a heart attack or having been seriously ill from another cardiac condition.

• Thoughts that you might die or remembering that you felt that way at the beginning of your illness. Your family also has this fear. Often, ac-

(continued)

knowledging that you have this feeling is too frightening to you; instead, you are angry or depressed. This is a normal reaction.
• Wondering if you will ever feel well again or like your old self when you hurt everywhere.
• Concerns about returning to work or being productive in some way or useful to someone.
• Wondering if new aches and pains mean you are getting sicker rather than well.

Fatigue and sleeplessness
Fatigue, lack of energy, and sleeplessness are all common and normal after hospitalization. Some of the reasons they occur may include the following:
• It takes time to recover from surgery or from having been in bed for a period of time after a heart attack.
• It takes time to regain your usual pattern of sleeping, especially if you have been taking a lot of sleeping pills. You may feel exhausted but are unable to sleep.
• Unexpressed or unacknowledged feelings create energy that can lead to fatigue if they are not released.
• Feelings of depression, anger, anxiety, fear, or worry, even if acknowledged, can cause fatigue and, especially, sleeplessness.

SEEKING ADDITIONAL HELP
If feelings of depression, anxiety, anger, worry, or any of the others mentioned above are so strong that you are unable to take care of yourself or participate in your usual activities, you need to seek additional help. This is especially true if these strong feelings last longer than 3 months.

Your nurse has mentioned several people who can be helpful to you, including your family doctor, clinical psychologist, psychiatrist, social worker, minister, rabbi, priest, family counselor, and psychiatric nurse specialist.

In the spaces below, list the names of people in your community you could consult if you need additional help.

_____

_____

_____

A FINAL NOTE
Try to be patient with yourself as you recover from your heart attack or surgery. After the few weeks of discomfort, like most patients, you'll begin to feel normal again. In fact, as you feel better, you might need to remind yourself that *it is all right to feel good* so that feeling down or bad doesn't become a habit to you.

Strategies for Dealing with Anxiety, Depression, and Other Strong Feelings

You have already discussed with your nurse the kinds of feelings you may expect to have after being discharged from the hospital as well as the length of time these feelings may last. This patient-teaching aid will give you different ways to expend the energy such feelings can cause.

All the physical activities mentioned in this aid should be done within the limits of your exercise prescription and your tolerance for performing the exercises. This is important because, in trying to solve one problem, you don't want to create additional problems for yourself.

Although a variety of activities are included in this aid, keep in mind that this is only a partial listing. Use the list to trigger your own imagination for activities to perform. Select your favorite activities, those which give you the most pleasure. Remember, these activities are to help you feel better about yourself, so enjoyment should be a primary consideration.

STRATEGIES PRESENTLY USED
In the spaces below, list activities you presently use to help reduce stress, anxiety, and anger or to feel better.

_____

_____

_____

_____

_____

_____

STRATEGIES TO TRY
Try any of the following strategies to help reduce anxiety, depression, and other strong feelings.

Anxiety, stress, edginess, and irritability
To help control and reduce feelings of anxiety, stress, edginess, and irritability, use one of the suggestions mentioned below.

(continued)

Relaxation
• Sit in a comfortable chair, preferably a recliner, with your feet up and head back. Or lie down on a bed or sofa, perhaps with a pillow under your knees to take the strain off your lower back.
• Make sure the room is quiet, at a comfortable temperature, and as free from distraction as possible.
• Close your eyes and take deep breaths. Clear your mind of intrusive thoughts; if such thoughts pop into your head, acknowledge them, then let them pass through.
• Starting at the head and moving to the feet, think about each of the following muscle groups, tensing and then relaxing them while breathing slowly and easily:
  —scalp muscles
  —facial muscles
  —throat and neck muscles
  —mouth muscles (separate your teeth about ¼″)
  —muscles in your right hand, wrist, lower arm, upper arm, and shoulder
  —muscles in your left hand, wrist, lower arm, upper arm, and shoulder
  —chest muscles
  —abdominal muscles
  —muscles in the right hip, thigh, leg, ankle, and foot
  —muscles in the left hip, thigh, leg, ankle, and foot
• When relaxed, maintain this position for 5 to 15 minutes.
• When ready to get up, slowly move your fingers and toes, then your legs and arms; sit up on the edge of the bed or chair for a few seconds, then get up and move around, remembering how pleasant it was to feel so calm and relaxed.
• Use this exercise once or twice a day as a regular routine and any time you can feel tension in your muscles, voice, or behavior.

Activities that release or use energy
• Take a walk at as vigorous a pace as your physical condition permits. Run if possible.
• Engage in other sports as your physical condition permits, including:
  —tennis
  —golf
  —swimming
  —bike riding.
• Work in the yard:
  —pulling weeds
  —raking
  —planting something beautiful.
• Perform household activities, including:
  —scrubbing
  —throwing things away.
• Perform interpersonal activities, such as:
  —calling a friend to chat
  —writing a letter
  —taking the children to the park

(continued)

—inviting a friend to lunch
—telling someone how you are feeling
—going out with a friend for lunch.
• Write out your feelings, trying to pinpoint the real, deep-rooted feelings, not just surface feelings. If you feel the emotions were caused by another person, write the person a letter mentioning it. You don't have to send the letter; rather, use it as a tool to help release your true feelings.

Doing something entirely different from your usual routine
• Learn to do something new, such as:
—taking a class for credit or fun
—reading a book on a new hobby and practicing from it.
• Volunteer somewhere, such as:
—church
—senior citizens organization
—Boy Scouts or Girl Scouts
—nursing home
—Meals on Wheels
—hospital
—nursery school.
Remember: Activities should be enjoyable or should release a lot of energy. Schedule them far enough apart to be able to relax between them. Give yourself permission to play, relax, or to do nothing. Set aside time to enjoy hobbies, music, reading, exercise, and playing with your children, grandchildren, or pets.

If your anxiety persists, worsens, or is unrelieved by distracting activities, seek the help of a counselor.

Depression and sadness
To help relieve depression, sadness, or just feeling down in the dumps, try using one of the following strategies.

Setting one goal per day and accomplishing it
• Read a chapter in a book.
• Accomplish one piece of yard work.
• Call one friend and talk for at least 2 minutes.
• Walk one unit more than yesterday. (For example, if you went around the block once yesterday, do it twice today.)
• Walk the prescribed distance and frequency each day if you are not yet increasing your activity.
• Stay at work 1 hour longer than yesterday. If you have not returned to work, discuss with your doctor how soon you will be able to (studies show that, after a heart attack, persons who return to work have less depression than those who do not).

Keeping up on your grooming and appearance
• Take a shower or a bath.
• Shave and dress in regular clothes each day.
• Stay out of bed.

Eating meals with the family
Eat at least half of each food served.

(continued)

Doing something you have been avoiding
Try to do whatever it is you keep putting off. The relief of having it out of the way will be noticeable. This includes making decisions, doing tasks, and contacting people.

If you are frequently thinking about what you "ought" to do, determine if doing it is realistic or not. If it is realistic and you want to do it, then start on it, if possible. If it seems unrealistic, or if you really don't want to do it and it can be left undone, try to let the thought go so that you don't feel guilty.

Sharing your feelings with others
Try talking with those having similar, mutual interests, such as members of:
• church groups
• senior citizens groups
• local Mended Hearts club
• community choir, orchestra, or band
• service clubs, such as Kiwanis, Rotary, or Lions.
Note: If you are having thoughts of suicide, share these thoughts with someone, such as a minister, crisis center counselor, trusted friend, family member, or psychiatrist. You need to talk with someone who will listen and help you get back to your usual way of feeling. Avoid talking with people whose only or usual response to you is "Don't worry," or "You have nothing to worry about." Although it may be true, you will need to determine this on your own.

If you are worrying about different things, try to analyze what is worrying you, then seek appropriate help. For example, if your worries are financial, discuss them with someone from your bank or the specific company involved, or contact the United Way for information on where you can go for help. If your worries are medical, talk with your doctor or a nurse practitioner. If your worries are spiritual, talk with your minister, priest, or rabbi. Whatever the problem, take measures to help the situation rather than just worrying about it.

Stress
Although you may not experience some of the stronger feelings mentioned earlier, you probably have a certain amount of stress in your life that you want to reduce. The following suggestions may help.

Determining whether specific problems can be realistically solved
If any of your problems can be solved, solve them as quickly as possible to get them out of your way. For problems that cannot be solved, admit to yourself that there is nothing you can do about them. Then tell yourself out loud to let them go.

Acknowledging your true feelings
Do not tell yourself how you ought to or should feel. Acknowledge how you actually do feel and let it go at that.

Finding ways to stimulate and challenge yourself
Take on only those activities and commitments you have time and energy for. Try to be realistic and to enjoy what you do. Include activities that

(continued)

stimulate and challenge you to learn something new. However, don't push yourself in a compulsive, driving way. That will only increase the stress, not relieve it.

Living for the present
Reflecting on and learning from the past and planning for the future are important aspects of your life. However, it is essential that you live each day in the present. Set goals for the future, then enjoy taking daily steps toward their realization. Don't dwell on the past.

Giving yourself permission to play, relax, or do nothing
Allow time to enjoy hobbies, music, reading, and exercise. Enjoy smelling the roses, noticing various cloud shapes in the sky, watching the progress of nearby construction, and feeling warm and cozy inside your home when the weather is cold and stormy outside.

Taking proper care of your body
Make sure you:
• follow a proper, nutritious diet
• get plenty of exercise (within your exercise prescription and tolerance level)
• get adequate sleep and relaxation.

Spending time alone
Give yourself privacy and space. Use this time alone to contemplate, meditate, exercise, relax, enjoy your own company, or to do absolutely nothing.

Being true to yourself and your beliefs
Live your life as true to your principles as you possibly can.

Redefining the situation
If a particular problem or situation continues to bother you, see if you can redefine it or look at it in a different light. Usually, people react to something based on their perceptions. Trying to see other perspectives of the same situation may help. Try saying to yourself, "I don't have to make myself miserable. I have a choice about being upset."

Keeping worries to a minimum
Find different things to be excited about or to laugh about. Try to keep your worries to a minimum.

When you go home from the hospital, use the spaces below to list the ways you have found to help yourself feel good about yourself, relaxed, and in control of yourself and your life.

_____

_____

_____

_____

PATIENT-TEACHING AID

Caregiver Guidelines: Dealing with the Patient's Emotions at Home

Your spouse (or loved one) is ready to come home from the hospital and you are probably very concerned about him, especially if he was extremely sick, or sick for a long time. You probably worried at some point that he might die. You may even still be afraid that will happen. He may have been irritable toward you while in the hospital and you may be wondering how to deal with such emotions at home. All your worries are legitimate and need to be addressed.

In the spaces below, list any worries you have and be sure to discuss them with the nurse, preferably in a private setting.

_____

_____

_____

_____

Your spouse will probably experience various emotions when he returns home. These feelings are normal and common to most patients who have undergone similar hospitalizations.

From the list below, check off any emotion or problem you think your spouse is likely to experience upon returning home:

☐ Wanting people to leave him alone

☐ Irritability

☐ Depression

☐ Soreness in incisional areas

☐ Sleeplessness

☐ Lack of sexual desire

☐ Unwillingness to adhere to doctor's instructions at times

☐ Worrying about everything

☐ Fear of being alone

☐ Crying all the time

☐ Lack of desire to do anything

☐ Fatigue

(continued)

Discuss with the nurse any feelings you have checked; she may be able to offer suggestions for dealing with some of them, such as sleeplessness or depression. *Note:* These emotions or problems usually last from 6 to 8 weeks and rarely last longer than 3 months. If they persist beyond 3 months, be sure to seek outside help.

HELPFUL GUIDELINES
Keep in mind the following guidelines to help care for your spouse at home:
• Because it takes a lot of energy to shower or bathe, make sure your spouse gives himself enough time so that he can rest afterward before doing anything else. It may take 2 or 3 months for this not to be so exhausting.
• Incisional soreness can last several months. During that time, the soreness will diminish somewhat; however, it may be noticeable for what seems like a long time. Suggest that your spouse take his pain medication so that he will be able to sleep or engage in other activities.

Although drug addiction is not likely to occur, talk with the doctor or nurse if you are concerned. If your spouse takes one or two doses of medication a day, you probably don't have to worry, especially if he has been active. And keep in mind that most of his pain will have disappeared by the end of 3 months.
• Having time to yourself is important, both for you and your spouse. If your spouse will be able to care for himself at home, you will have that much more time for yourself. However, if he will need a lot of care and attention, you should plan now to obtain periodic relief. If you do not have someone immediately available, talk with the nurse; she may be able to refer you to someone for additional assistance.

Use the spaces below for the names of persons who can help care for your spouse. You might even want to include here the times you would like to set aside for yourself and any activities you plan to do.

_____

_____

_____

_____

• It may be difficult for you to realize that your spouse is getting better and that he can do more for himself and be alone for longer periods of time. Make a point of noticing if this is happening, and let it happen. You may find that he is feeling better than he has in years, particularly if he has had valve surgery. He may even have no restrictions on his activity after recovery from surgery. Remember, his recovery is a good thing, so rejoice and try not to be afraid.

(continued)

IF COMPLIANCE IS A PROBLEM

Wanting to protect your spouse is normal, but it may not be helpful. This can become a source of irritation to both of you. Keep in mind that your spouse has to make his own decisions to adhere to the doctor's prescriptions for medication and exercise, and you may be distressed if he chooses to act contrary to those orders. Some reasons why he may be choosing to act against doctor's orders include the following:

• He may be trying to prove he is no longer sick.
• He may be trying to prove he is still in control.
• He may be trying to prove he can make his own decisions.
• He may be trying to prove he is independent.
• He may be trying to counteract his fears of dying or feeling helpless.
• He may feel that his drugs or other aspects of his medical care are making him sicker, but he can't tell you.

Ask him if he has any fears or concerns that may be preventing him from following doctor's orders. Specifically mention some of the reasons listed above; he may not be able to think of specific reasons on his own and your mentioning some specific fears may help him to open up to you.

You may find such a discussion difficult. If so, list your fears in the spaces below and discuss them with the nurse.

_____

_____

_____

Your spouse has the right to make his own decisions about following doctor's orders. You have an equal right to express your feelings about his decisions and to tell your spouse your reaction. Practice saying to the nurse what you might wish to say to your spouse if you are in this situation.

Consult another person—perhaps a trusted friend or one of the resources or support groups available to you and your spouse if you and your spouse are having difficulty discussing these concerns. Although that person may not be able to offer any new advice, you may find that just discussing the problem with someone who cares helps.

List the names of some persons or support groups you may wish to contact in the spaces below.

_____

_____

_____

Valve Replacement Surgery: Home Care

TEACHING PLAN
Assessment
• Assess the patient's and family's knowledge of home care after valve surgery, including medications, activity, diet, and complications.
• Determine the patient's and family's specific areas of concern about home care.
• Collaborate with the doctor to determine discharge orders.

Strategies to use
• Stimulate interest in the topic by beginning with the patient's and family's concerns.
• Assist the patient and his family to problem-solve the following:
  —how to manage the patient's diet at home
  —how to manage the patient's activity at home
  —how to recognize complications and what to do if they occur
  —how to manage the patient's postoperative pain
  —how to decrease the patient's risk of developing infectious endocarditis.

Patient-teaching aid
See *Guidelines for home care after valve replacement surgery*, page 424.

Evaluation method
• Have the patient and a family member explain, in their own words, home care measures and their specific plans for implementing each measure.

Interventions and outcome criteria
☑ **Intervention 1**
Discuss with the patient and family all the prescribed medications the patient will have to take.

Outcome criteria: Use the outcome criteria from "Medication Guidelines" in this section.

☑ **Intervention 2**
Discuss the patient's prescribed diet and fluid restrictions.

Outcome criteria: Use the outcome criteria from related teaching plans in this section.

☑ Intervention 3
Discuss the use of oxygen at home, if prescribed.

Outcome criteria: Use the outcome criteria from "Oxygen Use at Home" in this section.

☑ Intervention 4
Discuss with the patient and family the patient's activity at home, including:
• pacing activities
• managing activities of daily living
• the importance of sleep and rest
• how to make progress in activity.

Outcome criteria: The patient and family develop an appropriate plan for managing the patient's activity at home.

☑ Intervention 5
Discuss resumption of sexual activity at home.

Outcome criteria: Use the outcome criteria from "Sexual Activity and Heart Disease" in this section.

☑ Intervention 6
Discuss home management of incisional pain.

Outcome criteria: The patient and family state what measures to use to manage the patient's incisional pain at home.

☑ Intervention 7
Discuss how to care for incision lines and the sternum, including:
• daily care of incisions
• daily inspection for signs of infection
• precautions to take for 4 to 12 weeks until the sternum heals, such as:
   —no driving
   —limited lifting (less than 10 lb)
• avoiding activities that involve pushing or pulling heavy objects.

Outcome criteria: The patient and family state how to care for incision lines and sternum.

☑ Intervention 8
Discuss taking and recording daily weights.

Outcome criteria: The patient and family state how to correctly take and record daily weights.

☑ Intervention 9
Discuss how to count and record the radial pulse.

Outcome criteria: The patient and family demonstrate how to count and record the radial pulse.

☑ Intervention 10

Discuss the warning signs of complications, such as:
- signs of congestive heart failure, including:
  —increasing fatigue or dyspnea
  —edema in dependent sites
  —cough
  —weight gain of 2 lb or more in 24 hours
- signs of dysrhythmias, including:
  —significant changes in pulse rate and rhythm
  —signs of decreased cardiac output
- signs of pericarditis, including:
  —pain.

Also discuss how to obtain medical help for each complication listed.

Outcome criteria: The patient and family state signs of major complications and how to obtain appropriate medical care when indicated.

☑ Intervention 11

Discuss the risk of the patient's developing infectious endocarditis.

Outcome criteria: Use the outcome criteria from "Endocarditis, Infectious: Disease Process and Prevention" in this section.

☑ Intervention 12

Discuss the importance of follow-up care.

Outcome criteria: The patient and family state the importance of follow-up care.

Guidelines for Home Care after Valve Replacement Surgery

As you will soon be leaving the hospital, you may have questions about how to care for yourself at home. This teaching aid will discuss some of the most common questions patients and their families ask. If you have any additional questions not addressed in this aid, be sure to ask your nurse or doctor.

MEDICATIONS
Be sure to take all of your medications exactly as your doctor has ordered, as this is an important part of your home care. Your nurse will give you more information about each medication you will be taking at home.

DIET
Diet orders for patients who have recently undergone valve replacement surgery vary with the individual.

Your doctor has recommended that you follow this diet: _____

_____

    If you are on a restricted diet or if the amount you can drink each day is limited, your nurse will give you additional information to read.

OXYGEN
If your doctor wishes you to use oxygen at home, the nurse will give you information to read on home use of oxygen.

ACTIVITY
Activity levels for patients who have recently undergone valve replacement surgery vary depending on their age and overall medical condition and on how well their heart is pumping blood throughout the body.

Your prescribed activity level is: _____

_____

_____

    Regardless of your prescribed activity level, follow these general guidelines:
• When you get home, do about the same amount of activity at about the same pace as you were doing in the hospital.

(continued)

• Depending on doctor's orders, you may shower or bathe. If you bathe, you may need some help to get in and out of the tub for the first few days. If you shower, you may want to put a stool in the shower to sit on. Do not use extremely hot water in either the tub or the shower.

• Plan to get enough rest. Rest in between activities. Remember that rest does not always mean sleeping; it may include sitting quietly for 20 to 30 minutes.

• Plan to get enough sleep. It may be a good idea for you to take one or two brief naps during the day. However, be careful that you don't get too much sleep during the day, or you will not be able to sleep well at night. Plan on getting 8 to 10 hours of sleep at night.

• Stop any activity when you begin to feel tired. Do not let yourself become overtired.

• Stop any activity immediately if you become tired, feel more short of breath, have palpitations, feel dizzy, or break out in a cold sweat.

• Pace your activities, spreading them out during the day. Don't try to do too many things all at one time. Don't rush through any activity. Keep in mind that, when you first get home, "activities" include bathing, eating, walking, talking on the phone, and visiting with friends. A slow pace and plenty of rest are important.

• Increase your activity slowly, as prescribed by your doctor. Your nurse will give you additional information on how to progress your activity.

RESUMING SEXUAL ACTIVITY
Many patients are concerned that resuming sexual activity will hurt their heart. Sexual activity puts about the same stress on your heart as walking up a flight of stairs quickly or walking one or two blocks at a brisk pace. Your nurse will give you some guidelines on how to safely resume sex at home.

CARING FOR YOUR STERNUM
As you probably know, your sternum (or breastbone) was cut in two during surgery. It is now held together by wires; these wires will not be removed.

Your sternum should completely heal in 4 to 12 weeks. While it is healing, you may hear a slight clicking sound when you take a breath or turn. This is normal and will disappear when your sternum is completely healed.

While your sternum is healing, you need to be careful about putting too much strain on it. This means you should take the following precautions:

• Avoid any activities that involve lifting more than 10 lb. This includes carrying children, lifting or carrying bags of groceries, or carrying suitcases.

• Avoid any activities that involve pushing or pulling of heavy objects, such as mowing the grass, vacuuming, opening and closing heavy doors, and moving furniture.

• Avoid driving a car or riding a bicycle, motorcycle, horse, or lawn mower. An accident involving any of these could damage your sternum and slow its healing.

Your surgeon wants you to follow these precautions for _____ weeks.

(continued)

CARING FOR YOUR INCISION LINE

To care for your incision line, take the following measures:
• Gently wash the incision line with mild soap and warm water each day. Avoid vigorous scrubbing with a washcloth. Then, pat the area dry gently. Do not apply any lotions, creams, or powders on the incision line unless prescribed by your doctor.
• Inspect your incision line daily. You may need to use a mirror to see it well. You'll notice the incision begin to look better slowly over time. You may notice a touch of redness around the edges of the wound or a small area of swelling at the top of the incision; both are normal. Your incision may also itch while it heals.
• Check your incision line daily for any of the following trouble signs:
  —increasing tenderness of the incision line
  —increasing redness around the edges of the incision line
  —increasing swelling around the edges of the incision line
  —any drainage from the incision line.
If any of the above signs occur, call your doctor right away, as you may be developing an infection.

MANAGING INCISIONAL PAIN

You probably will experience some pain from your incision site at home just as you had in the hospital. It may be more noticeable when you take a deep breath, turn, or move. You may also notice it more at night when you are trying to fall asleep.

Decreasing your pain is an important part of your home care, as pain increases the stress on your heart and body. It can slow down your recovery.

To help decrease your pain, your doctor has prescribed the following

medication: _____

You may take _____ tablet every _____ hours as needed.

Below are some general guidelines for taking pain medication:
• Take your pain medication at night just before you try to fall asleep. Do not substitute sleeping pills for pain medication. If you are hurting, the sleeping pill will not work. The pain medication will relieve your pain and help you sleep at the same time.
• Take one tablet in the morning before you begin your day's activities.
• Take your pain medication often enough during the day to allow you to complete your planned activities comfortably. (Remember, you can only take your medication every _____ hours.)
• If you find that you are falling asleep frequently during the day, you may be taking too much pain medication. If you are taking two tablets, try taking only one. Or wait longer between taking pain medication.
• Try other methods of pain relief to help decrease the pain, including distraction techniques, watching television, listening to the radio, visiting with friends or family, or engaging in some other activity.
• Participate in your prescribed exercise and activity program to help decrease your incisional pain.

(continued)

PULSE RATE AND DAILY WEIGHTS

As part of your home care, weigh yourself daily. To weigh yourself correctly:
• weigh yourself at the same time in the morning using the same scale
• weigh yourself before breakfast and after urinating
• record the date and your weight
• notify your doctor if you gain 2 lb or more overnight.

You may also need to count your pulse rate each day. Your nurse will give you additional information on how to do this.

WARNING SIGNS

Sometimes, patients develop problems after valve replacement surgery. Knowing the warning signs lets you recognize the problems and get appropriate medical care quickly.

Heart failure

Notify your doctor immediately if you develop any of the following:
• increased shortness of breath (more than usual with your usual activity or at rest)
• increased tiredness (more than usual with your typical day's activities)
• shoes feeling too tight, swelling of the feet and ankles, or rings feeling too tight
• swelling in your lower back or hips (associated with spending most of the day in bed; usually noticed by a family member)
• development of a cough without flulike symptoms
• weight gain of 2 lb or more overnight.

Having any of these signs may indicate that your heart is not pumping well enough to meet your body's needs.

Problems with heart rhythm

Also notify your doctor immediately if any of the following occur:
• your pulse rate drops below _____ beats/minute or rises above _____ beats/minute
• your pulse rhythm changes from regular or slightly irregular to extremely irregular
• you feel dizzy, faint, or tired with any of the above changes in your pulse rate or rhythm.

These are warning signs that your heartbeat has become so irregular that your body is not getting enough blood and oxygen to meet its needs.

Pericarditis

Another possible complication is pericarditis (inflammation of the lining around the heart). Although this is usually not considered an emergency, you still need to contact your doctor if it develops. The major warning sign of pericarditis is pain. Typically located in the chest, shoulder, or neck, this pain usually worsens when you take a deep breath, swallow, or bend over.

Infectious endocarditis

Because you have an artificial valve in your heart, you have an increased chance of developing an infection in your heart called infectious endocarditis. Infectious endocarditis can be extremely serious; it can result in another surgery to replace the artificial valve. Your nurse will give you written information on how to reduce your chance of developing this infection.

(continued)

Plan now how you will get additional medical care if problems develop. In the spaces below, list any pertinent information.

Surgeon:_____

Phone: _____

Address: _____

Cardiologist: _____

Phone: _____

Address: _____

Family doctor: _____

Phone: _____

Address: _____

FOLLOW-UP
Be sure to keep all follow-up appointments with your surgeon, cardiologist, and family doctor. Your first appointment is:

Doctor: _____

Phone: _____

Date: _____

Time: _____

Location: _____

Vascular Bypass Surgery: Home Care

TEACHING PLAN
Assessment
Assess the patient's and family's knowledge of home management after vascular bypass surgery, including activity, monitoring for complications, and modification of risk factors for recurrent atherosclerosis.

Strategies to use
Assist the patient and family to problem-solve the following:
• how to identify risk factors the patient has for atherosclerosis and how to modify them
• how to prevent injury to the legs
• how to recognize complications
• how and when to obtain additional medical care.

Patient-teaching aid
See *Home care guidelines after vascular bypass surgery,* page 431.

Evaluation method
Have the patient or family member do the following:
• state major points of home management after vascular bypass surgery using their own words
• demonstrate correct foot care
• state plans for modifying the patient's risk factors for atherosclerosis.

Interventions and outcome criteria
☑ **Intervention 1**
Review the disease process of occlusive arterial disease, if necessary.

☑ **Intervention 2**
Discuss the patient's activity at home, including:
• use of walking as exercise
• avoidance of prolonged standing.
Outcome criteria: The patient and family state how to manage the patient's activity at home.

☑ **Intervention 3**
Teach the patient to assess circulation in the leg so he will know how to:
• check the pulse in his foot
• assess color and temperature
• notify the doctor about the development of acute arterial occlusions or occlusions from recurrent or continuing atherosclerotic disease.

Outcome criteria: The patient and family demonstrate how to assess circulation correctly; they state that the doctor should be notified for signs of decreased circulation.

☑ **Intervention 4**
Teach the patient to care for incision lines, including the following:
• how to wash and dry the incision lines gently, using warm water and mild soap
• how to assess the incision lines daily for signs of infection
• how to notify the doctor immediately if signs of infection develop.

Outcome criteria: The patient and family demonstrate correct care of incision lines; they also state that warmth, redness, or drainage are indications that the doctor should be called.

☑ **Intervention 5**
Discuss proper foot care (see "Occlusive Arterial Disease: Disease Process and Home Care" in this section).

Outcome criteria: Use the outcome criteria from "Occlusive Arterial Disease: Disease Process and Home Care" in this section.

☑ **Intervention 6**
Discuss atherosclerosis and identify the patient's risk factors.

Outcome criteria: The patient and family identify the patient's specific risk factors.

☑ **Intervention 7**
Help the patient develop plans to modify risk factors, including:
• decreasing the saturated fat or cholesterol in his diet
• stopping or reducing cigarette smoking
• controlling hypertension
• controlling diabetes mellitus.

Outcome criteria: The patient and family develop plans to modify his individual risk factors.

☑ **Intervention 8**
Discuss the importance of follow-up care.

Outcome criteria: The patient and family state that follow-up medical care is important.

Home Care Guidelines after Vascular Bypass Surgery

As you will soon be going home, you may have questions about how to manage your care at home. This patient-teaching aid answers some common questions patients ask after vascular bypass surgery. However, not all of the information may apply to you. The nurse will check off which sections you should read. If you have other questions that this teaching aid does not answer, be sure to ask your nurse or doctor.

INCISION LINE CARE
Gently wash your incision lines with warm (not hot) water and mild soap each day. Pat them dry gently. Do not put any lotions, creams, or powders on the incision lines unless prescribed by your doctor.

Look at your incision lines carefully each day. Depending on where they are located, you may need to use a mirror to see the entire incision well. Look carefully for any of the following trouble signs:
• increased tenderness of the incision lines
• increased redness around the edges of the incision lines
• increased swelling around the edges of the incision lines
• any drainage from the incision lines.
If any of these occur, call your doctor immediately. You may be developing an infection.

CHECKING CIRCULATION
Checking the circulation in your foot and leg on the side where you had the bypass surgery is very important.
• Begin by feeling for the pulse in your _____
(specify location). The nurse will show you how to find this pulse.
• Also, feel your leg and foot to see if they are warm to the touch.
• Finally, look at your leg and foot for any changes in color.

Notify your surgeon immediately if you have any of the following warning signs:
• the pulse in your _____
(specify location) becomes much more faint than usual or disappears so that you cannot feel it
• you notice your leg or foot has suddenly become cold to the touch
• you notice your leg or foot has changed from its normal color to pale or blue.

If you have any of the above symptoms, your bypass graft may be completely blocked so that no blood is getting to the lower part of your leg or foot. You will need to obtain immediate medical care.

(continued)

FOOT CARE
Good foot care is important in preventing injury to your feet. The nurse will give you another teaching aid on foot care.

ACTIVITY LEVEL
Activity levels after vascular bypass surgery can vary depending on your overall health. Your doctor has prescribed the following activity level for you at home:

_____

WALKING PROGRAM
Walking regularly every day is important. Walk on a level surface at a moderate pace. Stop when you start to get tired. Be sure to walk several times each day.

RECOGNIZING AND PREVENTING ATHEROSCLEROSIS
Because your surgery did not cure your atherosclerotic disease, you have a high chance of developing more blockages in your arteries. Signs and symptoms of more blockage include the following:
• you begin to have pain again in the calf of your leg with activity; this pain is relieved with rest
• you begin to have pain in your foot or lower leg at rest
• you develop an ulcer or injury to your leg that does not heal
• you develop any of the symptoms of decreased blood flow to your legs or feet that you had before surgery (list these symptoms in the spaces below).

_____

_____

Notify your doctor if you notice any of the signs listed above.
   Your nurse will give you more information about atherosclerosis, the factors that increase your risk for developing this again, and how you can change these factors to decrease your risk.

FOLLOW-UP
Keeping your follow-up appointments is very important. Your first appointment is written below.

Doctor: _____

Phone: _____

Address: _____

Date and Time: _____

APPENDIX, SELECTED REFERENCES, AND INDEX

APPENDIX: Resources for Teaching Patients with Cardiovascular Disease

American Cancer Society, local chapters

American Cancer Society publications:
"Fresh Start: Quit Smoking Program of the American Cancer Society"
"Quitter's Guide: Seven Day Plan to Help You Stop Smoking Cigarettes"

American Cancer Society
261 Madison Ave.
New York, N.Y. 10016

American Heart Association, local chapters

American Heart Association publications:
"About Your Heart and Diet"
"About Your Heart and Smoking"
"After a Heart Attack"
"American Heart Association Diet: An Eating Plan for Healthy
   Americans"
"Cholesterol and Your Heart"
"Coronary Risk Factor Statement for the American Public"
"Facts About Congestive Heart Failure"
"Heart Valve Surgery"
"Nutritious Nibbles"
"Recipes for Fat-Controlled Low Cholesterol Meals"
"Salt, Sodium, and Blood Pressure"
"Smoking and Heart Disease"
"Weight Control Guidance in Smoking Cessation"
"What You Should Know About Coronary Arteriography"
"What You Should Know About PTCA"

American Heart Association, National Center
7320 Greenville Ave.
Dallas, Tex. 75231

Cookbooks with recipes for low fat/low cholesterol and restricted-sodium meals available from local bookstores

Heart Attack: What's Ahead?
Available from Pritchett & Hull Assoc., Inc.
Suite 110
3440 Oakcliff Rd. NE
Atlanta, Ga. 30340

Moving Right Along After Open Heart Surgery
Available from Pritchett & Hull Assoc., Inc.
Suite 110
3440 Oakcliff Rd. NE
Atlanta, Ga. 30340

*Relax 1...2...3... A Workbook to Help You Manage Anxiety After a
Heart Attack.* By Carol Ann Healy
Available from Resource Applications, Inc.
720 Light Street
Baltimore, Md. 21230

SELECTED REFERENCES

Books

American Heart Association, Georgia Affiliate. *Heart Attack: What's Ahead?* Atlanta: Pritchett & Hull Assoc., Inc., 1980.

Bannerjee, S.N., ed. *Rehabilitation Management of Amputees.* Baltimore: Williams & Wilkins Co., 1982.

Becknell, E.P., and Smith, D.M. *System of Nursing Practice.* Philadelphia: F.A. Davis Co., 1975.

Benson, H. *Beyond the Relaxation Response.* New York: Berkley Publishing Group, 1984.

Braunwald, E., et al., eds. *Harrison's Principles of Internal Medicine,* 11th ed. St. Louis: C.V. Mosby Co., 1987.

Bray, G.A. "Overweight Is Risking Fate: Definition, Classification, Prevalence and Risks," in *Human Obesity: Annals of the New York Academy of Sciences.* Edited by Wurtman, R.J., and Wurtman, J.J., 1987.

Burrows, S., and Gassert, C. *Moving Right Along After Open Heart Surgery.* Atlanta: Pritchett & Hull Assoc., Inc., 1984.

Carpenito, L.J. *Nursing Diagnosis: Application to Clinical Practice,* 2nd ed. Philadelphia: J.B. Lippincott Co., 1987.

Drug Information for the Health Care Provider, vol. I, 6th ed. Rockville, Md.: United States Pharmacopeial Convention, Inc., 1986.

Epps, C. *Complications in Orthopaedic Surgery,* 2nd ed. Philadelphia: J.B. Lippincott Co., 1986.

Gordon, M. *Nursing Diagnosis: Process and Application,* 2nd ed. New York: McGraw-Hill Book Co., 1987.

Guzzetta, C., and Dossey, B. *Cardiovascular Nursing: Bodymind Tapestry.* St. Louis: C.V. Mosby Co., 1984.

Hurst, J.W., ed. *The Heart: Arteries and Veins,* 6th ed. New York: McGraw-Hill Book Co., 1986.

Jarrett, F., ed. *Vascular Surgery of the Lower Extremity.* St. Louis: C.V. Mosby Co., 1985.

Kadir, S. *Diagnostic Angiography.* Philadelphia: W.B. Saunders Co., 1986.

Kaplan, N.M. *Clinical Hypertension,* 4th ed. Baltimore: Williams and Wilkins Co., 1986.

Kempczinski, R. *The Ischemic Leg.* Chicago: Year Book Medical Publishers, 1985.

Kochar, M.S., and Woods, K.D. *Hypertension Control,* 2nd ed. New York: Springer Publishing Co., 1985.

Luckman, J., and Sorenson, K.C. *Medical-Surgical Nursing: A Psychophysiologic Approach,* 3rd ed. Philadelphia: W.B. Saunders Co., 1987.

Mathewson, M.K. *Pharmacotherapeutics: A Nursing Approach.* Philadelphia: F.A. Davis Co., 1986.

Pollock, M., and Schmidt, D. *Heart Disease and Rehabilitation,* 2nd ed. New York: John Wiley & Sons, 1986.

Quitter's Guide: Seven Day Plan to Help You Stop Smoking Cigarettes. New York: American Cancer Society, 1978.

Rando, T.A. *Grief, Dying and Death.* Champaign, Ill.: Research Press Co., 1984.

Sabiston, D., and Spencer, F. *Gibbon's Surgery of the Chest,* 4th ed. Philadelphia: W.B. Saunders Co., 1983.

Sanders, G. *Lower Limb Amputations: A Guide to Rehabilitation.* Philadelphia: F.A. Davis Co., 1986.

Sorenson, K.C., and Luckman, J. *Basic Nursing: A Psychophysiologic Approach.* Philadelphia: W.B. Saunders Co., 1986.

Strauss, A.L., et al. *Chronic Illness and the Quality of Life.* St. Louis: C.V. Mosby Co., 1984.

Weisman, A.D. *The Coping Capacity: On the Nature of Being Mortal.* New York: Human Sciences Press, 1984.

Wold, B. "Advances in Pacemaker Therapy," in *Advances in Cardiovascular Nursing.* Edited by Douglas, M., and Shinn, J. Rockville, Md.: Aspen Systems, 1985.

Periodicals

Altieri, C. "The Patient with Myocardial Infarction: Rest Prescriptions for Activities of Daily Living," *Heart & Lung* 13(4):355-60, 1984.

American College of Cardiology/American Heart Association. "Guidelines for Exercise Testing," *Journal of the American College of Cardiology* 8(3):725-37, 1986.

Appleton, D.L., and LaQuaglia, J.D. "Vascular Disease and Postoperative Nursing Management," *Critical Care Nurse* 5(5):34-42, 1985.

Barnathan, E., et al. "Aspirin and Dipyridamole in the Prevention of Acute Coronary Thrombosis Complicating Coronary Angioplasty," *Circulation* 76(1):125-34, 1987.

Chesebro, J.H., et al. "Thrombolysis in Myocardial Infarction (TIMI) Trial, Phase I: A Comparison Between Intravenous Tissue Plasminogen Activator and Intravenous Streptokinase," *Circulation* 76(1):142-54, 1987.

Christen, A.G., and McDonald, J.L., Jr., eds. "Management of Stress in the Dental Practitioner," *Dental Clinics of North America* 30(4): Supplement, 1986.

Codini, M. "Management of Acute Myocardial Infarction," *Medical Clinics of North America* 70(4):769-87, 1986.

Cohen, J. "Sexual Counseling of the Patient Following Myocardial Infarction," *Critical Care Nurse* 6(6):18-27, 1986.

Dalsing, M.C., et al. "Surgery of the Aorta," *Critical Care Quarterly* 8(2):25-37, 1985.

Finkelmeier, B., and Salinger, M. "Dual Chamber Cardiac Pacing: An Overview," *Critical Care Nurse* 6(5):12-26, 1986.

Griffin, J., et al. "Pacemaker Follow-Up: Its Role in the Detection and Correction of Pacemaker System Malfunction," *PACE* 9:387-91, 1986.

Hackett, T.P. "Depression Following Myocardial Infarction," *Psychosomatics* 26(11):Supplement, 23-28, 1985.

Hirsh, J., and Hull, R. "Treatment of Venous Thromboembolism," *Chest* 89(Supplement 5):426S-33S, 1986.

Johnson, J.E., and Leventhal, H. "Effects of Accurate Expectations and Behavioral Instructions on Reactions During a Noxious Medical Examination," *Journal of Personality and Social Psychology* 29(5):710-18, 1974.

"Joint National Committee on the Detection, Treatment and Evaluation of High Blood Pressure Report," *Archives of Internal Medicine* 144:1045-57, 1984.

Kaplan, N.M. "Non-Drug Treatment of Hypertension," *Annals of Internal Medicine* 102(3):359-73, 1985.

Loan, T. "Nursing Interaction with Patients Undergoing Coronary Angioplasty," *Heart & Lung* 15(4):368-75, 1986.

Magder, S. "Assessment of Myocardial Stress from Early Ambulatory Activities Following Myocardial Infarction," *Chest* 87:(4)442-47, 1985.

Marshall, J., et al. "Structured Postoperative Teaching and Knowledge and Compliance of Patients Who Had Coronary Artery Bypass Surgery," *Heart & Lung* 15(1):76-82, 1986.

National Institutes of Health Consensus Conference. "Prevention of Venous Thrombosis and Pulmonary Embolism," *Journal of the American Medical Association* 256(6):744-49, 1986.

O'Connor, A. "Factors Related to the Early Phase of Rehabilitation Following Aortocoronary Bypass Surgery," *Research in Nursing and Health* (6):107-16, 1983.

Osborne D. "Cardiovascular Responses of Patients Ambulated 32 and 56 Hours after Coronary Bypass Surgery," *Western Journal of Nursing Research* 6(3):321-24, 1984.

Papadopoulos, C., et al. "Sexual Activity after Coronary Bypass Surgery," *Chest* 90(5):681-85, 1986.

Purcell, J., and Burrows, S. "A Pacemaker Primer," *American Journal of Nursing* 85(5):553-68, 1985.

Remme, W. "Congestive Heart Failure—Pathophysiology and Medical Treatment," *Journal of Cardiovascular Pharmacology* 8(Supplement 1):S36-S52, 1986.

Ruggie, N. "Congestive Heart Failure," *Medical Clinics of North America* 70(4):829-51, 1986.

Sasahara, A., ed. "Symposium on Deep Vein Thrombosis," *American Journal of Surgery* 150(Supplement A):1-70, 1985.

Schwartz, L.P., and Brenner, Z.R. "Critical Care Unit Transfer: Reducing Patient Stress Through Nurse Interventions," *Heart & Lung* 8(3):540-46, 1979.

Sennott-Miller, L., and Miller, J.L. "Difficulty: A Neglected Factor in Health Promotion," *Nursing Research* 36(5):268-72, 1987.

Shurtz, J.D., et al. "Depression: Recognition and Control," *Dental Clinics of North America* 30(4)Supplement:S55-S65, 1986.

Stafford, M.J. "Monitoring Patients with Permanent Cardiac Pacemakers," *Nursing Clinics of North America* 22(2):503-19, 1987.

Stephens, C.R. "Stress: An Unnecessary Fact of Life," *Military Medicine* 152(1):19-24, 1987.

Stern, T.A. "The Management of Depression and Anxiety Following Myocardial Infarction," *Mount Sinai Journal of Medicine* 52(8):623-33, 1985.

Stern, T.A., et al. "Use of Benzodiazepines in a Coronary Care Unit," *Psychosomatics* 28(1):19-23, 1987.

"Symposium Proceedings. Nursing Interventions in Limiting Infarct Size in the Acute Myocardial Infarction Patient: Nursing Implications," *Heart & Lung* 16(6, Part 2):739-800, 1987.

Ujhely, G.B. "Grief and Depression: Implications for Preventive and Therapeutic Nursing Care," *Nursing Forum* V(2):23-35, 1966.

Velasquez, M.T., and Hoffman, R.G. "Overweight and Obesity in Hypertension," *Quarterly Journal of Medicine* 54(215):205-12, 1985.

Wagner, M., and Bower, B., eds. "Symposium on Peripheral Vascular Disease," *Nursing Clinics of North America* 21(2):195-272, 1986.

Weaver, R.C., and Rodnick, J.E. "Type A Behavior: Clinical Significance, Evaluation, and Management," *Journal of Family Practice* 23(3):255-61, 1986.

Weiner, D. "Predischarge Exercise Testing after Myocardial Infarction: Prognostic and Therapeutic Features," *Cardiovascular Clinics* 15(2):95-104, 1985.

Winters, W., and Cashion, W.R. "Imaging Techniques in Patients with Acute Myocardial Infarction," *Heart & Lung* 14(3):259-64, 1985.

INDEX

Nursing76®
Nursing77®
Nursing78®
Nursing79®
Nursing80®
Nursing81®
Nursing82®
Nursing83®
Nursing84®
Nursing85®
Nursing86®
Nursing87®
Nursing88®
Nursing89®

Year after year, one journal delivers more useful clinical information in less time than any other!

Over half a million nurses rely on their subscriptions to keep up with the flood of new drugs, treatments, equipment, and procedures that are changing nursing practice.

Each monthly issue is packed with thoroughly practical, accurate information in concise articles and departments that are clearly written and illustrated in step-by-step detail. You can read an article in minutes and come away with knowledge you can put to work with assurance.

Feature articles focus on demanding problems—ranging from hypertensive crises to cardiogenic shock—that require special skills. You'll quickly learn what to do, how to do it best, when (and when not) to do it.

Drug updates give you critical information quickly—indications, dosages, interactions, contraindications... all you need to administer drugs more confidently.

Assessment aids help you become more proficient in objectively assessing your patients, their conditions, and responses to nursing care.

Self-quizzes bring you the chance to test your knowledge of *current* nursing practices.

Patient-teaching aids help you prepare your patients to follow instructions at home.

Enter your own subscription today with the coupon below. It's a solid, career investment that pays big dividends for you and your patients.